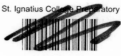
Teen Health Series

W9-CKJ-909

Women's Health Concerns SOURCEBOOK

Second Edition

Health Reference Series

Second Edition

Women's Health Concerns SOURCEBOOK

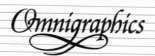

*Basic Consumer Health Information about the
Medical and Mental Concerns of Women, Including
Maintaining Health and Wellness, Gynecological
Concerns, Breast Health, Sexuality and Reproductive
Issues, Menopause, Cancer in Women, the Leading
Causes of Death and Disability among Women,
Physical Concerns of Special Significance to Women,
and Women's Mental and Emotional Health*

*Along with a Glossary of Related Terms and
Directories of Resources for Additional Help
and Information*

Edited by
Amy L. Sutton

Omnigraphics

615 Griswold Street • Detroit, MI 48226

Bibliographic Note

Because this page cannot legibly accommodate all the copyright notices, the Bibliographic Note portion of the Preface constitutes an extension of the copyright notice.

Edited by Amy L. Sutton

Health Reference Series

Karen Bellenir, *Managing Editor*
David A. Cooke, MD, *Medical Consultant*
Elizabeth Barbour, *Permissions Associate*
Dawn Matthews, *Verification Assistant*
Laura Pleva Nielsen, *Index Editor*
EdIndex, Services for Publishers, *Indexers*

* * *

Omnigraphics, Inc.

Matthew P. Barbour, *Senior Vice President*
Kay Gill, *Vice President—Directories*
Kevin Hayes, *Operations Manager*
Leif Gruenberg, *Development Manager*
David P. Bianco, *Marketing Consultant*

* * *

Peter E. Ruffner, *Publisher*
Frederick G. Ruffner, Jr., *Chairman*

Copyright © 2004 Omnigraphics, Inc.

ISBN 0-7808-0673-5

R
6 13.042
WOM

Library of Congress Cataloging-in-Publication Data

Women's health concerns sourcebook: basic information about health issues that affect women, featuring facts about menstruation and other gynecological concerns... / Amy L. Sutton, editor.–2nd ed.
  p. cm. – (Health reference series)
Previous ed. edited by Heather E. Aldred.
Includes index.
ISBN 0-7808-0673-5
  1. Women–Health and hygiene. 2. Women–Diseases. I. Sutton, Amy L. II. Health reference series (Unnumbered)

RA778.W7543 2004
613'04244–dc22

2004041493

22332

This book is printed on acid-free paper meeting the ANSI Z39.48 Standard. The infinity symbol that appears above indicates that the paper in this book meets that standard.

Printed in the United States

Table of Contents

Part II: Gynecological Concerns

Part III: Breast Health

Part IV: Sexuality and Reproductive Issues

Part VII: Other Leading Causes of Death and Disability among Women

Part VIII: Physical Concerns of Special Significance for Women

Part IX: Women's Emotional and Mental Health

Part X: Additional Help and Information

Preface

About This Book

Female-focused research in the last two decades has revealed that women experience disease and disability differently from men. By understanding their unique concerns, women can increase their quality of life and guard against premature death. For example:

- Heart attacks are just as common in women as they are in men, but women are much more likely to die from their first heart attack. One reason is that heart attack warning signs in women can be different from the warning signs in men. Women who know when to be concerned can seek medical care sooner.

- Although earlier research seemed to suggest that hormone replacement therapy (HRT) could protect women against post-menopausal disorders, recent studies show that HRT can actually increase a woman's risk of experiencing a heart attack, stroke, breast cancer, or blood clots. Women who have up-to-date information are able to discuss these issues with their physicians.

- Some disorders, including arthritis, osteoporosis, diabetes, depression, and chlamydia, are more prevalent among women than among men. Women who understand gender-associated risk factors are better able to make informed health care choices and adopt precautionary lifestyle changes.

This *Sourcebook* provides updated information about these and other women's health care topics, including gynecological concerns, breast health, sexuality and reproductive issues, menopause, cancer, the leading causes of death and disability, and other physical and mental concerns of special significance for women. Resource directories are included, along with a glossary of terms related to women's health.

Several other volumes within the *Health Reference Series* may also be of interest for those seeking comprehensive information about women's health issues:

- *Breast Cancer Sourcebook*
- *Breastfeeding Sourcebook*
- *Cancer Sourcebook for Women*
- *Domestic Violence Sourcebook*
- *Healthy Heart Sourcebook for Women*
- *Pregnancy and Birth Sourcebook*

How to Use This Book

This book is divided into parts and chapters. Parts focus on broad areas of interest. Chapters are devoted to single topics within a part.

Part I: A Women's Guide to Maintaining Health and Wellness describes general health concerns and preventive health care. It explains the female reproductive system and identifies the special needs of working women, women in various ethnic groups, and women with disabilities. Health maintenance topics, such as sleep, nutrition, weight management, and smoking, are also discussed.

Part II: Gynecological Concerns includes facts about common diseases and disorders of the female reproductive organs, including premenstrual syndrome, menstrual problems, pelvic pain, and other disorders of the uterus, ovaries, cervix, and vagina. A chapter on common gynecological surgeries and procedures explains laparoscopy, dilation and curettage (D&C), and hysterectomy.

Part III: Breast Health offers information about normal breast development, breastfeeding, breast changes during aging, and the prevention, diagnosis, and treatment of breast disorders. Breast cancer, however, is included in Part VI.

Part IV: Sexuality and Reproductive Issues describes conditions and disorders that affect sexually active women, including sexually transmitted diseases and sexual dysfunction. Other reproductive issues, including birth control (contraception), abortion infertility, and pregnancy are also discussed.

Part V: Menopause addresses the health considerations of aging women, examines the current debate surrounding hormone replacement therapy, and presents facts about alternative and complementary therapies for menopause symptoms.

Part VI: Cancer in Women presents facts about the risk factors, symptoms, treatment, and prevention of the most prevalent types of cancer in women, including lung, skin, thyroid, breast, and gynecological cancers.

Part VII: Other Leading Causes of Death and Disability among Women describes significant health problems in the female population, including cardiovascular disease, obesity, diabetes, respiratory disease, asthma, stroke, and osteoporosis.

Part VIII: Physical Concerns of Special Significance for Women offers information about conditions that affect women more often than men, including migraine pain, thyroid disease, chronic fatigue syndrome, fibromyalgia, lupus, urinary tract disorders, and spider and varicose veins. Health issues related to cosmetic concerns are also addressed.

Part IX: Women's Emotional and Mental Health details the symptoms, treatment, and prevention of emotional health problems that affect women, including stress, depressive disorders, anxiety disorders, and eating disorders. Information about violence against women and drug and alcohol abuse among women is also provided.

Part X: Additional Help and Information includes a glossary of important terms and directories of government agencies and private organizations that provide help and information to women.

Bibliographic Note

This volume contains documents and excerpts from publications issued by the following U.S. government agencies: Agency for Healthcare Research and Quality (AHRQ); Centers for Disease Control and

Prevention (CDC); Food and Drug Administration (FDA); Health Resources and Services Administration (HRSA); National Cancer Institute (NCI); National Center for Complementary and Alternative Medicine (NCCAM); National Heart, Lung, and Blood Institute (NHLBI); National Institute of Allergy and Infectious Diseases (NIAID); National Institute of Child Health and Human Development (NICHD); National Institute of Diabetes and Digestive and Kidney Disorders (NIDDK); National Institute of Environmental Health Sciences (NIEHS); National Institute of Mental Health (NIMH); National Institute on Aging (NIA); National Institutes of Health (NIH); National Women's Health Information Center (NWHIC); Office of Dietary Supplements, and the Office of Disease Prevention and Health Promotion (ODPHP).

In addition, this volume contains copyrighted documents from the following organizations: American Academy of Dermatology (AAD); American Academy of Orthopaedic Surgeons; American Association for Marriage and Family Therapy; American College of Obstetricians and Gynecologists (ACOG); American College of Surgeons; American Council for Headache Education; American Dietetic Association; American Lung Association; American Obesity Association; American Podiatric Medical Association; American Psychiatric Association; American Society for Dermatologic Surgery; American Society for Reproductive Medicine; American Society of Plastic Surgeons; Baylor College of Medicine Center for Research on Women with Disabilities; Breastcancer.org; Brigham and Women's Hospital Center for Uterine Fibroids; Cancer Research and Prevention Foundation; CancerSource; Childbirth Solutions, Inc.; Children's Hospital Medical Center of Akron; Cleveland Clinic Foundation; Community Breast Health Project; Gay and Lesbian Medical Association; HeartCenterOnline; Inlet Medical, Inc.; Interstitial Cystitis Association; Joslin Diabetes Center; Kaiser Family Foundation; Lange Productions; Magic Foundation for Children's Growth; March of Dimes; Medem, Inc.; National Alliance of Breast Cancer Organizations; National Anemia Action Council; National Breast Cancer Foundation; National Coalition for Women with Heart Disease; National Mental Health Association; National Sleep Foundation; National Women's Health Resource Center; Nemours Foundation/KidsHealth.org; Planned Parenthood; Society for Women's Health Research; Susan G. Komen Breast Cancer Foundation; and University of Pennsylvania Cancer Center/OncoLink.

Full citation information is provided on the first page of each chapter. Every effort has been made to secure all necessary rights to reprint the copyrighted material. If any omissions have been made, please contact Omnigraphics to make corrections for future editions.

Acknowledgements

Thanks go to the many organizations, agencies, and individuals who have contributed materials for this *Sourcebook* and to medical consultant Dr. David Cooke, verification assistant Dawn Matthews, and document engineer Bruce Bellenir. Special thanks go to managing editor Karen Bellenir and permissions specialist Liz Barbour for their help and support.

Note from the Editor

This book is part of Omnigraphics' *Health Reference Series*. The *Series* provides basic information about a broad range of medical concerns. It is not intended to serve as a tool for diagnosing illness, in prescribing treatments, or as a substitute for the physician/patient relationship. All persons concerned about medical symptoms or the possibility of disease are encouraged to seek professional care from an appropriate health care provider.

Our Advisory Board

The *Health Reference Series* is reviewed by an Advisory Board comprised of librarians from public, academic, and medical libraries. We would like to thank the following board members for providing guidance to the development of this *Series*:

Dr. Lynda Baker,
Associate Professor of Library and Information Science,
Wayne State University, Detroit, MI

Nancy Bulgarelli,
William Beaumont Hospital Library, Royal Oak, MI

Karen Imarisio,
Bloomfield Township Public Library, Bloomfield Township, MI

Karen Morgan,
Mardigian Library, University of Michigan-Dearborn,
Dearborn, MI

Rosemary Orlando,
St. Clair Shores Public Library, St. Clair Shores, MI

Medical Consultant

Medical consultation services are provided to the *Health Reference Series* editors by David A. Cooke, MD. Dr. Cooke is a graduate of Brandeis University, and he received his M.D. degree from the University of Michigan. He completed residency training at the University of Wisconsin Hospital and Clinics. He is board-certified in Internal Medicine. Dr. Cooke currently works as part of the University of Michigan Health System and practices in Brighton, MI. In his free time, he enjoys writing, science fiction, and spending time with his family.

Health Reference Series *Update Policy*

The inaugural book in the *Health Reference Series* was the first edition of *Cancer Sourcebook* published in 1989. Since then, the *Series* has been enthusiastically received by librarians and in the medical community. In order to maintain the standard of providing high-quality health information for the layperson the editorial staff at Omnigraphics felt it was necessary to implement a policy of updating volumes when warranted.

Medical researchers have been making tremendous strides, and it is the purpose of the *Health Reference Series* to stay current with the most recent advances. Each decision to update a volume will be made on an individual basis. Some of the considerations will include how much new information is available and the feedback we receive from people who use the books. If there is a topic you would like to see added to the update list, or an area of medical concern you feel has not been adequately addressed, please write to:

Editor
Health Reference Series
Omnigraphics, Inc.
615 Griswold Street
Detroit, MI 48226
E-mail: editorial@omnigraphics.com

Part One

A Women's Guide to Maintaining Health and Wellness

Chapter 1

Women's Health in the United States

Overview of Women's Health

At the start of the new millennium, women comprised more than half of the United States (U.S.) population. Indeed, women outnumber men in every age cohort over 25 years. Because women's life expectancy is now at a record 79.5 years, a majority of the rapidly growing aging population, particularly among those 85 years and older, are women. Ensuring good health in these years requires partnerships between women and their families, clinicians, employers, and community organizations.

The U.S. population is increasingly diverse. Over the decade 1990 to 2000, the proportion of the female population represented by White non-Hispanic women declined from 76 to 71.2 percent, while the Hispanic population grew from 8.6 to 11.6 percent and Asian/Pacific Islanders grew from 2.8 to 3.9 percent of U.S. females. Other racial and ethnic groups changed only slightly or remained constant.

"Overview of Women's Health" excerpted from the U.S. Department of Health and Human Services, Health Resources and Services Administration, Maternal and Child Health Bureau. *Women's Health USA 2002*. Rockville, Maryland: U.S. Department of Health and Human Services, 2002. "Health Coverage and Access to Care" excerpted with permission from Women's Health in the United States: Health Coverage and Access to Care, Kaiser Women's Health Survey, May 2002. © 2002 Henry J. Kaiser Family Foundation. All rights reserved. To obtain a free copy of this report, or additional information, call 800-656-4533, or visit www.kff.org.

The year 2000 census shows that men achieve higher levels of education than women. Data from the Bureau of Labor Statistics indicate that more than 56 percent of White, Black, and Hispanic women aged 16 and older are employed. Still, disparities exist in income between men and women, with women earning less than 75 cents for every dollar men earn.

Employment is a gateway for health insurance coverage. In 2000, nearly 87 percent of women had health insurance coverage and 13 percent of women lacked any health insurance coverage. Although women are more likely than men to have health insurance coverage, approximately one quarter of women aged 18 to 24 were without insurance in 2000.

Many women perform multiple roles—including caregiver to elderly relatives and young children—which affect their own health and economic stability. Data from The Commonwealth Fund's 1998 Survey of Women's Health indicate that 9 percent of women were caring for a sick or disabled relative, with 43 percent of these women providing more than 20 hours of care per week. Caregivers are more likely than non-caregivers to be in poor health.

Poverty continues to be a problem particularly affecting women in the U.S., with 11 percent of women living below the federal poverty level. Single women with young children or who are elderly are most likely to live in poverty, with Black and Hispanic women of all ages having particularly high poverty rates.

Preventive health care can help to promote good health throughout a woman's life span, and women are more likely than men to seek preventive care. In 1996, nearly a quarter (24 percent) of women's ambulatory care visits were for preventive services such as mammograms, Pap smears, and immunizations. Impressive gains have been made in closing the gap in the use of preventive services among women from all racial and ethnic groups, with Black women now having higher rates of Pap smears and comparable rates of mammography screenings as White women. Dental care is also an important component of preventive services. In 2000, the majority of women had visited a dentist in the last year. However, a substantial minority, approximately one third, had not visited a dentist for a year or more.

While these important preventive health services can detect diseases in early stages, the influence of medical care on women's health status is limited. Healthy behaviors, like regular physical activity and healthy nutritional choices, are critical to a long and healthy life. Women are less likely to engage in light or moderate leisure time physical activity than men. They are also less likely to consume recommended servings of fruit and vegetables. The percentage of women who smoke—a behavior associated with numerous chronic illnesses—has remained steady over the last several years at slightly more than 20 percent of the adult female population. Of particular concern is that adolescent girls report smoking cigarettes at slightly higher rates than boys (14.1 percent compared with 12.8 percent). Reducing the prevalence of smoking among women, particularly young women, is a public health priority. As prevention science continues to establish important relationships between lifestyle choices and chronic illnesses, education and activities that promote healthful behaviors become increasingly important.

Mental health is a critical component of a person's overall health. Though limited data are available to describe women's use of mental health care, it is apparent that depression significantly affects women. Women report a higher percentage of poor mental health days as compared to men and are more likely than men to be hospitalized for depression.

Substance abuse, which often occurs in people who suffer from mental illness, is also an important health concern among women. National survey data collected by the Substance Abuse and Mental Health Administration in 2000 found that more than a quarter of women 18 to 25 years old reported binge drinking in the past month and as many as 7.4 percent were found to drink heavily. This same survey also showed that approximately 24 percent of women aged 18 to 25 and 19 percent of females aged 12 to 17 had used some type of illicit drug in the past year, most commonly marijuana. In addition, approximately 8 percent of females aged 12 to 25 reported using psychotherapeutic prescription drugs for non-medical reasons in the past year. Rates of drug abuse for all types of drugs show that misuse declines significantly among women after age 25.

Women report a higher number of chronic conditions and have higher rates of disability and activity limitations than men. A person's self-report of health status provides an overall qualitative measure of health. A higher proportion of men than women rate their health as excellent or very good. Among women, Hispanic and Black women are more likely than White women to report their health as fair or poor.

For most major causes of death—heart disease, cancer, and stroke—women die at lower rates than men. However, heart disease remains the number one killer of women. More women are diagnosed each year with breast cancer than any other type of cancer, although lung cancer kills more women. Of the cancer deaths in 2001, it is estimated by the National Cancer Institute that 67,300 females died of

5

lung and bronchus cancers, compared with 40,200 deaths from breast cancer. Black women have the highest lung cancer death rates, and White women have the highest breast cancer death rates.

Women are disproportionately affected by such conditions as diabetes, asthma, and osteoporosis. The prevalence of diabetes increases with age and is higher among people who are overweight or obese. Women are also more likely to suffer from asthma, with 9.1 percent of women compared to 5.1 percent of men being afflicted by this condition. Osteoporosis, often called the silent disease because it frequently goes undiagnosed, is especially common in women aged 65 and older.

As the number of older Americans grows, attention is also focused on the care of senior citizens. The rate of women aged 65 and older in nursing homes fell between 1973 to 1974 and 1999, indicating that more women are living in the community, either independently or with relatives, in their older years. Women continue to make up the majority of nursing home residents.

As a result of these conditions and the utilization of the health care system, women have significant expenditures for health care. While most health care expense is paid by insurance, women bear about 20 percent of the costs out of pocket. The largest category of health care expenses for women in 1997 was inpatient services, followed by home health care costs.

Men and women alike will continue to benefit from advances in medical research and treatment. Perhaps the most important message that we have gained from these advances is that our health and quality of life are shaped by both our own health behaviors and our geographic and economic access to necessary preventive, primary, and acute care.

Health Coverage and Access to Care

Women are major consumers of health care services, in many cases negotiating not only their own care but also that of their family members. Their reproductive health needs, greater rate of health problems, and longer life spans compared with men make their relationships with the health system complex. Their access to care is often complicated by their disproportionately lower incomes and greater responsibilities juggling work and family. Because of their own health needs, limited financial resources, and family responsibilities, women have a vested interest in the scope and type of services offered by health plans, as well as in the mechanisms that fund health care services.

The Kaiser Family Foundation developed the Kaiser Women's Health Survey to learn more about the experiences of women with both their health plans and their health providers. This nationally representative telephone survey was administered to 3,966 women ages 18 to 64 in the spring and summer of 2001. Women who were nonelderly Latina, African American, uninsured, low income, or on Medicaid were oversampled to improve our understanding of the challenges facing women who are most likely to fall through the cracks in the health care system.

Key Findings

The health care system is not meeting the health needs of a sizable share of women. A significant portion of women cannot afford to go to the doctor and fill their prescriptions—even when they have insurance coverage. Women with health problems often have the hardest time getting care because of coverage restrictions, high costs, and logistical barriers, such as transportation. Women also have concerns about the quality of care they receive. A substantial proportion of women changed doctors because of dissatisfaction with care. For many women, coverage and access to care are unstable. Health coverage, involvement with health plans, and relationships with doctors are often short-lived, resulting in care that can be spotty and fragmented.

Selected survey findings include:

Health care costs present significant problems for nonelderly women.

- One-quarter (24%) of nonelderly women delayed or went without care in the past year because they could not afford it, compared with 16% of men.

- Almost three in 10 (28%) women found out-of pocket costs to be higher than they would have expected them to be when they went to their doctor, a rate similar to that of men.

- Nearly one-quarter (23%) of women gave their plan a low rating on the out-of-pocket costs they incurred.

Affordability of prescription drugs is a primary concern for a sizable share of nonelderly women.

- Half of nonelderly women used prescription drugs on a regular basis, compared with 31% of men.

7

- One in five (21%) nonelderly women did not fill a prescription because of the cost, compared with 13% of men. This was a problem for 40% of uninsured women, 27% of women with Medicaid, and 15% of privately insured women.

- About four in 10 women in fair or poor health (38%) did not fill a prescription in the past year due to cost; nor did one quarter (25%) of women who used prescription drugs on a regular basis.

Women in fair or poor health—who have the greatest need for health care services—often experience major problems gaining access to care.

- About one third of nonelderly women (32%) had a health condition that required ongoing medical treatment, such as asthma, allergies, or arthritis, compared with 26% of men.

- Of the 16% of women in fair or poor health, half (49%) reported they needed to see a doctor in the past year, but did not.

- Transportation difficulties resulted in delayed care for 21% of women in fair or poor health, four times the rate of women in better health (5%).

- Nearly one-quarter of women in fair or poor health (23%) reported that their health plan refused to approve or pay for needed tests or treatment in the past two years; 57% of them either delayed care or never got treatment.

Women have significant concerns about the quality of care they receive.

- Over one in five women (22%) expressed concerns about the quality of care they received from their physicians or health care providers, compared with 17% of men. This issue was a particular problem for women in fair or poor health (40%).

- Almost one in five women (18%) changed providers in the past five years due to dissatisfaction with care, twice the rate of men (9%).

- Overall, 14% of women gave their plan a low rating on the number and quality of physicians in the plan, as did the same share of men. This was a major concern for women with Medicaid (28%) and low-income women (21%).

Connection to the health system is unstable for many women.

- Nearly three in 10 women (28%) reported they were uninsured at some point in the past year.

- One in five (19%) were uninsured at the time of the survey, and one in 10 (9%) had coverage at the time of the survey, but were uninsured for some period in the past year. Rates were similar for men.

- Half of uninsured women (49%) lacked coverage for more than one year.

- Nearly half of nonelderly women had switched plans in the past five years. The leading reasons were employers changing plans (34%) or job changes for women or their spouses (30%). These statistics were similar for men.

- Among women who switched plans, 13% left their old provider and changed to a doctor affiliated with their new plan.

- Many women had relatively new relationships with their health care providers; one-third of women with a regular provider had been seeing that provider for two years or less.

These findings highlight the importance of viewing the health system through a woman's lens. Women's health is likely to be a silent victim of the recent economic downturn and rapidly increasing health care costs. In response to these major forces, employers may be more likely to drop dependent coverage, switch to less expensive or more limited plans, or raise worker costs for care. Because women are likely to be low-income and also rely on dependent coverage more often than men, they may have much to lose. Stable coverage likely will continue to elude many women.

With the rapid growth in prescription drug costs and limits on employer-based coverage, affordability barriers for women will undoubtedly rise. Fiscal pressures on employers, insurers, health plans, and providers are likely to create even more difficulties for women in affording and obtaining the range of health care services they require.

Chapter Highlights

The following section summarizes the highlights of each chapter of the report. It presents the findings on women's health status, their health insurance coverage, their satisfaction and experiences with their health plans and providers, and their access to and use of health care services.

Health Profile of Women

Women's health status is influenced by factors such as age, income, and race/ethnicity. This survey sought to document the health conditions that women face and the factors associated with poor health among women.

Many women have health conditions that require ongoing treatment. The prevalence of most of these chronic conditions increases with age.

- More than one in 10 women (13%) had a health problem that limited their ability to participate in everyday activities.

- Compared with women ages 18 to 44, women ages 45 to 64 were three times as likely to have cancer or heart disease and four times as likely to have arthritis or hypertension.

Low-income women are likely to have poor health status and activity limitations.

- Low-income women were twice as likely as those with higher incomes to have fair or poor health status (23% and 10%, respectively) and conditions that limit activity (19% and 9%).

- They were at higher risk for experiencing health problems in their older years, when the combination of age and economic hardship takes its toll. Among low-income women ages 45 to 64, 49% reported arthritis, 41% had hypertension, and 32% had mental health concerns such as anxiety or depression.

Health status differs by race and ethnicity.

- Latinas were the most likely to report fair or poor health (29%), and African-American women were the most likely to report a health condition that limited their activity (16%).

- Among African-American women ages 45 to 64, more than half (57%) reported hypertension and 40% had arthritis. One in six Latinas and African-American women in this age group were diagnosed with diabetes in the past five years.

Health Insurance Coverage

Health insurance facilitates women's access to care by reducing financial barriers to care. Unfortunately, many women lack insurance or face obstacles in securing health coverage. This survey was designed to learn more about the status of health coverage for nonelderly women, focusing on who has coverage and who is at greatest risk for being uninsured.

A significant portion of women lack health insurance coverage.

- One in five women ages 18 to 64 was uninsured, with the risk falling disproportionately on women with limited incomes; one third of low-income women lacked coverage.

- Latinas were at very high risk of being uninsured; nearly four in 10 (37%) were without coverage. Younger women (between the ages of 18 and 29), those who were foreign born, and those who lived in the South or West were the most likely to lack coverage.

- Half of uninsured women (51%) lacked coverage for more than one year.

- Six in 10 (57%) uninsured women worked either full- or part-time.

Most women with health insurance receive it through work.

- Employer-sponsored insurance was the predominant form of coverage for nonelderly women, with six in 10 covered by their own or their spouses' employer.

- Women were less likely than men to be covered by their own employers (33% vs. 53%, respectively) and more likely to be insured as a dependent (27% vs. 13%, respectively).

Medicaid, the state-federal health program for the poor, serves an important role for low-income women.

- Nearly one in 10 nonelderly women (9%) received Medicaid coverage.

- Medicaid played an especially important role for poor women, covering one third (34%).

11

Health Plans

A health plan's benefits and procedures can affect the types of pro-viders and services that women can obtain. This survey focused on women's concerns about their health plans and the factors that in-fluenced their decisions and determined their satisfaction with plans.

Women take a leading role in family coverage decisions.

- Nearly six in 10 women reported that they were the primary de-cision-makers in their families about health insurance; 22% made the decisions jointly with their spouses.

- In selecting health plans, more than half of women rated as "very important" the benefits offered, selection of doctors, cost of plan, and reputation of the plan.

- The overwhelming majority of nonelderly insured women (82%) were enrolled in a managed care plan, such as a health mainte-nance organization (HMO) or preferred provider organization (PPO), and 17% were in fee-for-service arrangements.

- Just over half of privately insured women (53%) were enrolled in a loosely controlled plan where they had some flexibility to see a spe-cialist without a referral or go out of network at higher cost. Al-most one third of women (30%) were in tightly controlled plans.

- Among women enrolled in Medicaid, 82% were members of a managed care plan.

The majority of women are generally satisfied with their health plans.

- Overall, few women gave their plans low ratings on issues such as the number of benefits (16%), ease of use (15%), and the number and quality of physicians in the plan (14%). Out-of-pocket costs were rated poorly by nearly one-quarter (23%) of nonelderly women.

- On many of these issues, women in poorer health, those on Med-icaid, and low-income women had higher rates of dissatisfaction than other women.

A sizable share of women face difficulties in getting needed care be-cause their plans deny payment or approval.

- One in seven women reported that their plans denied coverage for care they thought they needed.

- Lack of plan approval for treatment or tests resulted in nearly one-half of women who were denied care either delaying or never receiving the services they thought they needed.

- About half of women (53%) whose insurance denied payment for needed services disputed their plans' decisions.

- Low-income women (33%) were twice as likely as higher-income women (15%) not to obtain the treatment they thought they needed.

Health Providers

A woman's relationship and satisfaction with her provider is a critical component of her health care. This survey explored women's relationships with their providers, focusing on both what worked well and women's chief concerns.

Women's reproductive and general health care needs make their relationships with their health care providers complex.

- Nearly one in five women (17%) did not have a regular health provider, about half the rate of men (28%). Almost half of uninsured women (46%), one third of Latinas (31%), and one quarter of low-income women (24%) lacked a regular provider.

- About one half of women had at least two routine providers, typically a primary care provider such as an internist or a general practitioner, along with an obstetrician or gynecologist (ob/gyn). The other half of women saw just one provider for regular care, typically a primary care doctor. Only a small fraction of women (7%) relied exclusively on an ob/gyn for all of their routine care.

- Despite the increasing pool of women physicians, only about one third of women (31%) saw a female as their regular provider.

- Many women had relatively new relationships with their providers; one third of women with a regular provider had been seeing that provider for two years or less.

A sizable minority of women—particularly those that faced the greatest health challenges—reported that they have difficulty communicating with their providers.

- Women in poor health (18%) and Latinas (14%) were the most likely to feel that their doctor did not take the time to answer all their questions.

- Nearly two in 10 women (17%) reported that they did not understand or remember all of the information provided to them at their medical visit. This was particularly a problem for nearly one third of women in fair or poor health.

A significant portion of women have changed doctors because they were dissatisfied.

- Nearly one in five (18%) women had changed her doctor at some point in the past five years due to dissatisfaction, double the rate of men (9%).

Access to and Use of Health Care

Women's access to and use of the health system is influenced in part by their individual characteristics, health needs, and prior experience with both illness and the health system. It is also strongly influenced by insurance coverage and health system features. This survey examined the characteristics of women who faced the greatest challenges gaining access to health care and explored the factors that placed them at highest risk for experiencing barriers to care.

Most women (87%) had a health care visit in the past year, but where they got their care varied for different subgroups of women.

- Latinas and uninsured women, both groups at higher risk for experiencing access problems and barriers to care, were the least likely to have had a doctor visit in the past year (31% and 24%, respectively).

- Women on Medicaid or who were uninsured (about four in 10 each) as well as African American women and Latinas (27% and 38%, respectively) were more likely to rely on hospital clinics and health centers for medical care than other women.

Many women do not receive recommended screening tests.

- Only 35% of women 50 to 64 had a screening test for colon cancer in the past two years, 77% of women in the same age group had a mammogram in the past two years, and 56% percent of women 18 to 64 had a blood cholesterol test.

- Uninsured women and to a somewhat lesser extent, women on Medicaid were less likely than women with private coverage to obtain many of the recommended preventive screening tests.

Women experience multiple types of barriers to receiving health care.

- The cost of care was a significant barrier to obtaining medical attention for women. Nearly six in 10 (59%) uninsured women, 42% of women in fair or poor health, and 31% of Latinas delayed or went without care because they could not afford it.

- Transportation barriers were experienced by 7% of women, but were especially salient for women on Medicaid (23%), Latinas (18%), and uninsured women (12%).

- Child care problems contributed to delays and postponement of care for 10% of women with children, and ranged from 17% of women on Medicaid to just 8% of privately insured women.

Chapter 2

Female Reproductive System

Reproduction is the process by which organisms produce more organisms like themselves. All living things, including humans, reproduce: it's one of the things that set us apart from nonliving matter. And because all living things eventually die, new creatures of the same kind must constantly be born to perpetuate a particular species. Interestingly, although the reproductive system is essential to keeping a species alive, unlike other body systems, it is not essential to keeping an individual being alive.

How Is the Female Reproductive System Important for Living?

Without the female reproductive system, there would be no perpetuation of life. Although the female is dependent on the male for fertilization of her egg, it is she who carries the offspring through pregnancy and childbirth. Through the reproduction process, children are born, and families are continued. If people didn't reproduce, families would die out and the human race would cease to exist.

Humans, like other organisms, transmit certain characteristics of themselves to the next generation through their genes, the special

This information was provided by KidsHealth, one of the largest resources online for medically reviewed health information written for parents, kids, and teens. For more articles like this one, visit www.KidsHealth.org, or www.TeensHealth.org. © 2001 The Nemours Center for Children's Health Media, a division of The Nemours Foundation.

carriers of human traits. The genes parents pass along to their children are what make children similar to others in their family, but they are also what make each child unique. These genes come from the father's sperm and the mother's egg, which are produced by their respective reproductive systems.

Basic Anatomy

Most species have male and female organisms. Each sex has its own unique reproductive system. They are different in shape and structure, but both are specifically designed to produce, nourish, and transport either the egg or sperm.

Unlike its male counterpart, the female reproductive system is almost entirely hidden within the pelvis. It consists of organs that enable a woman to produce eggs (ova), to have sexual intercourse, to nourish and house the fertilized egg (ovum) until it is fully developed, and to give birth.

Females also have external organs collectively called the vulva (which means "covering"). Located between the legs, the outer parts of the vulva cover the opening to a narrow canal called the vagina. The fleshy area located just above the top of the vaginal opening is called the mons pubis. A thin sheet of tissue called the hymen partially covers the opening of the vagina. Two pairs of skin flaps, the labia (which means "lips") surround the vaginal opening. The clitoris, which is located toward the front of the vulva where the folds of the labia join, is a small cylindrical structure similar to the male penis; it also contains erectile tissue. Inside the labia are openings to the urethra (the canal that carries urine from the bladder to the exterior of the body) and vagina. The outer labia and the mons pubis are covered by pubic hair in the sexually mature female.

The female internal organs are the vagina, uterus, fallopian tubes, and ovaries. The vagina is a 3- to 6-inch-long tubular structure that extends from the vaginal opening to the uterus. It has muscular walls lined with mucous membrane, and it serves as the female organ of copulation (sexual intercourse) as well as the birth canal. It connects with the uterus, or womb, which houses the fetus during pregnancy. About 3 inches long and 2 inches wide and shaped like an inverted pear, the uterus is a muscular, expandable organ with thick walls.

At the lower part of the uterus is the cervix, which opens into the vagina. At the upper part, the fallopian tubes connect the uterus with the ovaries, two oval-shaped organs that lie to the right and left of the uterus. They produce, store, and release eggs through the fallopian tubes into the uterus. The ovaries also produce the hormones estrogen and progesterone. Also part of the reproductive system are the breasts. Mammary glands inside the breasts secrete milk after childbirth.

Normal Physiology

The organs of sexual reproduction are the gonads, which are the ovaries in females and the testes in males. Females produce female gametes, or eggs; males produce male gametes, or sperm. Sexual reproduction is the fertilization of a female gamete by a male gamete. When a female is born, each of her ovaries has hundreds of thousands of eggs, but they remain dormant until her first menstrual cycle, which occurs during puberty. At this time, during adolescence, the pituitary gland secretes hormones that stimulate the ovaries to produce female sex hormones, including estrogen, which helps the female develop into a sexually mature woman.

Also at this time, females begin releasing eggs as part of a monthly period called the menstrual cycle. Approximately once a month, during ovulation, an ovary discharges a tiny egg that reaches the uterus through one of the fallopian tubes. Unless fertilized by a sperm while in the fallopian tube, the egg dries up and is expelled about 2 weeks later from the uterus during menstruation. Blood and tissues from the inner lining of the uterus combine to form the menstrual flow, which usually lasts from 3 to 5 days.

If a female and male have sexual intercourse within several days of ovulation, fertilization can occur. When the male ejaculates, about one tenth of an ounce of semen is deposited into the vagina. Between 200 and 300 million sperm are in this small amount of semen, and they "swim" up from the vagina through the cervix and uterus to meet the egg in the fallopian tube. It takes only one sperm to fertilize the egg.

About a week after the sperm fertilizes the egg, the fertilized egg has become a multicelled blastocyst, a pinhead-sized hollow ball with fluid inside, now housed in the uterus. The blastocyst burrows itself into the lining of the uterus, called the endometrium. Estrogen causes the endometrium to thicken and become rich with blood, and progesterone, another hormone released by the ovaries, maintains the thickness of the endometrium so that the blastocyst can attach to the uterus and absorb nutrients from it. This process is called implantation.

As cells from the blastocyst take in nourishment, the embryonic stage of development begins. The inner cells form a flattened circular

19

shape called the embryonic disk, which will develop into a baby. The outer cells become thin membranes that form around the baby. The embryonic cells multiply thousands of times, move to new positions, and eventually become the embryo. After approximately 8 weeks, the embryo is about the size of an adult's thumb, but all of its parts—the brain and nerves, the heart and blood, the stomach and intestines, and the muscles and skin—have formed.

During the fetal stage, which lasts from 9 weeks after fertilization to birth, development continues as cells multiply, move, and differentiate. The fetus floats in amniotic fluid inside the amniotic sac. Its oxygen and nourishment come from the mother's blood via the placenta, a disk-like structure that adheres to the inner lining of the uterus and is connected to the umbilical cord. The umbilical cord attaches the embryo at its navel to the mother's uterus. The umbilical arteries in the cord carry blood from the fetus to the placenta, and an umbilical vein returns blood from the placenta to the fetus. The amniotic fluid and membrane cushion the fetus against bumps and jolts to the mother's body.

Pregnancy lasts an average of 266 days. When the baby is ready for birth, its head presses on the cervix, which begins to relax and widen to get ready for the baby to pass into and through the vagina, which has enlarged to become the birth canal. The mucus that has formed a plug in the cervix loosens, and with amniotic fluid, comes out through the vagina when the mother's "water" breaks.

When contractions begin, the uterine walls contract as they are stimulated by the pituitary hormone oxytocin. The contractions cause the cervix to widen and begin to open. After several hours of this widening, the cervix is dilated (opened) enough for the baby to come through. The baby is pushed out of the uterus, through the cervix, and along the birth canal. The baby's head usually comes first; the umbilical cord comes out with the baby and is cut after the baby is delivered.

The last stage of the birth process involves the delivery of the placenta, which is now called the afterbirth. It has separated from the inner lining of the uterus, and through further contractions of the uterus it is expelled with its membranes and fluids.

Diseases, Conditions, Disorders, and Dysfunctions

Like all body systems, the female reproductive system is at risk for certain diseases and conditions. The following are some examples.

Disorders of the Vulva and Vagina

Vulvovaginitis, an inflammation of the vulva and/or vagina, is the most common childhood gynecological problem. In young girls, it is most often caused by irritating substances (such as laundry soaps or bubble baths), and may be exacerbated by poor personal hygiene (such as wiping from back to front after a bowel movement). Symptoms include redness and itching in the vaginal area and sometimes vaginal discharge. Vulvovaginitis can also be caused by an overgrowth of *Candida*, a yeast-like fungus normally present in the vagina, although yeast infections are more common in teenagers and adults.

Vaginal bleeding, when it occurs in premenstrual girls, is most commonly due to the presence of a foreign body in the vagina, such as wadded-up toilet paper. Less often it may be due to urethral prolapse, a condition in which the mucous membranes of the urethra protrude into the vagina and form a mass that bleeds easily. It can also be due to an injury or sexual abuse.

Labial adhesions, the adherence (sticking together) of the labia in the midline, usually appears in infants and young girls. Although there are usually no symptoms associated with the condition, labial adhesions can lead to an increased risk of urinary tract infection. It is sometimes treated with a topical estrogen cream to help separate the labia.

Disorders of the Ovaries

Tumors, although relatively rare in childhood, can occur. In adolescents, the most common type of gynecological tumor is the ovarian teratoma, and it may be either benign or malignant. Tumors are usually detectable as masses in the abdomen and may be accompanied by abdominal pain; they are usually removed surgically.

Ovarian cysts are noncancerous sacs filled with fluid or semi-solid material. Although they are common and generally harmless, they can become a problem if they grow very large. Large cysts may push on surrounding organs, causing abdominal pain. In most cases, cysts will disappear spontaneously and treatment is unnecessary. However, if the cysts are painful, birth control pills may be used to alter their growth, or they may be removed surgically.

Ovarian torsion, or twisting of the ovary, is a fairly uncommon condition that can occur when an ovary becomes twisted or because of a developmental abnormality or disease. This blocks blood from flowing through the blood vessels that supply and nourish the ovaries. The most common symptom is lower abdominal pain. Surgery is usually necessary to correct the condition.

Polycystic ovary syndrome is a hormonal disorder in which an over-production of male hormones (androgens) by the ovaries causes the ovaries to become enlarged and develop fluid-filled sacs, or cysts. It often first appears during adolescence, and associated problems may include obesity, acne, erratic menstrual periods, and the appearance of masculine characteristics such as hair growth on the face and chest. Depending on the type and severity of the condition, it may be treated with drugs that work against the effects of the male hormones and possibly birth control pills to regulate hormone balance and menstruation. It is associated with a higher risk of infertility later in life, particularly if untreated.

Menstrual Problems

Both common and varied, menstrual problems range from dysmenorrhea (painful periods) and menorrhagia (heavy periods) to oligomenorrhea (missed and/or infrequent periods). Treatments may include pain medication and hormone pills.

Sexually Transmitted Diseases

These include infections and diseases such as HIV/AIDS (human immunodeficiency virus/acquired immune deficiency syndrome), human papilloma virus (HPV, or genital warts), syphilis, chlamydia, gonorrhea, and herpes genitalis. They are spread from one person to another by sexual intercourse and other genital contact involving the sexual organs and other body parts.

Toxic Shock Syndrome

This rare illness is caused by a bacterial infection that is more likely to develop if a tampon is left in too long. It can produce high fever, diarrhea, vomiting, and shock.

Glossary

afterbirth: Placenta and fetal membranes that are expelled after delivery.

amniotic fluid: Fluid in the amniotic sac, the membrane that surrounds the developing fetus.

blastocyst: Early stage of embryo development; pinhead-sized hollow ball with fluid inside.

cervix: Lower end of the uterus that opens into the vagina.

clitoris: Small cylindrical structure at the top of the vaginal opening; contains erectile tissue similar to the male penis.

egg: Female sex cell; also called an ovum.

embryo: The developing human from the time of implantation to the end of the eighth week after conception.

endometrium: Inner lining of the uterus.

fallopian tubes: Tubes through which eggs (ova) pass from the ovaries to the uterus.

fertilization: The joining of male and female sex cells (ovum and sperm) to form a new organism.

fetus: Developing human from the ninth week after conception until birth.

gamete: Sex cell that joins with another gamete of the opposite sex to produce a new organism.

gonads: Sex organs that contain the gametes and produce sex hormones.

hymen: Thin tissue that partially covers the vaginal opening.

implantation: The process of attachment of the embryo to the inner wall of the uterus.

labia: Two pairs of skin flaps surrounding the vaginal opening.

mammary glands: Milk-producing glands in the female breasts.

menstrual cycle: Monthly maturation and release of an egg (ovum) from an ovary.

mons pubis: Fleshy area located just above the top of the vaginal opening.

ovaries: Structures in which female eggs (ova) are located.

ovulation: Release of a mature egg (ovum) from an ovary.

oxytocin: Hormone that stimulates contractions in the uterus during the birth process.

placenta: Structure attached to the umbilical cord that provides nourishment for the developing fetus and removes its waste by an exchange with the mother's bloodstream.

semen: Fluid containing sperm that is ejaculated by the male sperm: Male sex cell(s).

urethra: Canal that carries urine from the bladder to the exterior of the body.

uterus: Muscular, pear-shaped internal female reproductive organ in which the embryo and fetus develop during pregnancy; also called the womb.

vagina: Muscle-walled tube that serves as the birth canal and entrance to the internal female reproductive tract.

vulva: Female external sex organs.

Note: All information on KidsHealth is for educational purposes only. For specific medical advice, diagnoses, and treatment, consult your doctor.

Chapter 3

Feeling Good about Growing Up

When we think of sexuality, we might just think about our bodies. We might just think about our sex organs. But our sexuality has as much to do with how we think and feel as it does with how we behave. Sexuality is a basic part of our physical, mental, emotional, and spiritual lives.

Our sexuality should be enjoyed and celebrated. It is not something to be ashamed of or embarrassed about. Healthy sexuality allows us to be open, flexible, creative, safe, and responsible as we explore our sexual thoughts and feelings. It lets us recognize that sex can be fun and can also fulfill many emotional needs. Sex also has risks.

Having a healthy attitude about sexuality means knowing our values, beliefs, attitudes, limits, and boundaries, and respecting that knowledge by being responsible. It allows us to feel attractive, regardless of our age, gender, sexual orientation, race, religion, height, weight, or physical or mental ability. It lets us be ourselves.

Knowing as much as possible about our sexual selves, in terms of our beliefs, values, and physical needs will help us create responsible, healthy, and satisfying sexual lives.

Our Sexual Bodies

Girls and boys have different sex organs. Only girls and women have vulvas. Only boys and men have penises. Vulvas and penises are located in the front of the body between the legs.

"The Facts of Life: A Guide for Teens and Their Families: As Girls Become Women." Reprinted with permission from Planned Parenthood ® Federation of America, Inc. © 2002 PPFA. All rights reserved.

The labia, urethra, clitoris, and opening to the vagina are all part of the vulva. Sometimes, girls use mirrors to see the parts of their vulvas.

The labia majora and labia minora are two folds of fleshy tissue on the outermost parts of the vulva. The labia majora—the outer lips—are closer to the legs. Pubic hair grows there on most adolescents and adult women. The labia minora protect the inner vulva. They do not have pubic hair.

The opening of the vagina is in the middle of the vulva. It is a passageway to a woman's reproductive organs. Above it, the opening of the urethra is not easy to see. It provides a passageway for urine to flow from the bladder to the outside of the body.

Only the tip of the clitoris is visible at the top of the vulva in the soft folds where the labia meet. The rest of the clitoris reaches inside the body.

Puberty Happens to Everybody

But it doesn't happen to everybody at the same time. Generally, girls start puberty earlier than boys. The bodies of some girls begin changing at age eight. Others don't start changing until they are 14.

Some of the changes are the same for girls and boys. We get taller. We begin to grow hair under our arms and around our vulvas or penises. We sweat more, too, mostly under the arms. That's when a lot of people start washing more often and start using deodorants. Also, our voices deepen. This usually happens more suddenly in boys than in girls.

Many of us get pimples during puberty on the face, back, chest, or buttocks. We get them as our skin starts growing thicker and the glands under it start making more oil. Our pores become clogged and infected. That's another good reason to wash and shampoo often.

Hormones Make Our Bodies Grow Up

Our bodies make chemicals called hormones that guide our growth into women and men—estrogen and progesterone in girls and testosterone in boys. Often we grow so fast that we feel clumsy. We even may have uncomfortable growing pains, usually in our arms and legs.

Estrogen causes lots of the changes. Girls' breasts begin to get fuller. Often one breast grows faster than the other. Their hips get rounder. Their waists get narrower. Their vulvas and clitorises grow slightly, too.

Girls may have a white, sticky discharge from their vaginas called leukorrhea. They shouldn't worry about it unless the vulva becomes itchy or irritated. If it does, a girl should visit her doctor or clinician.

We inherit our size, eye color, and skin color from our parents. We also inherit large breasts or small breasts, thin legs or thick legs, big penises or small penises, and thick beards or thin beards. Most of the time we inherit average breasts, legs, penises, or beards. But we are all very different, no matter what—and that's normal.

Clitorises, labia, penises, and breasts vary in shape and size. The appearance of the outer folds of the labia—the labia majora—varies in size, shape, and color from woman to woman. The color of the labia minora is also different for every woman. In some women, the labia are smooth—in others, they are wrinkled. The clitoris may be smaller than a pea or bigger than a fingertip. It reaches inside the body up to five inches.

Women's breasts are different in shape and size. The nipples may be flat or raised. They, and the area around them—the aureole—differ in color from woman to woman. A woman's breasts can give her sexual pleasure when touched. Small or large, her breasts can also produce milk after she has a baby.

Some people prefer big penises or big breasts. However, being attractive depends more on personality—how we think of ourselves, present ourselves, take care of ourselves, and respect ourselves and other people.

During puberty, things happen inside the body, too. Most girls start having periods. Most boys start having wet dreams. And girls and boys begin having a lot more thoughts and feelings about sex.

Important changes are happening inside the body. The reproductive system is maturing. Boys begin producing sperm—the male reproductive cells. Girls' ovaries begin to ripen eggs—the female reproductive cells.

Pregnancy can happen if only one sperm joins with an egg. The sperm can reach the egg if a boy or man puts his penis in or near the vagina. Often our reproductive systems grow up faster than we do. That's why girls can get pregnant and boys can cause pregnancy before they finish growing up.

As Girls Become Women

Girls and women have orgasms during sexual dreams. Women and girls become sexually excited by sexual thoughts and dreams or sex play with themselves or another person. Their vaginas become wet, their clitorises become erect, and if they become very sexually excited,

27

they may have orgasms or a series of orgasms. In some women, a clear fluid spurts out of the urethra during sexual excitement or orgasm. This is also called ejaculation.

The vagina connects the sex organs of the vulva to the other reproductive organs inside the body. The soft folds of the walls of the vagina adjust to the size of the penis during vaginal intercourse and stretch during childbirth. Girls and women also have two ovaries, a cervix, a uterus, and two fallopian tubes.

Each ovary holds hundreds of thousands of pinpoint-sized eggs. Girls are born with all the eggs they will ever have. One ovary releases a mature egg about once a month. This is called ovulation. Before ovulation, the uterus builds up a spongy, soft lining. It is made of tissue and blood. This lining is like a nest for the egg if pregnancy happens.

After ovulation, the egg moves through a fallopian tube toward the uterus. Most of the time, the egg breaks apart before it gets there. Then

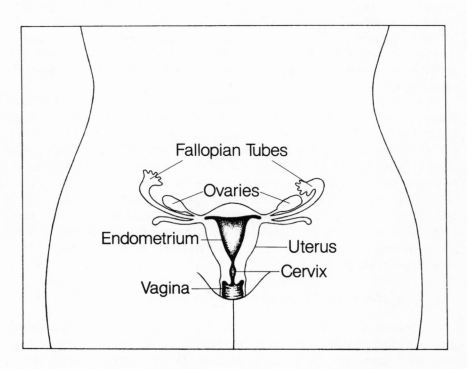

Figure 3.1. *Female reproductive system. Source: National Cancer Institute.*

the tissue and blood aren't needed. They flow out of the uterus, through the cervix and vagina out of the body. This is called menstrual flow or a period. Different women have different amounts of flow during their periods. About only three or four tablespoonfuls of it are blood—although it may seem like more.

But the egg doesn't always break apart. If the egg meets a sperm in the fallopian tube, they can join together. The joining of the egg and sperm is called fertilization. Pregnancy begins if a fertilized egg attaches itself to the lining of the uterus. The lining stays in place until the pregnancy ends. That's why pregnant women do not have periods.

The first time menstruation happens is called menarche. Some families celebrate menarche as the time when a girl becomes a woman. Other families are more private about it. But whether or not menarche is celebrated, it is an exciting and important moment in a girl's life. It is also normal for girls to feel nervous or scared when they start getting their periods.

The time from the first day of one period to the first day of the next is called a menstrual cycle. On average, menstrual cycles begin between the ages of 12 and 13. They end when women are between 45 and 55 years old.

Periods last about five days. It may be seven to 21 days from the beginning of a woman's period to ovulation. Then there are usually 14 to 16 days from ovulation to the beginning of the next period.

During puberty, it's not unusual for three, four, five, or six months to go by between periods. Eventually, they happen every four or five weeks. Sometimes there is a spotting of blood between periods. Some women know when they are going to have their periods by the way their bodies feel. Others don't. Some women keep a record of their periods on a calendar to become more familiar with their cycle.

Some girls and women may have physical or emotional discomfort up to two weeks before menstruating. This is called premenstrual syndrome (PMS). Usually mild, PMS happens in fewer than half of all women.

Women use sanitary pads or tampons to absorb menstrual flow. Every package has instructions. Tampons and sanitary pads come in different sizes and varieties. Some are for lighter flows. Some are for heavier flows.

Pads stay in place by sticking inside the underwear. A tampon fits inside the vagina. The walls of the vagina hold it in place. Each tampon has a string that hangs out of the vagina. The tampon is removed easily by pulling the string slowly. Tampons or pads and regular bathing are all a woman or girl needs to stay clean during her period. Douches, vaginal deodorants, and perfumed pads and tampons are unnecessary and may irritate the vulva and vagina.

Some girls wonder if tampons will stretch the hymen and make them lose their virginity. The hymen is a thin skin that stretches across the opening of the vagina. There is usually an opening in it to let menstrual flow out of the body.

The hymen is very important to some people. They believe that a girl without a hymen is no longer a virgin—that a boy has put his penis in her vagina. Girls are born with various sizes and openings of the hymen. Some may even appear to have no hymen. Others stretch theirs open during certain kinds of exercise like bicycling or horseback riding. Tampons don't usually stretch the hymen open all the way.

Girls and women who use tampons change them every three or four hours, or more often if bleeding is heavy. Too many bacteria can develop if a tampon is left in place too long. This can cause a rare illness called toxic shock syndrome (TSS). Although very rare, TSS is very serious. If you vomit and develop a high fever, diarrhea, muscle aches, sore throat, dizziness, faintness, or weakness, and a sunburn type rash while using a tampon, take it out and see your clinician—fast. You can reduce your risk by using a pad or less absorbent tampon while sleeping.

Usually, women and girls do not have serious problems with their periods. Some feel depressed or moody. Some have cramps on the first day or two of their periods. Exercise and a healthy diet may reduce cramps. Putting a hot-water bottle or heating pad on the abdomen can help, too.

Usually cramps aren't severe enough to prevent normal activities. If they are, a girl should talk with her parent, the school nurse, a teacher, or a clinician. There are very good medicines that lessen the pain of menstrual cramps.

Chapter 4

As Girls Become Women

Chapter Contents

Section 4.1

Female Puberty

Reprinted with permission from "Female Puberty," part of the *Tips to Grow By*© series produced as a public service by the Children's Medical Center of Akron, Ohio. © 2001 Children's Medical Center of Akron. For additional information, visit www.akronchildrens.org/kids-teens.

Puberty is the process of growing from a girl into a woman that every girl will go through sometime between the ages of 9 to 16. Your body changes at its own pace, which is largely determined by your genes. Ask your mom at what age she started puberty. Some girls begin puberty earlier or later than their friends do. Puberty usually starts earlier for girls than boys. For a few years, you may be bigger and seem more mature than boys your age.

Will I look different?

Physically your body will begin to look more like an adult woman. Sometime between the ages of 9 to 16 special glands in your brain send a signal to your ovaries. This signal tells them to increase production of the female sex hormones. This causes big changes in your body that can last from two to six years. During this time you'll start your menstrual cycle or period and you'll have the ability to get pregnant. During puberty, your ovaries begin releasing eggs for the first time. If the egg isn't fertilized by a male's sperm, the uterine lining isn't needed. It flows out through the cervix and vagina in a process called menstruation or more commonly referred to as your period.

Your body will change in other ways too:

- Your breasts will develop. It's normal for one breast to grow more quickly than the other and to stay uneven in size.

- You'll grow taller.

- You'll develop curves. Your hips and thighs widen and your pelvis expands into a more womanly shape.

- You get hair in new places. Hair grows under your armpits and in the pubic area between your legs (it looks like an upside down triangle of hair). Fine hair will also grow on your legs. All of this hair isn't usually the same color or texture of the hair that grows on your head so don't be alarmed!

- Your skin becomes thicker and more oily as your oil glands become more active. Keep your hair and skin clean to help avoid pimples.

- Your sweat glands become more active which means you sweat more. Wear deodorant to eliminate body odor. Bathe daily and keep your clothes clean.

- Your feet and hands grow bigger. Your feet are most likely to reach their full adult size long before the rest of you does.

- Your appetite and weight increase. You need more calories while your body is growing. If you are gaining weight, don't panic and start dieting.

- Eat well-balanced meals and try to stay away from junk food. Once you stop growing, your weight will level off.

- You may have vaginal discharge. Six months to a year before you start your period, you may notice a clear, milky white discharge that may turn yellow on your underwear. It's normal. If it bothers you, you may feel more comfortable wearing a panty-liner.

Section 4.2

Questions and Answers about Puberty

Reprinted with permission from "Female Puberty," part of the *Tips to Grow By*© series produced as a public service by the Children's Medical Center of Akron, Ohio. © 2001 Children's Medical Center of Akron. For additional information, visit www.akronchildrens.org/kids-teens.

How will I feel about puberty?

Puberty can be a very emotional time. You'll begin to have more intense feelings of love and joy and also of loneliness and sadness. As you get older you'll also have more responsibilities at home and at school. You'll also begin to decide what's important to you, what kinds of friends you want to have, and the kind of person you want be. You'll probably want some independence from your parents, yet still find comfort in the security they provide. Your parents are proud that you're maturing into a young adult, yet they may get their feelings hurt because you'd rather spend time with your friends than with them. You may also argue with them over the fairness of house rules, family obligations, chores, etc. Try sharing your feelings with your parents and coming up with solutions that all of you can live with.

The teenage years can also make you feel insecure. Being popular and belonging to a group may be very important to you; having friends can help you feel secure. If you aren't accepted by a particular group, try and seek out friends elsewhere. Remember that you are a valuable and important person and you shouldn't have to change or do things you don't want to do just to be accepted as someone's friend. If you feel pressure from your friends to do something you don't want to, ask yourself whether what they want you to do could hurt you or help you.

Does sex play a role in puberty?

Your body is now physically able to have sexual intercourse and produce a baby. Actions you take now could affect your health and happiness in the future. Sexually transmitted diseases (STDs) are spread by sex. Many are silent infections, which means there aren't any signs or symptoms to let you know anything is wrong. Some STDs increase your risk of cancer or your ability to have a baby in the future and some, like AIDS, can kill you.

Never let anyone pressure you into having sex. If you have sex before you're ready, you may experience anger or regret. It's best to wait until you're sure of your feelings, you're able to accept any possible results, and you're ready to make a lifelong commitment to one person. Being a parent of an unplanned-for baby will limit your social life and change your future. Parents must work hard for many years to provide a home, food, clothing, health care, education, and guidance to their children. This is a huge responsibility even for married adult couples who plan the timing of their families.

When should I see a medical professional?

If you do decide to become sexually active, it's important to talk to a trusted adult and your pediatrician, family doctor, nurse practitioner, or gynecologist, a doctor who specializes in women's reproductive health, before you act. All can counsel you on the use of birth control, or contraception, which refers to methods used to prevent pregnancy. The only method that is 100 percent effective at preventing pregnancy or sexually transmitted disease is abstinence (not having sex at all).

Even if you choose to wait to become sexually active, it's still important to make an appointment once a year, beginning at age 18, to see your family doctor or a gynecologist. Decide whether you are more comfortable with a male or female doctor. Ask around for recommendations. Your mom probably goes to someone she likes or you can ask your friends or school nurse. When you meet with the doctor, make sure you answer his or her questions truthfully about your medical and personal history. The information you give will stay private. He or she won't discuss it with your parents or others. It is considered confidential patient information.

At your annual exam you may feel a little embarrassed, but the exam shouldn't hurt. You can expect your doctor to check your breasts for lumps and your nipples for abnormal discharge. He or she will also show you how to perform monthly breast self examinations. The doctor will do a Pap smear to check your cervix for signs of cancer or abnormal cells and a pelvic exam to check for cysts on your ovaries and fibroids in your uterus. These are all important preventive measures to keep you healthy.

Pay attention to your body. Easy to treat infections can become serious problems if left untreated. Call the doctor or nurse practitioner right away if you have:

- Been a victim of rape or sexual abuse (also contact the police or victim abuse center)

- Vaginal discharge that's heavier than usual or has a strong color or odor

- Genital lumps or sores

- Vaginal redness, itching, or burning

- A breast lump, abnormal nipple discharge, pain, or change in your breasts

- Abdominal pain aside from usual cramps associated with your period

- Changes in your period after you've been menstruating for more than a year

- A sexual partner who tells you he or she has an STD

Also, see a health care provider if your breasts and pubic and underarm hair haven't begun to develop by age 14, or if you haven't started your period by age 16. This may mean your body isn't producing enough estrogen (a female hormone) on its own. Your doctor should be able to treat this problem.

How can I take care of myself during puberty?

When you feel good, you look good. During puberty it's extra important to take care of your body by eating a healthy diet consisting of a variety of foods from the five basic food groups. Get enough rest and exercise. Both will help increase your energy and reduce your stress levels. Bathe and shower regularly to help prevent body odor and acne breakouts.

If you have questions about the changes your body is going through, find an adult you trust. Remember he or she went through puberty too.

Section 4.3

Precocious Puberty

The Pituitary Gland: The Master Gland

The pituitary gland, which is often referred to as the master gland, regulates the release of most of the body's hormones (chemical messengers that send information to different parts of the body). It is a pea-sized gland that is located underneath the brain. The pituitary gland controls the release of thyroid, adrenal, growth, and sex hormones. The hypothalamus, located in the brain above the pituitary gland, regulates the release of hormones from the pituitary gland.

Hormones: The Chemical Messengers

Hormones are chemical messengers that carry information from one cell to another in the body. Hormones are carried throughout body by the blood, and are responsible for regulating many body functions. The body makes many hormones (e.g., thyroid, growth, sex, and adrenal hormones) that work together to maintain normal bodily function. Hormones involved in the control of puberty include:

- GnRH: Gonadotropin releasing hormone, which comes from the brain in boys and in girls. Other androgens from the adrenal glands (located near the kidneys) produce pubic and axillary hair at the time of puberty.

- Estrogen: A female sex hormone, which is responsible for breast development in girls. It is made mainly by the ovaries, but is also present in boys in smaller amounts.

- Sex Hormones: Responsible for the development of pubertal signs as well as changes in behavior and the ability to have children.

37

Precocious Puberty

Precocious puberty means having signs of puberty (e.g., pubic hair or breast development) at an earlier age than usual.

Normal Puberty

There is a wide range of ages at which individuals normally start puberty. Girls usually develop breasts and then pubic hair between the ages of 8 and 13 years. Menstrual periods typically start at 12 to 13 years of age. Girls will often experience moodiness and become more irritable during puberty. Boys normally develop testicular enlargement and then pubic hair between the ages of 9 and 14 years. Underarm and facial hair, as well as deepening of the voice, typically occur between the ages of 13 and 16 years. Your child may be taller than the other children in his/her class. This is because the hormones that increase at the time of puberty also cause a spurt in growth.

Causes of Precocious Puberty

In the majority of cases of precocious puberty, the cause is unknown. In some instances, the pituitary signals the ovaries and testicles to make female and male hormones at an earlier than usual time. In other cases, signs of puberty occur prematurely because of abnormalities in the ovaries, testicles, or adrenal glands. Tests are usually necessary to determine whether the cause of precocious puberty is in the brain or in another area of the body.

Treatment

If your child's doctor determines that treatment is necessary, your child may receive a medication (analog or modified form of GnRH). The goals of treatment with this drug are to temporarily stop puberty and to decrease the rate of bone maturation. Rapid bone maturation will cause your child's adult height to be shorter than his or her potential height. After the first couple of months of treatment, your child's rapid growth should slow and his or her pubertal stage will remain the same or possibly regress. Many children are too young to deal with the psychological aspects of early puberty and by stopping further advances, your child may feel more like his or her friends.

GnRH analogs are given by injection daily, or at intervals of every 3 or 4 weeks. If your child receives daily medication, then a nurse will teach you how to safely give injections at home. If your child receives the medication once a month, your local physician or a visiting nurse will most likely give the injection.

Possible Treatment Side Effects

During the first 6 weeks of treatment your child may experience the following side effects: Girls may have mood changes, acne, an increase in breast size, and menses. Boys may have an increase in pubic hair and testicular development as well as acne. These effects are only temporary and should be controlled by the seventh week of treatment. Other side effects your child may experience include redness and slight pain at the site of the injection. Rarely, a sterile abscess may occur. Use of a filter needle to reconstitute the depot form of the analog will help prevent this. Your child will receive medication until it is appropriate for puberty to resume. Research to date indicates that when the treatment is stopped puberty should resume and advance normally.

Follow-Up Clinic Visits

It will be important for your child to be seen every 3 months. This will allow the doctor to adjust the GnRH analog dose to ensure that your child is receiving the appropriate amount. Your child's height will be measured in order to determine his or her growth rate. If treatment is successful, your child's growth rate should decrease. A physical exam will be done at each visit to evaluate development, and a bone age X-ray will be done at least once a year. Hormone levels occasionally need to be checked.

Due to early puberty, your child may be taller than other children of his/her age. It is important to treat children according to their actual age rather than their size, or apparent age, since children tend to develop self-esteem and behave according to how they are treated. Parents of children with precocious puberty should remind teachers, relatives, and friends about this important relationship.

Your child may feel embarrassed by the physical effects of puberty. All children want to look and act like their friends. It is helpful to emphasize to your child that all girls and boys normally experience puberty but in his or her case it has occurred sooner than usual. It is important to tell your child that the changes in her or his body are normal. Your child should be allowed to participate in his or her usual activities, which may include spending the night with a friend, athletics, and extracurricular events. Encourage your child to discuss with you worries that he or she may be having.

Questions Many Parents Have

How should I explain this disorder to my child?

Your child may have several questions regarding early puberty and its treatment. It is often helpful to reassure your child that the pubertal changes in his or her body are normal, and that most individuals will eventually have these changes but that in his/her body they happened sooner than usual.

What should we tell friends and relatives?

It is not necessary to tell anyone about your child's problem; if, however, they ask about the problem and you wish to discuss this with them, explain that your child is perfectly normal but has started puberty at an earlier than normal age. If your child is receiving injections, you can explain that they are given to temporarily stop puberty, which assists these children in achieving an acceptable adult height.

What will my child's final adult height be?

Final adult height depends on multiple factors. Parental heights play a significant role in the height of a child. The relationship between bone age and chronological age is also important since excessive skeletal maturation for age provides less time for growth. If puberty was detected at an early stage, then your child will have a better chance of reaching his/her expected height. If, however, puberty was detected at a later stage, then his/her bones will be more advanced and this will limit the time remaining for growth and, therefore, final adult height.

Chapter 5

Health Care Visits

Chapter Contents

41

Section 5.1

Choosing a Health Plan

Excerpted from "Your Guide to Choosing Quality Health Care," Agency for Healthcare Research and Quality, AHRQ Pub. No. 99-0012; published July 1999; updated July 2001. Available online at http://www.ahcpr.gov; accessed July 2003.

Today there are more health plans to choose from than ever before. Not everyone has a choice. But if you do, this section can help you choose the plan that offers the best quality for you and your family.

The quality of health plans varies widely. In 1997, a study published by the National Committee for Quality Assurance (NCQA) showed differences in the ways managed care organizations provide access to care, keep people healthy, treat illness, deliver high-quality service, and satisfy patients. For example, studies show that treating heart attack patients with beta blocker drugs saves lives. The NCQA found that in some health plans, most heart attack patients got beta blockers. In other health plans, only one in three did.

Research shows that Americans say that quality is the most important thing they think about when choosing a health plan. But research also shows that few people understand their options well enough to make an informed choice.

What Are Your Choices?

The two major types of health plans are fee-for-service and managed care. Managed care plans can go by many names: Health Maintenance Organization (HMO); Preferred Provider Organization (PPO); Individual Practice Association (IPA); and Point of Service (POS) plan, to name a few. But different groups do not always define these names the same way.

Do not be confused by whether the plan is a fee-for-service plan, or whether the plan is one of the many kinds of managed care plans. What you need to understand is not the plan's label, but the characteristics of the plan. Research shows that it is important to understand your options and how they affect your choice of providers and services, costs, and quality of care.

Before you join a plan, it is hard to know what kind of care you will get. One way to find out is to learn what members of the plan say about it. This kind of information is called consumer ratings or consumer satisfaction information.

More and more states, businesses, health plans, Medicare, and even the Federal Government's personnel office are starting to use a survey called Consumer Assessment of Health Plans (CAHPS). It tells them what members think of the plans they are in. CAHPS was designed by national experts in healthcare quality, under a project funded by the Agency for Healthcare Research and Quality.

Also, NCQA has added CAHPS survey questions to its own member satisfaction survey. The NCQA survey is part of its performance measurement program, called HEDIS.

The information from the CAHPS surveys is summarized in reports to help you compare health plans and decide which one is best for you. Here are examples of the kind of information you will find in a report that is based on CAHPS survey questions:

- Do members get the health services they need? Without long waits?

- How easy is it for members to get a doctor they are happy with?

- How easy is it to see a specialist?

- Do doctors in the plan listen carefully?

- Do they explain things well?

- Are office staff polite and helpful?

- Is the health plan's customer service good at giving information and helping with problems?

- Do members have too many forms to fill out?

- How do members rate the care from the doctors and other health care providers in the plan?

- How do they rate their plan overall?

You also may want to check your phone book for your state's department of health, or the insurance commissioner's office. For more help in finding your state health insurance contact, write or call the National Association of Insurance Commissioners, Executive Headquarters,

2301 McGee, Suite 800, Kansas City, MO 64108-2604; telephone 816-842-3600 or, if busy 816-374-7175. The information also is available at its Web site: http://www.naic.org.

Section 5.2

Choosing a Doctor

Excerpted from "Your Guide to Choosing Quality Health Care," Agency for Healthcare Research and Quality, AHRQ Pub. No. 99-0012; published July 1999; updated July 2001. Available online at http://www.ahcpr.gov; accessed July 2003.

It is important to choose your doctor with care, because quality varies. For example, the Pacific Business Group on Health asked patients of California doctors' groups how they rated their care. The results? More than 80 percent of the patients said they were satisfied with their care. But fewer than two-thirds were happy with the ease of getting that care.

This section can help you choose a primary care doctor who will meet your needs and give you quality care. The information also may be useful in choosing any specialists you might need.

Primary care doctors are specially trained to serve as your main doctor over the long term. They provide your medical and health care, help you stay healthy, and help to manage your care. Your primary care doctor can refer you to specialists (doctors who treat only certain parts of the body, conditions, or age groups) if you need them.

Internists and family physicians are the two largest groups of primary care doctors for adults. Many women see obstetricians/gynecologists for some or all of their primary care needs. Pediatricians and family practitioners are primary care doctors for many children.

Physician assistants, nurse practitioners, and certified nurse midwives are trained to deliver many aspects of primary care. Physician assistants must practice in partnership with doctors. Nurse practitioners and certified nurse midwives can work independently in some states, but not others.

Doctors and Health Plans

If you already are in a health plan, your choices may be limited to doctors who participate in the plan. But if you have a choice of plans, you may want to first think about which doctor(s) you would like to use. Then, you may be able to choose a plan that has your choice of doctor(s).

Decide What You Want and Need in a Doctor

What is most important to you in a doctor? A few ideas are listed below. Add your own to create a list that will help you choose a doctor who is right for you.

- My doctor must be highly rated by a consumer or other group. (You will want to find out who did the ratings. Is the information reliable? Who collected it? Does the group have something to gain from the ratings?)

- My doctor needs to have experience with my condition(s): (Research shows that doctors who have a lot of experience with a condition tend to have better success with it.)

- I want a doctor who has privileges (is permitted to practice) at the hospital of my choice:

- My doctor must be part of my health plan.

Check on Quality

Once you have a list of doctors, there are several ways to check on their skills and knowledge, and the quality of care they provide:

- Find out if a consumer or other group has rated doctors in the area where you live. (Again you will want to find out how reliable the ratings are.)

- Information on doctors in some states is available on the Internet at http://www.docboard.org. This Website is run by Administrators in Medicine—a group of state medical board directors.

- The American Board of Medical Specialties (800-733-2267) can tell you if the doctor is board certified. Certified means that the doctor has completed a training program in a specialty and has passed an exam (board) to assess his or her knowledge, skills, and experience to provide quality patient care in that specialty. Primary care doctors also may be certified as specialists. You can also check the website at http://www.certifacts.org. (Note: While board certification is a good measure of a doctor's knowledge, it is possible to receive quality care from doctors who are not board certified.)

- Call the American Medical Association (AMA) at 312-464-5000 for information on training, specialties, and board certification about many licensed doctors in the United States. This information also can be found in Physician Select at AMA's website: http://www.ama-assn.org.

Trust your own reactions when deciding whether this doctor is the right one for you. But you also may want to give the relationship some time to develop. It takes more than one visit for you and your doctor to get to know each other.

Section 5.3

General Preventive Care for Women

Excerpted from "A Lifetime of Good Health: Your Guide to Staying Healthy," by the U.S. Department of Health and Human Services, National Women's Health Information Center (NWHIC), 2002. Available online at http://www.4woman.gov/faq/PreventionGuide.pdf; accessed August 2003.

Prevention is key to living long and living well. Getting preventive screenings and immunizations are among the most important things you can do for yourself. Take time to review these guidelines for screening tests and immunizations. Use the charts on the next few pages to remind yourself of when you need to see your health care provider based on your personal health profile. Make an appointment today.

Table 5.1. Recommended Screenings and Immunizations for Women at Average Risk for Most Diseases

Screening Tests	Ages 18-39	Ages 40-49	Ages 50-64	Ages 65 and Older
General Health:				
Full Check-Up, including weight and height	Discuss with your health care provider	Discuss with your health care provider	Discuss with your health care provider	Discuss with your health care provider
Thyroid test (TSH)	Starting at age 35, then every 5 years	Every 5 years	Every 5 years	Every 5 years
Heart Health:				
Blood pressure test	Starting at age 21, then once every 1–2 years if normal	Every 1–2 years	Every 1–2 years	Every 1–2 years
Cholesterol test	Starting at age 20, then every 5 years	Every 5 years	Every 5 years	Every 5 years
Bone Health:				
Bone mineral density test		Discuss with your health care provider	Discuss with your health care provider	Discuss with your health care provider
Diabetes:				
Blood sugar test		Starting at age 45, then every 3 years	Every 3 years	Every 3 years
Breast Health:				
Breast exam	Yearly by a health care provider; monthly self-breast exam.	Yearly by a health care provider; monthly self-breast exam.	Yearly by a health care provider; monthly self-breast exam.	Yearly by a health care provider; monthly self-breast exam.
Mammogram (x-ray of breast)		Every 1–2 years. Discuss with your health care provider.	Yearly	Yearly

47

Table 5.1. Continued. Recommended Screenings and Immunizations for Women at Average Risk for Most Diseases

Screening Tests	Ages 18-39	Ages 40-49	Ages 50-64	Ages 65 and Older
Reproductive Health:				
Pap test and pelvic exam	Every 1–3 years after 3 consecutive normal tests. Discuss with your health care provider.	Every 1–3 years after 3 consecutive normal tests. Discuss with your health care provider.	Every 1–3 years after 3 consecutive normal tests. Discuss with your health care provider.	Every 1–3 years after 3 consecutive normal tests. Discuss with your health care provider.
Chlamydia test	If sexually active, yearly until age 25	If you are at high risk for chlamydia or other sexually transmitted diseases (STDs) you may need this test.	If you are at high risk for chlamydia or other sexually transmitted diseases (STDs) you may need this test	If you are at high risk for chlamydia or other sexually transmitted diseases (STDs) you may need this test
Sexually transmitted diseases (STD) tests	If you have multiple sexual partners; or a partner with multiple sexual partners; or a partner with an STD or sexual contact with STDs; or a personal history of STDs.	If you have multiple sexual partners; or a partner with multiple sexual partners; or a partner with an STD or sexual contact with STDs; or a personal history of STDs.	If you have multiple sexual partners; or a partner with multiple sexual partners; or a partner with an STD or sexual contact with STDs; or a personal history of STDs.	If you have multiple sexual partners; or a partner with multiple sexual partners; or a partner with an STD or sexual contact with STDs; or a personal history of STDs.
Colorectal Health:				
Colonoscopy		Every 5–10 years	Every 5–10 years	Every 5–10 years
Double contrast barium enema (DCBE)		Every 5–10 years (only if not having colonoscopy every 10 years)	Every 5–10 years (only if not having colonoscopy every 10 years)	Every 5–10 years (only if not having colonoscopy every 10 years)
Flexible sigmoidoscopy		Every 5 years	Every 5 years	Every 5 years
Fecal occult blood test test			Yearly	Yearly

Rectal exam	Discuss with your health care provider	Every 5–10 years at time of each screening (sigmoidoscopy, colonoscopy, or DCBE)	Every 5–10 years at time of each screening (sigmoidoscopy, colonoscopy, or DCBE)	Every 5–10 years at time of each screening (sigmoidoscopy, colonoscopy, or DCBE)
Eye and Ear Health:				
Vision exam with eye care provider	Once initially between age 20 and 39	Every 2–4 years	Every 2–4 years	Every 1–2 years
Hearing test (discuss with your health care provider)	Starting at age 18, then every 10 years	Every 10 years	Discuss with your health care provider.	Discuss with your health care provider.
Skin Health:				
Mole Exam	Monthly mole self-exam; starting at age 20, by a health care provider every 3 years.	Monthly mole self-exam; by a health care provider every year.	Monthly mole self-exam; by a health care provider every year.	Monthly mole self-exam; by a health care provider every year.
Oral Health:				
Dental (Oral Exam)	One to two times every year	One to two times every year	One to two times every year	One to two times every year
Mental Health Screening	Discuss with your health care provider.	Discuss with your health care provider.	Discuss with your health care provider.	Discuss with your health care provider.
Immunizations:				
Influenza vaccine	Discuss with your health care provider	Discuss with your health care provider	Discuss with your health care provider	Recommended yearly
Pneumococcal vaccine				One time only
Tetanus-Diphtheria Booster Vaccine	Every 10 years	Every 10 years	Every 10 years	Every 10 years

Note: These charts are guidelines only. Your health care provider will personalize the timing of each test and immunization to best meet your health care needs.

49

Section 5.4

Recommended Screenings and Immunizations for Women with High Risk Factors

U.S. Department of Health and Human Services, National Women's Health Information Center (NWHIC), December 2002. Available online at http://www.4woman.gov; accessed July 2003.

Each table lists screenings or tests you might need more often or earlier due to having high risk factors, or things in your life that increase your chances of developing a condition or disease.

Table 5.2. Risk Factors Associated with Family History **(continued on next page)**

Does your family history include?	Then ask your health care provider if you need the following screenings or tests more often or at a younger age:
High blood pressure	Blood pressure test
High cholesterol	Cholesterol test
Diabetes	Blood sugar test
Heart disease; premature heart disease or heart attack	Blood pressure test; cholesterol test; exercise stress test
Breast cancer	Mammogram; ovarian screening tests
Cervical, uterine, or vaginal cancer	Pap test; pelvic exam; ovarian screening tests; colon screening
Ovarian cancer	Pelvic exam; ovarian screening tests; colon screening; clinical breast exam
Osteoporosis; bone fracture in adulthood	Bone mineral density test
Thyroid disease or thyroid cancer	Thyroid test and/or genetic counseling

Table 5.2. Risk Factors Associated with Family History **(continued from previous page)**

Does your family history include?	Then ask your health care provider if you need the following screenings or tests more often or at a younger age:
Gum (periodontal) disease	Oral exam
Hearing problems; deafness	Hearing test
Vision problems; eye disease; blindness	Vision exam
Inflammatory bowel disease; colon polyps; colon, ovarian, or endometrial cancer	Colonoscopy; sigmoidoscopy; DCBE; rectal exam; fecal occult blood test
Cancer, heart disease, or any illness at an unusually young age (50 or under)	Genetic counseling, possible early screening tests
Two relatives with the same kind of cancer	Genetic counseling, possible early screening tests
Birth defects or genetic disorder (you or your partner)	Genetic counseling, possible early screening tests. If you want to become pregnant, genetic counseling for you and your partner.

Table 5.3. Health Risk Factors Associated with Ethnicity, Age, Pregnancy, Weight, or Work and Living Conditions **(continued on next page)**

Are you?	Then ask your health care provider if you need the following screenings or tests more often or at a younger age:
African American	Blood pressure test; cholesterol test; blood sugar test; vision exam; colonoscopy; genetic counseling for sickle cell anemia
Hispanic American	Blood pressure test; cholesterol test; blood sugar test; colonoscopy
Alaska Native/Pacific Islander	Blood sugar test
American Indian	Blood sugar test
Ashkenazi Jewish Descent	Genetic counseling for Tay-Sachs disease, if you want to become pregnant

51

Table 5.3. Health Risk Factors Associated with Ethnicity, Age, Pregnancy, Weight, or Work and Living Conditions **(continued from previous page)**

Are you?	Then ask your health care provider if you need the following screenings or tests more often or at a younger age:
Ashkenazi Jewish with family history of breast or ovarian cancer	Genetic counseling for possible BRCA 1/2 mutation
Asian American	Blood sugar test
Age 65 or older	Bone mineral density test; flu vaccine; pneumococcal vaccine
Between the ages of 60 and 64, weigh less than 154 pounds, and not taking estrogen	Bone mineral density test
College age	MMR vaccine; varicella vaccine
Postmenopausal	Bone mineral density test
Pregnant	Blood pressure test; blood sugar test; urine test; HIV test; STD tests; MMR vaccine
A non-pregnant woman of childbearing age	MMR vaccine; varicella vaccine
A smoker	Blood pressure test; cholesterol test; bone mineral density test; oral exam; vision exam
Overweight	Blood pressure test; blood sugar test; weight
Living in prison	Tuberculosis (TB) test; HIV test; STD tests
Living in long-term care	TB test; influenza vaccine; pneumococcal vaccine
A health care worker	TB test; influenza vaccine; pneumococcal vaccine; MMR vaccine; varicella vaccine
A health care worker exposed to blood	HIV test; hepatitis screening; hepatitis A, B vaccines

Table 5.4. Current and Previous Health Risk Factors **(continued on next page)**

Do you have or have you had?	Then ask your health care provider if you need the following screenings or tests more often or at a younger age:
High blood pressure	Blood pressure test; cholesterol test; blood sugar test
High cholesterol	Blood pressure test; cholesterol test; blood sugar test
Heart disease	Blood pressure test; cholesterol test; blood sugar test; influenza vaccine; pneumococcal vaccine
Diabetes	Blood pressure test; cholesterol test; blood sugar test; vision exam; urine test
Gestational diabetes (diabetes during pregnancy)	Blood sugar test
Breast cancer	Mammogram; ovarian screening tests
Cervical, uterine, vaginal cancer	Pap test; pelvic exam; ovarian screening tests; colon screening
Ovarian cancer	Pelvic exam; ovarian screening tests; mammogram; colon screening
Previous abnormal Pap tests	Pap test; pelvic exam
Early menopause (natural or surgically induced); absent or infrequent menstrual periods; advanced age; a personal history of bone fracture in adulthood; lifelong low calcium intake; lifelong inactive lifestyle, or little physical activity; low body weight (less than 154 pounds) or a history of an eating disorder such as anorexia nervosa	Bone mineral density test
An autoimmune disease (including lupus, rheumatoid arthritis, scleroderma, multiple sclerosis, psoriasis)	Thyroid test; TB test; influenza vaccine; MMR vaccine; pneumococcal vaccine; autoimmune screening test; bone mineral density test
Chronic lung disease	Influenza vaccine; pneumococcal vaccine
Chronic liver disease	Hepatitis A vaccine

Table 5.4. Current and Previous Health Risk Factors **(continued from previous page)**

Do you have or have you had?	Then ask your health care provider if you need the following screenings or tests more often or at a younger age:
Thyroid disease	Thyroid test; influenza vaccine; pneumococcal vaccine; bone mineral density test (of hyperthyroid)
Gum (periodontal disease)	Oral exam
Colon polyps; Inflammatory bowel disease	Colonoscopy
A developmental delay	Vision exam; hearing test
Eye injury or disease	Vision exam
Ear injury or prolonged exposure to loud noise	Hearing test
HIV/AIDS	Oral exam; vision exam; Pap test; pelvic exam; TB test; thyroid test; STDs tests; influenza vaccine; pneumococcal vaccine; hepatitis screening; hepatitis A, B vaccines
A blood transfusion form 1978-1985	HIV test; hepatitis screening
Multiple sex partners (or a partner who has multiple sex partners)	STD tests; HIV test; hepatitis B test; Pap test; pelvic exam
Alcoholism	Pneumococcal vaccine; TB test; psychological screening; liver tests
Intravenous (IV) drug use or addiction	Hepatitis screening; hepatitis A, B vaccines; TB test; STD tests; HIV test; psychological screening
A sexually transmitted disease (STD)	STD tests; HIV test; Pap test; pelvic exam
Lived or worked with someone exposed to tuberculosis (TB)	TB test
A serious injury (cut or laceration)	Tetanus-Diphtheria booster vaccine
A baby recently (within the last few weeks or months)	Postpartum depression screening

Chapter 6

Maintaining Gynecological Health

Chapter Contents

Section 6.1

Your Obstetrician/Gynecologist: Your Partner in Health Care

American College of Obstetricians and Gynecologists. *Your Ob-Gyn: Your Partner in Health Care.* (Patient Education Pamphlet No. AP109). Washington, DC. © ACOG 2000.

Your health is a concern shared by you and your doctor. Your doctor takes care of your basic health needs and treats problems. This includes telling you about leading a healthy lifestyle and doing tests and exams to look for disease. It is up to you to follow a healthy lifestyle and be aware of any changes in your body that may signal a problem. Even if you are not having any problems, you should see your obstetrician-gynecologist, or ob-gyn, for routine checkups.

This section will explain:

- The role of your ob-gyn
- The kind of care you can expect to receive
- How you can work with your doctor for better health

What Is an Obstetrician-Gynecologist?

An ob-gyn is a doctor who specializes in the care of women. He or she is trained in obstetrics—the care of pregnant women. This includes:

- Preconceptional period (before pregnancy)
- Pregnancy
- Labor and childbirth
- Postpartum period (after a baby is born)

Ob-gyns also are trained in gynecology. Gynecology covers a woman's general health care. This includes care of her:

- Reproductive organs

56

- Breasts
- Sexual function

It also includes treating hormone disorders and infections. Your ob-gyn also is trained in surgery to correct or treat pelvic organ or urinary tract problems.

Your ob-gyn offers preventive health care, too. This can help you to make choices that will prevent health problems. Preventive health care includes exams and routine tests that look for problems before you are sick. It also includes immunizations to prevent disease.

Your doctor can evaluate your health and provide care for a range of medical problems, not just those of the reproductive system. For many women, the ob-gyn is their primary care physician—the doctor they turn to first for health care.

Your Ob-Gyn's Qualifications

All ob-gyns receive complete medical training. Their training equips them to give general care to women, as well as care that relates to pregnancy and the reproductive organs. Ob-gyns have earned degrees from college and medical school. They also have completed a four-year course of special training—a residency—in obstetrics and gynecology.

After residency, a doctor may be board certified by the American Board of Obstetrics and Gynecology. To become board certified, the doctor must pass two tests. The first is a written test. This test shows that he or she has the knowledge and skills required to treat women. It covers both medical and surgical care.

He or she also must show experience in treating women's health conditions for two years in practice after residency. At this point, he or she takes a second test—an oral exam given by a panel of experts. This exam reviews the skills, knowledge, and ability to treat many conditions. It includes a review of cases treated during the past year. Doctors certified after 1986 must be recertified in 10 years.

There are three subspecialty areas in obstetrics and gynecology:

- Gynecologic oncology (care of women with cancers of the reproductive system)

- Maternal-fetal medicine (care of women whose pregnancies are complicated by medical or obstetric problems)

- Reproductive endocrinology (care of women who have hormonal or infertility problems)

All certified ob-gyns can treat patients with these disorders. Some doctors have special training that qualifies them to take a test to be certified in these areas. Such doctors often teach other doctors.

If the letters FACOG are written after your ob-gyn's name, it means that he or she is a Fellow (full member) of the American College of Obstetricians and Gynecologists (ACOG). All ACOG Fellows are board certified. ACOG is a national group of more than 36,000 ob-gyns. It supports women's health care issues and offers a range of teaching programs to help doctors keep up with the latest advances in women's health care.

Your doctor may be a Junior Fellow in ACOG. Junior Fellows are in a training program or have just finished training. They are in practice preparing to pass the final oral exam.

Your ob-gyn may work as part of a health care team of other professionals. This is known as a collaborative practice. This health care team is led by the ob-gyn and may consist of:

- Residents—Provide care to patients at teaching hospitals after graduation from medical school.

- Certified nurse-midwives—Care for women during pregnancy and childbirth. They have an extra 12 to 18 months of schooling after graduating from an accredited nursing program and must pass a national certification exam.

- Nurses—Assist doctors in providing patient care and education. They have completed accredited nursing programs and passed tests.

- Nurse practitioners—Provide a wide range of services, which includes obtaining medical histories, doing physical exams, and diagnosing and treating common illnesses and diseases. They are licensed registered nurses who have advanced education. In some states, they must pass a national certification exam.

- Physician assistants—Handle various medical duties. They have completed at least a two-year educational program after college.

- Dietitians—Give advice and guidance on diet and nutrition.

- Social workers—Provide counseling and information on community services. They have studied in a special program and must be licensed.

- Childbirth educators—Teach parents-to-be about conception, pregnancy, birth, and parenting.

Collaborative practice brings together health care professionals with different knowledge and skills. They work as a team, and each member has a role. In this type of practice, patients receive care from many types of professionals. Each person does what he or she does best. Services are provided in a cost-effective manner that may save you waiting time, too. The contributions of each member are key to the care of the patient.

What Kind of Care Does Your Ob-Gyn Provide?

The care provided by your ob-gyn can range from a basic gynecologic exam to complete health care of reproductive or other disorders. The type of care depends on your needs and options available.

Well-Woman Visit

The well-woman visit is a key part of preventive care. This consists of an evaluation of your general health and an exam of your breasts and pelvic (reproductive) organs. With this exam, your ob-gyn:

- Looks for health problems in their early stages

- Detects risks to your health

- Tells you how you can change your lifestyle to lower these risks

- You also may have certain tests and immunizations. It depends on your age.

You should have a well-woman exam on a routine basis if you are sexually active or age 18 or older. Most women should see their ob-gyn once a year. More frequent exams may be needed based on your health risk factors. If you have a health problem or notice any changes in your body, such as an unusual vaginal discharge or genital itching, you should contact your doctor right away.

Health History

During your exam, one of the first things your doctor does is obtain a history of your health. This will include information about:

- Your past illnesses

- Family health history

- Your menstrual periods

- Use of medications and birth control
- Whether you are or ever have been pregnant

The Pap Test

During the Pap test, cells are taken from the cervix to look for changes that could be a sign of cervical cancer or changes that could lead to cervical cancer. The test detects possible signs of disease in women who do not have symptoms such as bleeding, pelvic pain, or discharge.

Table 6.1. Your Periodic Health Evaluation

Routine Tests/Immunizations	How Often
Ages 13 to 18 years	
Pap test	Yearly when sexually active or by age 18 years
Tetanus-diphtheria booster	Once between ages 11 and 16 years
Hepatitis B vaccine	One series for those not previously immunized
Ages 19 to 39 years	
Pap test	Annually
Tetanus-diphtheria booster	Every 10 years
Ages 40 to 64 years All the above (in each category), plus:	
Mammography	Every 1 to 2 years until age 50, then yearly
Cholesterol testing	Every 5 years starting at age 45 years
Fecal occult blood testing	Yearly starting at age 50 years
Sigmoidoscopy	Every 3 to 5 years after age 50 years
Fasting glucose testing	Every 3 years after age 45 years
Ages 65 years & older All the above (in each category), plus:	
Urinalysis	Yearly
Influenza (flu) vaccine	Yearly
Pneumococcal vaccine	Once

You should have your first Pap test by age 18 or when you become sexually active. Women are advised to have a Pap test once a year. Based on test results and the presence of any risk factors for cervical cancer, this test may need to be done more or less often. It's best to check with your doctor.

The doctor performs the Pap test during your pelvic exam. To ensure accurate results, you should arrange to have the test when you're not having your period. Do not douche or use vaginal medication for two to three days beforehand.

First, a speculum is inserted into the vagina so the cervix can be seen. Then a small brush or swab and applicator are used to remove cells from the cervix. You may have some spotting for a day or two after the test, especially if you're pregnant. Cells will be taken from inside the opening of the cervix and from the outer part of the cervix. They are sent to a lab to be tested. A trained technician or doctor looks for cells that do not appear normal. Results are based on how the cells look.

The Pap test is the best way to detect conditions that may lead to cervical cancer. By treating these conditions, cancer often can be avoided or treated early.

The doctor also may ask about your job, level of stress, health habits, sexual activity, and any risks to your health (such as an abusive relationship). Your answers should be honest and open. This will help your doctor look after your health. Anything you tell your doctor will be kept secret—no one else will know.

If you have any poor health habits, such as smoking, a high-fat diet, or drug or alcohol abuse, you should discuss these with your doctor. These habits can increase the risk of disease and have a bad effect on your overall health. Also, smoking and substance use can harm the health of your baby if you are pregnant.

Your doctor can help you break poor habits and replace them with healthier ones. If you are sexually active or planning to be, your doctor also can talk to you about contraception and prevention of sexually transmitted diseases (STDs), including human immunodeficiency virus (HIV).

Physical Exam

The general physical exam often begins with a check of your weight and blood pressure. Your doctor also may listen to your heartbeat and feel your abdomen and neck. The exam is based on your age and any risk factors you may have. The gynecologic exam is done to assess the health of your reproductive organs.

Your ob-gyn will first check your breasts for signs of lumps. You should do a breast self-exam regularly. If you are not sure how to do this exam, your doctor or nurse can teach you.

After examining your breasts, the doctor does an exam of your pelvic organs. You will be asked to lie on a table with your legs raised and your knees bent and spread apart. The doctor first examines the outside genitals (vulva). He or she then will insert a slender device called a speculum into the vagina to view the vagina and cervix and take a sample of cells for testing. After the speculum is removed, the doctor inserts one or two gloved fingers into the vagina and reaches up to the cervix. The uterus and ovaries can be felt from the inside with this hand while the other hand presses on the abdomen from the outside. This allows the size, position and, shape of these organs to be checked.

During the exam, your doctor also may examine your rectum using a gloved finger. The exam can help your doctor detect any tumors or lumps or other problems that may be present.

Tests

The type of tests you receive and how often they are done depend on your age and whether you are at risk for any disease. One test that all women should have on a regular basis is the Pap test. This is done during the pelvic exam. The doctor uses a cotton swab or brush to take a sample of cells from the cervix. These are studied in a lab for signs that could signal cancer of the cervix.

Other tests also may be part of your well-woman exam:

- Cholesterol test is a blood test done to check levels of cholesterol, a substance that helps carry fat through the blood.

- Patients with a high cholesterol count are advised about diet and other preventive health measures.

- Mammography is an X-ray of the breasts to detect breast cancer.

- Fecal occult blood test is a test of a stool sample for hidden blood that may detect colon or rectal cancer.

- Sigmoidoscopy is the use of a slender device placed into the rectum and lower colon to look for cancer.

- Urinalysis is a test done on urine to look for changes that might be a sign of illness.

• Blood count is a test to detect anemia and infection.

If you are concerned about being exposed to STDs, including HIV, tell your doctor. He or she may suggest you have certain tests done.

Care of Reproductive System and Other Conditions

Your ob-gyn can detect and treat a number of medical conditions that affect the reproductive system. An ob-gyn also may treat certain medical conditions that do not involve the breasts or reproductive organs. This is key for women who don't regularly see a doctor other than their ob-gyn.

In some cases, the ob-gyn will diagnose a medical problem and refer the patient to another doctor for treatment. In others, the ob-gyn can treat the problem and provide routine health care. The decision on how to treat a disorder depends on how severe it is, whether it is getting worse or is under control, and the comfort level of a woman and her doctor.

Finally

You and your ob-gyn can work as a team to ensure your good health. If you take proper care of yourself, visit your doctor regularly, and report any symptoms that may signal a problem, you will increase your chances of staying healthy. It is always better to prevent illness— through a healthy lifestyle and preventive care—than to treat it.

Glossary

Collaborative Practice: A type of practice where care is given by a team of professionals.

Gynecology: The branch of medicine that involves care of women's health, including the reproductive system and breasts.

Obstetrician-Gynecologist: A doctor with special skills, training, and education in women's health care.

Obstetrics: The branch of medicine that involves care of a woman during pregnancy, labor, childbirth, and after the baby is born.

Pap Test: A test in which cells are taken from the cervix and examined in a lab for abnormalities that could signal cancer.

Sexually Transmitted Disease (STD): A disease that is spread by sexual contact, including chlamydia infection, gonorrhea, genital warts, herpes, syphilis and infection with human immunodeficiency virus (HIV, the cause of acquired immunodeficiency syndrome [AIDS]).

Vulva: The lips of the external female genital area.

Section 6.2

Mammograms

U.S. Department of Health and Human Services, National Women's Health Information Center (NWHIC), March 2002. Available online at http://www.4woman.gov; accessed June 2003.

What is a mammogram?

A mammogram is a test that is done to look for any abnormalities, or problems, with a woman's breasts. The test uses a special x-ray machine to take pictures of both breasts. The results are recorded on film that your health care provider can examine.

Mammograms look for breast lumps and changes in breast tissue that may develop into problems over time. They can find small lumps or growths that a health care provider or woman can't feel when doing a physical breast exam. Breast lumps or growths can be benign (not cancer) or malignant (cancer). If a lump is found, a health care provider will order a biopsy, a test where a small amount of tissue is taken from the lump and area around the lump. The tissue is sent to a lab to look for cancer or changes that may mean cancer is likely to develop. Finding breast cancer early means that a woman has a better chance of surviving the disease. There are also more choices for treatment when breast cancer is found early.

How is a mammogram done?

You stand in front of a special x-ray machine. The person who takes the x-rays (always a woman) places your breasts (one at a time) between two plastic plates. The plates press your breast and make it flat. You will feel pressure on your breast for a few seconds. It may cause you some discomfort, feeling like squeezing or pinching. But, the flatter your breasts, the better the picture. Most often, two pictures are taken of each breast—one from the side and one from above. The whole thing takes only a few minutes.

How often should I get a mammogram?

Women over 40 should get a mammogram every 1 to 2 years. This guideline was just re-issued by the federal government's U.S. Preventive Services Task Force. And, it is also the position of the Secretary of the U.S. Department of Health and Human Services. Women who have had breast cancer or breast problems, or with a family history of breast cancer may need to start having mammograms at a younger age or more often. Talk to your health care provider about how often you should get a mammogram. Be aware that mammograms don't take the place of getting breast exams from a health care provider and examining your own breasts.

If you find a lump or see changes in your breast, talk to your health care provider right away no matter what your age. Your health care provider may order a mammogram for you to get a better look at your breast changes.

Where can I get a mammogram?

Be sure to get a mammogram from a facility certified by the Food and Drug Administration (FDA). These places must meet high standards for their x-ray machines and staff. Some of these facilities also offer digital mammograms.

Your health care provider, local medical clinic, or local or state health department can tell you where to get no-cost or low-cost mammograms. Also, call the National Cancer Institute's toll free number 1-800-422-6237 for information on no-cost or low-cost mammograms.

Section 6.3

Pap Tests

Excerpted from the publication by the U.S. Department of Health and Human Services, National Women's Health Information Center (NWHIC), July 2002. Available online at http://www.4woman.gov; accessed July 2003.

What is a Pap test?

The Pap test (also called a Pap smear) checks for changes in the cells of your cervix. The cervix is the lower part of the uterus (womb) that opens into the vagina (birth canal). The Pap test can tell if you have an infection, abnormal (unhealthy) cells, or cancer.

Why do I need a Pap test?

A Pap test can save your life. It can find cancer of the cervix—a common cancer in women—before it moves to other parts of your body (becomes invasive). If caught early, treatment for cancer of the cervix can be easier and the chances of curing it are far greater. Pap tests can also pick up infections and inflammation and abnormal cells that can change into cancer cells.

Do all women need Pap tests?

It is important for all women to make Pap tests, along with pelvic exams, a part of their routine health care. You need to have a Pap test if you are over 18 years old. If you are under 18 years old and are or have been sexually active, you also need a Pap test. There is no age limit for the Pap test. Even women who have gone through menopause (the change of life, or when a woman's periods stop) need to get Pap tests.

Women who are living with HIV, the virus that causes AIDS, are more at risk for developing cancer of the cervix and other cervical diseases. The U.S. Centers for Disease Control and Prevention recommends that HIV positive women have an initial Pap test, and then another one 6 months later. If both of these Pap tests show

66

no cancer or other problems, then a Pap test can be done only once a year.

How often do I need to get a Pap test?

Many health care providers tell women to get a Pap test every year. But, your health care provider may recommend a Pap test every 1 to 3 years after you have had 3 normal Pap tests for 3 years in a row. Talk with your health care provider about what is best for you.

Is there anything special I need to do before going for a Pap test?

For two days before the test, you should not douche or use vaginal creams, suppositories, foams, or vaginal medications (like for a yeast infection). It is also best to not use any vaginal deodorant sprays or powders for two days before your test. And, do not have sexual intercourse within 24 hours of your test. All of these can cause inaccurate test results by washing away or hiding abnormal cells. You should not have a Pap test when you have your period. The best time to have one is between 10 and 20 days after the first day of your last period.

How is a Pap test done?

Your health care provider can do a Pap test during a pelvic exam. It is a quick test that takes only a few minutes. You will be asked to lie down on an exam table and put your feet in holders called stirrups, letting your knees fall to the side. A sheet will cover your legs and stomach. The health care provider will put an instrument called a speculum into your vagina, opening it to see the cervix and to do the Pap test. She or he will use a special stick, brush, or swab to take a few cells from inside and around the cervix. The cells are placed on a small glass slide, then checked by a lab to make sure they are healthy. While painless for most women, a Pap test can cause discomfort for some women.

What happens after the Pap test is done?

If the cells are okay, no treatment is needed. If an infection is present, treatment is prescribed. If the cells look abnormal, or not healthy, more tests may be needed. A Pap test is not 100% right all the time, so it is always important to talk to your health care provider about your results.

What will happen if my Pap test finds something that is not normal?

If the Pap test shows something confusing or a minor change in the cells of the cervix, the test may be done again. If the test shows a major change in the cells of the cervix, the health care provider may perform a colposcopy. This is a procedure done in an office or clinic with an instrument (called a colposcope) that acts like a microscope, allowing the health care provider to closely see the vagina and the cervix. Your health care provider may also take a small amount of tissue from the cervix (called a biopsy) to examine for any abnormal cells, which can be a sign of cancer.

Section 6.4

Breast Self-Exam

"Early Detection," © 2003 National Breast Cancer Foundation. Graphics and text reprinted with permission of the National Breast Cancer Foundation (www.nationalbreastcancer.org).

Early Signs of Breast Cancer

- A lump is detected, which is usually single, firm, and most often painless.

- A portion of the skin on the breast or underarm swells and has an unusual appearance.

- Veins on the skin surface become more prominent on one breast.

- The breast nipple becomes inverted, develops a rash, changes in skin texture, or has a discharge other than breast milk.

- A depression is found in an area of the breast surface.

Women's breasts can develop some degree of lumpiness, but only a small percentage of lumps are malignant.

While a history of breast cancer in the family may lead to increased risk, most breast cancers are diagnosed in women with no family history. If you have a family history of breast cancer, this should be discussed with your doctor.

Facts about Breast Cancer

- Every three minutes a woman is diagnosed with breast cancer.

- This year 182,000 new cases of breast cancer are expected in the United States.

- One woman in eight who lives to age 85 will develop breast cancer during her lifetime.

- Breast cancer is the leading cause of death in women between the ages of 40 and 55.

- Seventy percent of all breast cancers are found through breast self-exams. Not all lumps are detectable by touch. We recommend regular mammograms and monthly breast self-exams.

- Eight out of ten breast lumps are not cancerous. If you find a lump, don't panic—call your doctor for an appointment.

- Mammography is a low-dose X-ray examination that can detect breast cancer up to two years before it is large enough to be felt.

- When breast cancer is found early, the five-year survival rate is 96%. This is good news! Over 2 million breast cancer survivors are alive in America today.

Detection Plan

An early breast cancer detection plan should include:

- Clinical breast examinations every three years from ages 20 to 39, then every year thereafter.

- Monthly breast self-examinations beginning at age 20. Look for any changes in your breasts.

- Baseline mammogram by the age of 40.

- Mammogram every one to two years for women 40 to 49, depending on previous findings.

- Mammogram every year for women 50 and older.

- A personal calendar to record your self-exams, mammograms, and doctor appointments.

- A low-fat diet, regular exercise, and no smoking or drinking.

How to Do a Breast Self-Examination

- In the shower. Fingers flat, move gently over every part of each breast. Use your right hand to examine left breast, left hand for right breast. Check for any lump, hard knot, or thickening. Carefully observe any changes in your breasts.

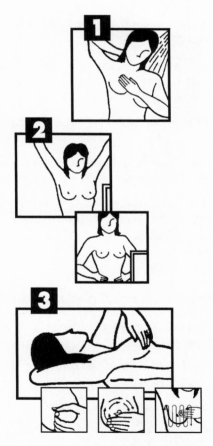

Figure 6.1. How to do a breast self-examination: 1—In the shower; 2—Before a mirror; 3—Lying down.

- Before a mirror. Inspect your breasts with arms at your sides. Next, raise your arms high overhead. Look for any changes in contour of each breast, a swelling, a dimpling of skin or changes in the nipple. Then rest palm on hips and press firmly to flex your chest muscles. Left and right breasts will not exactly match—few women's breasts do.

- Lying down. Place pillow under right shoulder, right arm behind your head. With fingers of left hand flat, press right breast gently in small circular motions, moving vertically or in a circular pattern covering the entire breast. Use light, medium, and firm pressure. Squeeze nipple; check for discharge and lumps. Repeat these steps for your left breast.

Section 6.5

Douching

U.S. Department of Health and Human Services, National Women's Health Information Center (NWHIC); November 2002. Available online at http://www.4woman.gov; accessed July 2003.

What is douching?

Douching is rinsing or cleaning out the vagina (also called the birth canal) by squirting water or other solutions (such as vinegar, baking soda, or douching solutions you can buy at drug and grocery stores) into the vagina. The water or solutions are held in a bottle and squirted into the vagina through tubing and a nozzle.

Why do women douche?

Reasons women have given for using douches include to: rinse away blood after a menstrual period, clean the vagina after sex to avoid sexually transmitted diseases (STDs) and wash away semen to prevent pregnancy; and reduce odors.

71

How common is douching?

Douching is a common practice among women in the United States—37% of American women between the ages of 15 to 44 douche regularly. Of these women, about half douche on a weekly basis.

Is douching safe?

Health care providers do not recommend douching to clean the vagina. Douching changes the delicate chemical balance in the vagina (and the vaginal flora), which can make a woman more prone to bacterial infections. It also can spread existing vaginal or cervical infections up into the pelvic organs (uterus, fallopian tubes, and ovaries).

Research shows that women who douche on a routine basis tend to have more problems than women who do not douche or who rarely douche. These problems include vaginal irritation, infections (called bacterial vaginosis or BV), and sexually transmitted diseases (STDs). Women who douche often are also more at risk for getting pelvic inflammatory disease (PID). PID is an infection of a woman's pelvic organs. It is caused by bacteria, which can travel from a woman's vagina and cervix up into her pelvic organs. If left untreated, PID can lead to infertility (not being able to get pregnant) and ectopic pregnancy (pregnancy in the fallopian tube instead of the uterus). Both BV and PID can lead to serious problems during pregnancy, such as infection in the baby, problems with labor, and early delivery.

What is the healthiest and safest way to clean the vagina?

Because the chemical balance of the vagina is very sensitive, it is best to let the vagina clean itself. The vagina takes care of cleaning itself naturally through secretions of mucous. Warm water and gentle, unscented soap during the bath or shower is the best way to clean the outside areas of the vagina. Products like feminine hygiene soaps, powders, and sprays are not necessary, and may be harmful.

It is important to see your health care provider right away when you have any vaginal pain, itching, burning, or a foul odor; pain when urinating; a vaginal discharge that is not normal, such as thick and white (like cottage cheese) or yellowish-green. You may have a yeast infection, urinary tract infection, or bacterial infection, all of which can be treated. Do not clean the vagina or douche before an exam with a health care provider. This will wash away the vaginal discharge, which helps the health care provider to determine the type of infection.

Chapter 7

Lesbian Health Concerns

Chapter Contents

Section 7.1

Unique Health Care Concerns of Lesbians

"Lesbian Health," U.S. Department of Health and Human Services, National Women's Health Information Center (NWHIC); published 1998, updated 2000. Available online at http://www.4woman.gov; accessed July 2003.

Do lesbians have unique health care concerns?

Fundamentally, lesbian health concerns are women's health concerns and as such lesbians need access to the same high quality health screening and preventive care that is appropriate for all women throughout the life cycle. Unfortunately, the unique health care needs of lesbians are often ignored by a medical world that assumes heterosexuality. Lesbians and their providers often remain uninformed about important health issues including the need for: cervical and breast cancer screening, reducing the risk of sexually transmitted diseases and HIV, caring for mental health issues including depression, diagnosing and treating substance abuse, lesbian pregnancy and parenting assistance, and understanding domestic/intimate violence.

Two substantial barriers to care include (1) lack of financial resources or insurance, including no access to coverage under their partner's policy, and (2) past negative experience in the health care setting. As such, the unique health care needs of lesbians can only be met by increasing access to important health care services and informing lesbians and health care providers of the importance of obtaining appropriate care.

Finding a provider that is lesbian-sensitive, seeking lesbian-specific health information, and supporting research on issues of relevance to the lesbian population are important steps to ensuring that the unique health care needs of lesbians are addressed. Several resources exist to promote these goals.

Do lesbians need Pap smears?

Research has shown that lesbians are less likely to receive Pap smears than heterosexual women are. Reasons for this include lack of access to health care services and lack of information among both lesbians and health professionals about lesbian health needs. It is also possible that lesbians seek obstetrician-gynecologists less frequently than do heterosexual women, so they have less exposure to screening services traditionally offered by ob-gyn. Many health care providers and patients share the false assumption that because lesbians are not currently sexually active with men, they are not at risk for developing dysplasia (abnormal cells in the cervix). As a result of this misinformation, lesbians may avoid medical services and health care providers may give incorrect advice and underutilized appropriate health screenings for these patients. However, lesbians, like all women, need regular Pap smears.

Pap smears are one of the most effective methods of cancer prevention for women. The Pap smear tests for abnormal changes in the cells of the cervix that may become cancerous if left untreated. If detected early, these changes can be treated with minimal intervention, discomfort, and cost.

While it is thought that lesbians who have never had heterosexual intercourse have less cervical cancer, no research has been conducted to quantify the actual risk to this population. We know that one of the viruses that are associated with cervical cancer, the human papillomavirus (HPV), can be transmitted from woman to woman. Also, lesbians who have had heterosexual intercourse at some point in their lives may have been exposed to HPV. Therefore, lesbians need Pap smears on a regular basis, even if they have never or have rarely been sexually active with men.

Are lesbians at risk for STDs and HIV?

Lesbians are at risk for many sexually transmitted diseases, as well as for HIV.

Genital warts, usually associated with the Human Papillomavirus (HPV), can be transmitted sexually from woman to woman. The herpes virus can be transmitted when a lesion from one woman comes into contact with the oral mucosa or the genital mucosa of her female partner. Hepatitis B can also be transmitted between women. Any sexually active person should be immunized against hepatitis B (a three shot series).

There is no evidence at this time that gonorrhea, syphilis, or chlamydia is sexually transmitted between women who are sexually active with women, but large studies have not been done. The majority of lesbian women are sexually exclusive with women (although 90%

have been heterosexually active at some time): however, there are some lesbians who do have male partners, and this subpopulation of lesbians is at risk for gonorrhea, chlamydia and syphilis.

At this time, we have no documentation of HIV transmission between lesbians, and HIV does occur in lesbians, usually due to two factors 1) sharing of needles and 2) when lesbians sleep with men who have been exposed to HIV. However, because there is a theoretical risk of HIV transmission between lesbians, safe sex guidelines are recommended. Small studies are currently underway to study the risk of HIV infection in lesbians.

Section 7.2

Ten Things Lesbians Should Discuss with Their Health Care Providers

Reprinted with permission from "Ten Things Lesbians Should Discuss With Their Health Care Providers," Gay and Lesbian Medical Association, July 17, 2002. © Gay and Lesbian Medical Association. For more information, visit www.glma.org.

A survey of members of the Gay and Lesbian Medical Association (GLMA) listed 10 health care concerns lesbians should include in discussions with their physicians or other health care providers.

"We did the survey," said GLMA Executive Director Maureen S. O'Leary, RN, "because many lesbians and far too many health professionals are not comfortable or do not know how to discuss health issues related to sexual orientation. Unfortunately, there are some health risks that are of greater concern to lesbians, and we need to make sure they are addressed."

Gynecologist and former GLMA President Kathleen O'Hanlan, MD, said that the medical community must look at all factors—gender, age, family history, and current health—but that there are cultural competence issues involved in treatment of lesbians that many do not understand.

"We in the medical community need to find remedies for all the factors that reduce utilization of medical services and screening compliance among lesbians," she said. "Short of changing the laws of the country to reduce the sting of ubiquitous disdain, clinicians need to provide a safe haven for medical care for all women."

"We know from research," said O'Hanlan, "that lesbians are less likely to seek medical care than other women because of the stigma they experience everywhere in society. They also experience it when they go for medical care. Health care providers may feel uncomfortable asking questions they feel to be personal. They then limit their visit and dash out without counseling the patient."

"Although more research is needed to understand the prevalence and causes," O'Hanlan continued, "there is evidence that lesbians smoke more and drink more. It is also more likely they are overweight, which adds significant health risks. Unfortunately, some health care providers make the presumption of heterosexuality or they may offend the lesbian patient in their conversations since they lack understanding of the salient cultural issues. Either way, it reduces the likelihood that the lesbian patient will return for care."

"We need to get the discussions going," O'Leary said. "Most health care professionals understand that there are certain risks that come with being a woman or with the aging process. However, need to make sure that lesbians get equal care and that means incorporating this kind of understanding into the regular approach to treatment."

Lesbian Health Concerns

Breast Cancer: Lesbians have the richest concentration of risk factors for this cancer than any subset of women in the world. Combine this with the fact that many lesbians over 40 do not get routine mammograms, do breast self-exams, or have a clinical breast exam, and the cancer may not be diagnosed early when it is most curable.

Depression/Anxiety: Lesbians have been shown to experience chronic stress from homophobic discrimination. This stress is compounded by the need that some still have to hide their orientation from work colleagues, and by the fact that many lesbians have lost the important emotional support others get from their families due to alienation stemming from their sexual orientation.

Gynecological Cancer: Lesbians have higher risks for some of the gynecologic cancers. What they may not know is that having a yearly exam by a gynecologist can significantly facilitate early diagnosis associated with higher rates of curability if they ever develop.

Fitness: Research confirms that lesbians have higher body mass than heterosexual women. Obesity is associated with higher rates of heart disease, cancers, and premature death. What lesbians need is competent advice about healthy living and healthy eating, as well as healthy exercise.

Substance Use: Research indicates that illicit drugs may be used more often among lesbians than heterosexual women. There may be added stressors in lesbian lives from homophobic discrimination, and lesbians need support from each other and from health care providers to find healthy releases, quality recreation, stress reduction, and coping techniques.

Tobacco: Research also indicates that tobacco and smoking products may be used more often by lesbians than by heterosexual women. Whether smoking is used as a tension reducer or for social interactions, addiction often follows and is associated with higher rates of cancers, heart disease, and emphysema—the three major causes of death among all women.

Alcohol: Alcohol use and abuse may be higher among lesbians. While one drink daily may be good for the heart and not increase cancer or osteoporosis risks, more than that can be a risk factor for disease.

Domestic Violence: Domestic violence is reported to occur in about 11 percent of lesbian homes, about half the rate of 20 percent reported by heterosexual women. But the question is where do lesbians go when they are battered? Shelters need to welcome and include battered lesbians, and offer counseling to the offending partners.

Osteoporosis: The rates and risks of osteoporosis among lesbians have not been well characterized yet. Calcium and weight-bearing exercise as well as the avoidance of tobacco and alcohol are the mainstays of prevention. Getting bone density tests every few years to see if medication is needed to prevent fracture is also important.

Heart Health: Smoking and obesity are the most prevalent risk factors for heart disease among lesbians; but all lesbians need to also get an annual clinical exam because this is when blood pressure is checked, cholesterol is measured, diabetes is diagnosed, and exercise is discussed. Preventing heart disease, which kills 45 percent of women, should be paramount to every clinical visit.

Chapter 8

Nutrition and Weight Management

Chapter Contents

Section 8.1

Diet and Nutrition

Excerpted and reprinted with permission from the *Journal of the American Dietetic Association,* Volume 99, Number 6, 738-751, June 1999, Reaffirmed, American Dietetic Association and Dietitians of Canada Joint Position. The complete text of this position paper, including references, is available at http://www.eatright.org. An updated paper will be available in 2004.

Until recently, women's health only involved issues of the reproductive system. However, within the past 10 years it has evolved to a much broader paradigm, well beyond reproduction. From a physiological perspective, women's health now refers to the prevention, diagnosis, and management of conditions or diseases that may:

- be unique to women (e.g., menstruation, pregnancy, menopause, diseases of the reproductive tract)

- be more prevalent in women than in men (e.g., bone, joint, and rheumatic diseases; diabetes mellitus; eating disorders; breast cancer; and specific thyroid, neurologic, gastrointestinal, and psychiatric diseases)

- manifest differently in women than men (e.g., heart disease, substance abuse, acquired immunodeficiency syndrome [AIDS], violence)

Women's health goes well beyond the physiological differences noted above. Women's health involves their emotional, social, cultural, spiritual, and physical well-being. It is determined not only by biology, but by the social, political, and economic context of their lives. A woman's health is shaped by her environment; that is, where she lives, works, learns, and plays.

Despite living 6.4 years longer, on average, than men, women suffer poorer health outcomes and greater disability from disease. The 10 leading causes of deaths in U.S. women of all ages and races are (in descending order): diseases of the heart, malignant neoplasms, cerebrovascular disease, chronic obstructive pulmonary disease, pneumonia and influenza, diabetes, accidents, Alzheimer's disease, kidney disease, and septicemia. Similarly, the 2 most prevalent causes of death in Canadian women are heart disease and cancer.

In women aged 25 to 44 years, immunodeficiency virus infection is ranked as the first cause of death in black women and the fifth in white women. For women over the age of 45, the first and second leading causes of death are the same for black and white women; however, average life expectancy is 79.6 years for white women and 73.9 years for black women.

Nutrition is involved in the etiology or treatment of half of the 10 leading causes of death in women. Although not appearing in the top 10 causes of mortality, the incidence of osteoporosis and extremes in body weight are approaching epidemic proportions in women and are addressed in this chapter. Dietetics professionals are in the perfect position to understand the issues surrounding women's health in order to deliver a message to women to allow them to make wise decisions regarding their health.

This chapter focuses on five of the leading nutrition-related causes of morbidity and mortality in North American adult women: cardiovascular disease, cancer, osteoporosis, weight control, and diabetes. In addition, this chapter summarizes other issues that affect women's nutritional health.

Cardiovascular Disease

Coronary heart disease (CHD) and stroke are the most frequent causes of death in the United States, killing around half a million women over the age of 45 years annually. More women die from cardiovascular disease than all cancers combined. Yet the belief that heart problems only strike men still lingers. Forty-six percent of women responding to a U.S. Gallup poll perceived breast cancer as their major health threat; only 4% believed heart disease was the major threat. Similar perceptions are observed in Canadian women.

Modifiable risk factors in women include smoking, hypercholesterolemia, obesity and central adiposity, diabetes, hypertension, physical inactivity, and diet. Elevated serum triglycerides, low levels of high-density lipoproteins (HDLs), and central obesity are strong discriminators of heart disease in women. In fact, young women who gain 20 pounds or more in early adulthood double their risk of heart disease. Because they have more risk factors, premenopausal black women have a 2- to 3-fold greater rate of heart disease than premenopausal white women.

81

The cornerstone to preventing cardiovascular disease is lifestyle change, of which nutrition is a major component. Suggestions for using medical nutrition therapy to prevent cardiovascular disease include maintaining weight control (the most important strategy); limiting quantity of dietary fat; limiting animal sources rich in saturated fatty acids and cholesterol; eating an abundance of fruits, vegetables, complex carbohydrates, and whole grains; consuming adequate amounts of fish containing fatty acids; using vegetable oils rich in monounsaturated fatty acids; controlling blood pressure with dietary intervention; increasing physical activity; and stopping smoking.

Cancer

Cancer is the second leading cause of mortality in women residing in the United States and Canada. The incidence of cancers in Canadian women is similar to that in U.S. women. Factors such as heredity, smoking, diet, body mass, estrogen replacement therapy, and physical inactivity affect cancer occurrence. In women, the leading cause of cancer deaths is lung cancer, succeeded by breast, and then colorectal.

Collectively, gynecologic cancers such as cervical, endometrial, and ovarian cancer are the third most common cause of cancer in women. Between the ages of 50 to 74 years, cancer is the leading cause of death in women in Canada.

Lung Cancer

Lung cancer rates among U.S. and Canadian women are rising. Between 1973 and 1994, lung cancer mortality in U.S. women increased 143.7% due to increased exposure to environmental carcinogens and increased smoking, especially in white and African-American women who are less educated. In addition, many young women rely on smoking as a means of weight control, putting them at increased risk of developing cancer. National data demonstrate that white and African-American women smoke at higher rates (25%) than do Latinas (15%) or Asian-American women (8%). Tobacco smoke, whether active or passive, is the most important epidemiologic factor contributing to the development of lung cancer. Compared with men, women are more susceptible to tobacco carcinogens, due to physiological differences in how they detoxify lung carcinogens.

Epidemiologic studies generally support the hypotheses that diet may affect lung cancer risk. Diets high in fruits and vegetables provide protection against lung carcinoma due to their carotenoid, flavonoid, and/or phytochemical content. Data are inconsistent regarding the effect of dietary fat and cholesterol on lung cancer risk. Diets high in fat, saturated fat, and cholesterol have been shown to increase lung cancer risk. However, in a recent investigation of lung cancer risk among U.S. women, dietary fats and red meat were not associated with lung cancer risk after adjusting for potential cofounders such as body mass index (BMI), and frequency of vegetable and fruit intake.

Breast Cancer

In North American women, breast cancer is the most frequently diagnosed carcinoma and the second most common cause of cancer death. Established and probable risk factors for breast cancer include family history of breast cancer, early menarche, older age at birth of first child, late menopause (after the age of 55), some forms of benign breast disease, oral contraceptive use for more than 5 to 10 years, postmenopausal estrogen-replacement therapy, and excessive alcohol use. Dietary and other factors potentially have a role in its etiology. More specifically, the amount and type of fat consumed; the carotenoid, phytochemical, and flavonoid content of the diet; and lifestyle conditions, such as overeating and physical inactivity may affect breast cancer risk.

Osteoporosis

Osteoporosis is a bone disease characterized by reduced bone mass leading to increased susceptibility to fractures. Women are 4 times more likely to suffer from osteoporosis than men. Osteoporosis is currently defined as bone mineral density (BMD) more than 2.5 standard deviations below the mean value of peak bone mass in young normal women.

Osteoporosis is irreversible; however, it may be prevented by maximizing peak bone mass during the first 2 to 3 decades of life in order to sustain bone health during natural periods of bone loss (menopause and aging). The nutrients or food components that are linked to bone health include calcium, vitamin D, sodium, caffeine, protein, phosphorus, magnesium, fluoride, and phytoestrogens. Other nutrients may affect bone, such as vitamin K, vitamin C, vitamin A, manganese, copper, iron, zinc, and fatty acids; however, there is currently insufficient evidence for establishing recommended levels for bone health for the latter nutrients.

The goal is to maximize bone mass early in adulthood and to minimize bone loss in life. The recommendations to do both are essentially the same: maintenance of adequate estrogen status; regular physical activity; adequate intakes of calcium, vitamin D, and magnesium; and avoidance of excessive dietary sodium, protein, alcohol, and cigarette smoking.

Body Weight Abnormalities

Societal norms for the ideal female body weight and shape have changed over the past several decades. As women age, they experience a larger increase in body fat and greater declines in basal metabolic rate compared with men. Despite the physiological changes such as menarche, pregnancy, lactation, and menopause that increase fat storage in women, women are faced with social pressures to be thin.

BMI (calculated as kg/m^2) is the standard population-based measure of overweight and obesity. In the United States, healthy body weight refers to a body weight that is within a BMI range of 19 to 25, which is similar to Canadian guidelines of a BMI within the range of 20 to 25. According to recent U.S. federal guidelines, overweight is defined as a BMI of 25 to 29.9, and obesity as a BMI of 30 or above. In addition, a waist circumference of more than 35 inches in women signifies increased risk of cardiovascular disease and diabetes mellitus. Compared to waist-to-hip ratio, the traditional anthropometric method for measuring regional fat distribution, waist girth, is a better predictor of central adiposity.

The regulation of body-fat distribution is different in women than men because of hormonal changes that occur with reproductive cycling and childbearing. Menopause is accompanied by a notable increase in the waist-hip ratio in women.

Obesity is linked with increased incidence of dyslipidemia, hypertension, and type 2 diabetes, all of which are major contributors to mortality in women. Women who are obese are at greater risk for hypertension, gallbladder disease, respiratory disease, gout, sleep apnea, osteoarthritis, and several forms of cancer. Furthermore, obesity is associated with poor pregnancy outcome, miscarriage, infertility, and polycystic ovarian syndrome.

Not only does obesity increase the risk of several diseases, but it also places a great psychological burden on women. People who are obese suffer from prejudice in society and a reduced quality of life. Disordered eating patterns and altered body image perceptions begin early in a woman's life and continue across her life span. Many women are dissatisfied with their bodies, have low self-esteem, and engage in phases of dieting throughout their life span.

Diabetes Mellitus

In the United States, the prevalence of self-reported diabetes is approximately 6.6% of women aged 45 to 64 years. African-American women have the highest age-adjusted prevalence of diabetes followed by African-American men, white women, and white men (in descending order). African-American women have a high incidence of diabetes, in part because of high rates of obesity. In Canada, the overall prevalence of self-reported diabetes mellitus is 5.1% in adults aged 18 to 74 years. Women aged 50 years or older living in Ontario, Canada, reported a 5.4% rate of diabetes mellitus. In 1995, diabetes mellitus was the sixth leading cause of death in women in the United States.

The risk factors for diabetes mellitus depend on its classification. Autoimmune, genetic, and environmental factors are involved in the development of type 1 diabetes. Type 2 diabetes accounts for 90% to 95% of diagnosed diabetes. The risk factors for type 2 diabetes include older age, obesity, central adiposity, family history of diabetes, prior history of gestational diabetes, impaired glucose tolerance, physical inactivity, race/ethnicity, hypertension, and dyslipidemia. Gestational diabetes mellitus complicates approximately 4% of all pregnancies in the United States and 8.4% in Native Canadian women. Gestational diabetes mellitus occurs more frequently in African-Americans, Hispanic/Latino Americans, American Indians, Asians, and persons with a family history of diabetes or obesity.

Women with diabetes are susceptible to health-related conditions. An increased occurrence of cardiovascular disease occurs in women with diabetes because of enhanced platelet adhesion and aggregation, altered vascular endothelium, hyperinsulinemia, hyperglycemia, and dyslipidemia. Diabetes affects a woman's reproductive health. For example, poor glycemic control during pregnancy is associated with higher maternal and infant morbidity. Lactation presents a challenge in terms of metabolic control. However, breast-feeding should be encouraged, especially in women with type 2 diabetes who tend to be overweight, because it is associated with reduction of maternal fat stores and positive outcomes for the child.

Diabetes and its long-term complications are affected by weight and metabolic control. Because obesity is associated with glucose intolerance and cardiovascular disease, women with diabetes who are obese need to achieve a healthy weight. Control of total energy intake, and intake of total grams of fat, in combination with increased physical activity, can assist in weight loss and maintenance.

As a vital member of the diabetes management team, dietetics professionals should have an understanding of the health issues that affect women with diabetes to assist in the achievement of glycemic control throughout the life span. Medical nutrition therapy should individualize dietary carbohydrate and fat requirements to optimize blood glucose and lipid concentrations.

Section 8.2

Exercise and Weight Control

"Physical Activity and Weight Control," National Institutes of Health, National Institute of Diabetes and Digestive and Kidney Diseases, Weight-control Information Network, NIH Pub. No. 03-4031, March 2003. Available online at http://www.niddk.nih.gov; accessed July 2003.

Physical activity helps you control your weight by using excess calories that would otherwise be stored as fat. Most foods you eat contain calories, and everything you do uses calories, including sleeping, breathing, and digesting food. Balancing the calories you eat with the calories you use through physical activity will help you reach and maintain a healthy weight.

Becoming Physically Active

Experts recommend at least 30 minutes of moderate-intensity physical activity on most, if not all, days of the week. To achieve and maintain a healthy weight, particularly after you have lost a large amount of weight, you may need to do 60 minutes or more of moderate-intensity physical activity each day.

Physical activity may include structured activities such as walking, running, basketball, or other sports. It may also include daily activities such as household chores, yard work, or walking the dog. Pick a combination of structured and daily activities that fit your schedule.

If you have been inactive for a while, start slowly and work up to 30 minutes a day at a pace that is comfortable for you. If you are unable to be active for 30 minutes at one time, accumulate activity over the course of the day in 10- to 15-minute sessions.

Health Benefits of Physical Activity

Regular physical activity helps control your weight and may help:

- Reduce your risk of or manage chronic diseases such as type 2 diabetes, high blood pressure and cholesterol, heart disease, osteoporosis, arthritis, and some cancers;
- Build strong muscles, bones, and joints;
- Improve flexibility and balance;
- Ward off depression; and
- Improve mood and sense of well-being.

Aerobic Activity

You can meet your goal of at least 30 minutes of moderate-intensity physical activity by participating in aerobic activities. Aerobic exercise includes any activity that makes you breathe harder than when you are resting and increases your heart rate.

Experts recommend moderate-intensity exercise. At this pace, you may breathe harder and find it more difficult to talk, but you should still be able to carry on a conversation. If you are just beginning, slowly work up to moving at a moderate-intensity pace.

Strength Training

Strength training is another way for you to meet the recommended minimum of 30 minutes of moderate-intensity physical activity each day. Strength training will also help you burn extra calories and build strong muscles, bones, and joints.

Experts recommend strength training 2 to 3 days each week, with 1 full day of rest between workouts to allow your muscles to recover. If you are new to strength training, or physical activity in general, consider hiring a certified personal trainer who can plan an individualized program to help you work out safely and effectively. A personal trainer who has a degree in exercise physiology or is certified through a national certification program such as the American College of

Sports Medicine or National Strength and Conditioning Association may be able to help you reach your physical activity goals.

Mind and Body Exercise

In addition to aerobic activity and strength training, you may wish to include other forms of exercise in your physical activity program. Alternatives to traditional exercise provide variety and fun. They may also help reduce stress, increase muscular strength and flexibility, and increase energy levels. Examples of these exercises include yoga, Pilates, and tai chi.

Regular physical activity will help you feel, move, and look better. Whether your goal is to achieve and maintain a healthy weight or improve your health, becoming physically active is a step in the right direction. Take advantage of the health benefits of physical activity and make it a part of your life.

Section 8.3

Losing Weight: More Than Counting Calories

"Losing Weight—More Than Counting Calories," *FDA Consumer*, by Linda Bren. Published January-February 2002; revised March 2003. Available online at http://www.fda.gov; accessed July 2003.

Are You Overweight?

Overweight refers to an excess of body weight, but not necessarily body fat. Obesity means an excessively high proportion of body fat. Health professionals use a measurement called body mass index (BMI) to classify an adult's weight as healthy, overweight, or obese. BMI describes body weight relative to height and is correlated with total body fat content in most adults.

To get your approximate BMI, multiply your weight in pounds by 703, then divide the result by your height in inches, and divide that result by your height in inches a second time.

A BMI from 18.5 up to 25 is considered in the healthy range, from 25 up to 30 is overweight, and 30 or higher is obese. Generally, the higher a person's BMI, the greater the risk for health problems, according to the National Heart, Lung and Blood Institute (NHLBI). However, there are some exceptions. For example, very muscular people, like body builders, may have a BMI greater than 25 or even 30, but this reflects increased muscle rather than fat. "It is excess body fat that leads to the health problems such as type 2 diabetes, high blood pressure, and high cholesterol," says Eric Colman, M.D., of the Food and Drug Administration's Division of Metabolic and Endocrine Drug Products.

Successful Losers

A popular weight-loss myth is that everyone who loses weight eventually gains it back, says Rena Wing, Ph.D., a professor of psychiatry at Brown Medical School in Providence, RI. Wing, the co-developer of a research study known as the National Weight Control Registry, has worked to deflate this myth.

Successful losers report four common behaviors, says Wing. They eat a low-fat, high-carbohydrate diet, they monitor themselves by weighing in frequently, they are very physically active, and they eat breakfast. Eating breakfast every day is contrary to the typical pattern for the average overweight person who is trying to diet, says Wing. "They get up in the morning and say 'I'm going to start my diet today,' and they eat little or no breakfast and a light lunch. Then they get hungry and consume most of their calories late in the day. Successful weight losers have managed to change this pattern."

Six years after their weight loss, most of the registry's successful losers still report eating a low-calorie, low-fat diet, with about 24 percent of calories from fat. (The Dietary Guidelines for Americans recommend no more than 30 percent of daily calories from fat.) They also exercise for about an hour or more a day, expending about 2,800 calories per week on a variety of activities. This is equivalent to walking 28 miles a week, or four miles a day, says Wing.

Setting a Goal

The first step to weight loss is setting a realistic goal. By using a BMI chart and consulting with your health-care provider, you can determine what is a healthy weight for you.

Studies show that you can improve your health with just a small amount of weight loss. "We know that physical activity in combination with reduced calorie consumption can lead to the 5 to 10 percent weight loss necessary to achieve remission of the obesity-associated complications," says William Dietz, M.D., Ph.D., director of the Division of Nutrition and Physical Activity at the CDC.

"Even these moderate weight losses can improve blood pressure and help control diabetes and high cholesterol in obese or overweight adults."

To reach your goal safely, plan to lose weight gradually. A weight loss of one-half to 2 pounds a week is usually safe, according to the Dietary Guidelines for Americans. This can be achieved by decreasing the calories eaten or increasing the calories used by 250 to 1,000 calories per day, depending on current calorie intake. (Some people with serious health problems due to obesity may lose weight more rapidly under a doctor's supervision.) If you plan to lose more than 15 to 20 pounds, have any health problems, or take medication on a regular basis, a doctor should evaluate you before you begin a weight-loss program.

Changing Eating Habits

Dieting may conjure up visions of eating little but lettuce and sprouts—but you can enjoy all foods as part of a healthy diet as long as you don't overdo it on fat (especially saturated fat), protein, sugars, and alcohol. To be successful at losing weight, you need to change your lifestyle—not just go on a diet, experts say.

Limit portion sizes, especially of foods high in calories, such as cookies, cakes and other sweets; french fries; and fats, oils and spreads. Reducing dietary fat alone—without reducing calories—will not produce weight loss.

Choose a healthful assortment of foods that includes vegetables, fruits, grains (especially whole grains), fat-free milk, and fish, lean meat, poultry, or beans. Choose foods naturally high in fiber, such as fruits, vegetables, legumes (such as beans and lentils), and whole grains. The high fiber content of many of these foods may help you to feel full with fewer calories.

All calorie sources are not created equal. Carbohydrate and protein have about 4 calories per gram, but fat has more than twice that amount (9 calories per gram). Just as for the general population, weight-conscious consumers should aim for a daily fat intake of no more than 30 percent of total calories.

Keep your intake of saturated fat at less than 10 percent of calories. Saturated fats increase the risk for heart disease by raising blood cholesterol.

If you drink alcoholic beverages, do so in moderation. Alcoholic beverages supply calories but few nutrients.

Limit your use of beverages and foods that are high in added sugars—those added to foods in processing or preparation, not the naturally occurring sugars in foods such as fruit or milk. Foods containing added sugars provide calories, but may have few vitamins and minerals.

Increasing Physical Activity

Most health experts recommend a combination of a reduced-calorie diet and increased physical activity for weight loss. Most adults should get at least 30 minutes and children should get 60 minutes of moderate physical activity on most, and preferably all, days of the week. But fewer than 1 in 3 U.S. adults gets the recommended amount of physical activity, according to The Surgeon General's *Call To Action To Prevent and Decrease Overweight and Obesity*.

Prescription Weight-Loss Drugs

For obese people who have difficulty losing weight through diet and exercise alone, there are a number of FDA-approved prescription drugs that may help. "On average, individuals who use weight-loss drugs lose about 5 percent to 10 percent of their original weight, though some will lose less and some more," says the FDA's Colman.

All of the prescription weight-loss drugs work by suppressing the appetite except for Xenical (orlistat). Xenical is the first in a new class of anti-obesity drugs known as lipase inhibitors. Xenical interferes with lipase function, decreasing dietary fat absorption by 30 percent. Because the undigested fats are not absorbed, fewer calories are available to the body. The main side effects of Xenical are cramping, diarrhea, flatulence, intestinal discomfort, and leakage of oily stool.

Meridia (sibutramine), approved by the FDA in 1997, increases the levels of certain brain chemicals that help reduce appetite. Because it may increase blood pressure and heart rate, Meridia should not be used by people with uncontrolled high blood pressure, a history of heart disease, congestive heart failure, irregular heartbeat, or stroke. Other common side effects of Meridia include headache, dry mouth, constipation and insomnia.

Other anti-obesity prescription drugs that were approved by the FDA many years ago based on very short-term, limited data include: Bontril (phendimetrazine tartrate), Desoxyn (methamphetamine) and Ionamin and Adipex-P (phentermine). They are speed-like drugs that should not be used by people with heart disease, high blood pressure, an overactive thyroid gland, or glaucoma. These drugs are approved only for short-term use, such as a few weeks. They generally don't cause weight loss beyond several weeks, and they have significant potential for physical dependence or addiction.

Until September 1997, two other drugs, fenfluramine (Pondimin and others) and dexfenfluramine (Redux), were available for treating obesity. But at the FDA's request, the manufacturers of these drugs voluntarily withdrew them from the market after newer findings suggested that they were the likely cause of heart valve problems. The FDA recommended that people taking the drugs stop and that they contact their doctor to discuss their treatment.

Prescription weight-loss drugs are approved only for those with a BMI of 30 and above, or 27 and above if they have other risk factors, such as high blood pressure or diabetes. People should contact a doctor before using any kind of drug, including a weight-loss drug.

Over-the-Counter Drugs

Until recently, weight-control drugs containing the active ingredient phenylpropanolamine (also used as a nasal decongestant) were available over-the-counter (OTC). However, based on evidence linking this ingredient to an increased risk of hemorrhagic stroke (bleeding in the brain), the FDA asked drug manufacturers to discontinue marketing products containing phenylpropanolamine.

Some dietary supplement makers claim their products work for weight loss. These products are not reviewed by the FDA before they are marketed. "Under our existing laws, manufacturers have the responsibility for ensuring that their dietary supplement products are safe and effective," says Christine Lewis Taylor, Ph.D., R.D., director of the FDA's Office of Nutritional Products.

Many weight-loss products claim to be natural or herbal, but this does not necessarily mean that they're safe. These ingredients may interact with drugs or may be dangerous for people with certain medical conditions. If you are unsure about a product's claims or the safety of any weight-loss product, check with your doctor before using it.

Linda Bren is a staff writer for *FDA Consumer*.

Chapter 9

Special Nutritional Concerns

Chapter Contents

Section 9.1

Anemia

Excerpted with permission from *Anemia: A Hidden Epidemic*, a publication of the National Anemia Action Council, supported by an unrestricted
educational grant from Amgen, Inc. © 2002 HealthVizion Communications, Inc. All rights reserved. For additional information, or to view the
complete text of *Anemia: A Hidden Epidemic*, visit the website of the
National Anemia Action Council at www.anemia.org.

Key Points

- Anemia is often underrecognized and undertreated.
- Anemia is associated with many chronic diseases and other con-
  ditions.
- If left untreated, anemia can have serious consequences.
- Anemia can be readily managed by current therapies.

A Hidden Epidemic

Traditionally, the health care community has not focused on anemia as a serious and common condition. However, findings from the
National Center for Health Statistics and the recent identification of
anemia as a significant public health concern by the United States
Department of Health and Human Services in Healthy People 2010
have sounded a call for a re-examination of the impact of anemia on
the health of Americans.

Based on a national household interview survey, the National Center for Health Statistics estimated in 1996 that 3.4 million Americans
were living with anemia. The actual number of individuals with the
condition may be far greater, as anemia is often underdiagnosed and
undertreated. Anemia's signs and symptoms may be vague, and it is
present in a substantial number of patients with a variety of chronic
and serious diseases.

Frequently, however, anemia remains undetected because it is masked
by symptoms of the diseases with which it is associated, including chronic

94

kidney disease, cancer, diabetes, cardiovascular disease, HIV/AIDS, rheumatoid arthritis, and inflammatory bowel disease.

The National Kidney Foundation's Kidney Disease Outcomes Quality Initiative (NKF-K/DOQI) new clinical practice guideline on the classification system for chronic kidney disease (CKD) estimates that more than 19.5 million Americans have CKD. Anemia is a common and early complication of CKD and worsens as the disease progresses.

The estimated 50 million Americans with hypertension and 17 million with diabetes are at increased risk for CKD—and subsequently anemia.

Not only is anemia a consequence of many diseases, it may also occur from the treatment of the disease itself, such as in patients with cancer, HIV/AIDS, and hepatitis C. Candidates for surgery may be anemic due to underlying disease or become so due to blood loss during the perioperative period. Anemia also occurs more frequently among the elderly, and its prevalence in this group is expected to increase as baby-boomers become senior citizens.

At least 3.4 million Americans have been diagnosed as anemic, and millions more may be undiagnosed or at increased risk of developing anemia. Anemia is a hidden epidemic in this nation, and a condition that can have serious consequences if left untreated. However, it is also a condition that can be readily managed by current therapies.

Anemia Defined

Anemia is defined as a reduction in the number of circulating red blood cells, the hemoglobin concentration, or the volume of packed red cells (hematocrit) in the blood. In the laboratory, anemia is identified when a patient's hemoglobin (Hb)/hematocrit (Hct) values fall below the lower end of a normal range of values for age- and sex-matched subjects.

The likelihood and severity of anemia is based on the patient's deviation from normal values. Women in their childbearing years normally have a lower Hb value by about 1 gm/dL than men of the same age, likely due to hormonal influences. After menopause, the gender difference virtually disappears.

The three major categories of anemia are hypoproliferative, maturation defects, and hemolysis/blood loss. The most common anemia in the United States is hypoproliferative anemia, which includes iron deficiency, chronic kidney disease (CKD), and the inflammation-associated anemia of chronic disease, which is found in patients with chronic conditions, such as rheumatoid arthritis, inflammatory bowel disease, HIV/AIDS, and cancer.

Anemia may be acquired (e.g., through blood loss, inflammation, and malignancy) or inherited (e.g., by patients with sickle cell disease, thalassemia, and other hemoglobinopathies).

Diagnosing Anemia

Since anemia is a sign of a wide range of underlying disorders, and, in itself, is associated with morbidity and even an increased risk of mortality, it is critical that the underlying pathophysiologic mechanism be identified for any given patient.

The hypoproliferative anemias may be associated with inadequate erythroid marrow stimulation by erythropoietin for red blood cell production and with inadequate iron availability for Hb synthesis. Because it is the most common cause of anemia, iron deficiency must be ruled out in the evaluation of any anemic patient.

Anemia is almost always discovered through abnormal laboratory screening test results. It is unusual for patients to present with anemia so advanced that the clinical manifestations (e.g., pallor, palpitations, weakness, etc.) predominate.

Anemia Management

A correct diagnosis of the cause is key to managing anemia. Once the cause is determined, the approach is to implement the appropriate treatment to correct the anemia. In most medical practices, the identification of iron deficiency should be foremost, since it may be associated with occult bleeding or other serious conditions, and it can be quickly and easily treated with iron supplementation.

Other less common but reversible anemias include vitamin B_{12} and folate deficiency, and some cases of anemia associated with inflammation. Each of these requires a slightly different therapeutic approach.

Section 9.2

Caffeine

Excerpted from National Institutes of Health, Center for the Evaluation of Risks to Human Reproduction; published May 17, 2002; updated June 24, 2003. The full text is available online at http://cerhr.niehs.nih.gov; accessed July 2003.

Caffeine and Fertility

Numerous studies have been conducted to determine the effects of caffeine intake on fertility in women. One small study in 1988 suggested that caffeine, equivalent to the amount consumed in 1-to 2-cups of coffee daily, might decrease female fertility. However, the researchers acknowledged that delayed conception could be due to other factors they did not consider, such as exercise, stress, or other dietary habits. Since then, larger, well-designed studies have failed to support these findings.

In 1990, researchers at the Centers for Disease Control and Prevention and Harvard University found that caffeine consumption had little or no effect on the reported time to conceive. Supporting those findings, a 1991 study of 11,000 Danish women examined the relationship among number of months to conceive, cigarette smoking and coffee and tea consumption. Although smokers who consumed eight or more cups of coffee per day experienced delayed conception, non-smokers did not, regardless of caffeine consumption.

The Organization of Teratology Information Services (OTIS, 2001) reviewed the studies examining caffeine effects on fertility and concluded that, "Low to moderate caffeine consumption (<300mg/day) does not seem to reduce a woman's chance of becoming pregnant."

Caffeine and Pregnancy

The March of Dimes (MOD, 2002) notes that during pregnancy, caffeine easily passes from the mother to her unborn child through the placenta. Because the systems for breaking down and eliminating chemicals are not fully developed in the unborn child, blood levels of caffeine may remain elevated for longer periods in the unborn child compared to the mother. OTIS (OTIS, 2001) notes that, " . . .higher amounts of caffeine could affect babies in the same way as it does adults. Some reports have stated that children born to mothers who consumed >500mg/day were more likely to have faster heart rates, tremors, increased breathing rate, and spend more time awake in the days following birth."

The effects of caffeine intake on miscarriages, birth defects, and low birth weight have been studied, and different results were obtained in the various studies. Major studies over the last decade have shown no association between birth defects and caffeine consumption. Even offspring of the heaviest coffee drinkers were not found to be at higher risk of birth defects.

Groups such as OTIS, March of Dimes, and Motherisk reviewed studies examining caffeine intake during pregnancy and are in agreement that high caffeine intake (>300 mg/day, equivalent to more than 3 cups of coffee/day) should be avoided during pregnancy. There is also general agreement that low caffeine intake (<150 mg/day, about 1-½ cups of coffee) during pregnancy is not likely to harm the unborn child. However, there is some disagreement regarding moderate caffeine intake.

Following a statistical analysis of studies examining caffeine intake in pregnant woman, Motherisk (Motherisk, 2000) stated, "Our results suggest a small but statistically significant increase in risk of spontaneous abortion and low birth weight babies in pregnant women consuming more than 150 mg of caffeine per day. Pregnant women should be encouraged to be aware of dietary caffeine intake and to consume less than 150 mg of caffeine a day from all sources throughout pregnancy."

Subsequent to their review of caffeine studies, OTIS (OTIS, 2001) stated that "Recent reports suggest that low to moderate consumption of caffeine does not increase the risk for miscarriage. A few studies have shown that there may be an increased risk for miscarriage with high caffeine consumption (>300 mg/day), particularly in combination with smoking or alcohol, or with very high levels of caffeine consumption (>800 mg/day). OTIS (OTIS, 2001) goes on to say that, "In humans, even large amounts of caffeine have not been shown to cause an increased chance for birth defects." OTIS concluded that (OTIS, 2001), "Most experts agree that moderation and common sense are the keys for consuming caffeinated items during pregnancy. "Moderate" caffeine consumption is approximately 300mg/day, which is similar to 3 cups of coffee. It is also important for pregnant women to drink sufficient quantities of water, milk, and juice. These fluids should not be replaced with caffeinated beverages."

Caffeine and Breastfeeding

Caffeine can enter the breast milk of nursing mothers (IFIC, July 1998). According to the American Academy of Pediatrics (AAP 2002), "Caffeine tends to build up in babies' systems because their bodies cannot get rid of it very easily. A morning cup of coffee is not likely to harm your baby, but too much caffeine can cause problems such as poor sleeping, nervousness, irritability, and poor feeding. Try using decaffeinated coffee and tea and avoid colas and other carbonated drinks that have added caffeine." OTIS (OTIS, 2001) states that, "women should remain well hydrated with water, juice, and milk while breastfeeding."

Section 9.3

Female Athletic Triad

Sports and exercise are healthy activities for girls and women of all ages. But a female athlete who focuses on being thin or lightweight may eat too little and exercise too much. Doing this can cause long-term damage to your health or even death. It can also hurt your athletic performance or make it necessary to limit or stop exercise. Three interrelated illnesses may develop when a girl or young woman goes to extremes in dieting or exercise. Together these conditions are known as the female athletic triad:

- Disordered eating: Abnormal eating habits (i.e., crash diets, binge eating) or excessive exercise keeps your body from getting enough nutrition.

- Menstrual dysfunction: Poor nutrition, low calorie intake, high energy demands, physical and emotional stress, or low percentage of body fat can lead to hormonal changes that stop your menstrual periods (amenorrhea).

- Osteoporosis: Lack of periods disrupts your body's bone-building processes and weakens the skeleton, making your bones more likely to break.

Females at Risk

Females in any sport can develop one or more parts of the triad. At greatest risk are those in sports that reward being thin for appearance (i.e., figure skating, gymnastics) or improved performance (i.e., distance running, rowing). Fashion trends and advertising often encourage women to try to reach unhealthy weight levels. Some female athletes suffer low self-esteem or depression, and may focus on weight loss because they think they are heavier than they actually are. Others feel pressure to lose weight from athletic coaches or parents. Female athletes should consider these questions:

- Are you dissatisfied with your body?
- Do you strive to be thin?
- Do you continuously focus on your weight?

If the answers are yes, you may be at risk for developing abnormal patterns of eating food (disordered eating), which can lead to menstrual dysfunction and early osteoporosis.

Disordered Eating

Although they usually don't realize or admit that they are ill, people with disordered eating have serious and complex disturbances in eating behaviors. They are preoccupied with body shape and weight and have poor nutritional habits. Females are 10 times more likely to have disordered eating compared with males, and the problem is especially common in females who are athletic. The illness takes many forms. Some people starve themselves (anorexia nervosa) or engage in cycles of overeating and purging (bulimia). Others severely restrict the amount of food they eat, fast for prolonged periods of time or misuse diet pills, diuretics, or laxatives. People with disordered eating may also exercise excessively to keep their weight down.

Disordered eating can cause many problems including dehydration, muscle fatigue and weakness, an erratic heartbeat, kidney damage and other serious conditions. You may not get enough calcium, which can lead to bone loss. It's especially bad to lose bone when you are a child or teenager because that's when your body should be building bone. You may also get hormone imbalances that lead to more bone loss through menstrual dysfunction.

Menstrual Dysfunction

Missing three or more periods in a row is cause for concern. With normal menstruation, your body has estrogen, a hormone that helps to keep bones strong. With amenorrhea, you may not get the estrogen you need and may lose bone density and strength (premature osteoporosis). If this happens during youth, you may also get serious problems later in life when the natural process of bone mineral loss begins after menopause. Amenorrhea may also cause stress fractures and make it difficult to get pregnant if you ever want to have a baby.

Osteoporosis

Bone tissue wears away, making your skeleton fragile. Low bone mass puts you at increased risk for fractures.

Get Treatment

Recognizing the female athletic triad is the first step toward treating it. See your doctor right away if you think you might have disordered eating, miss several menstrual periods, or get a stress fracture in sports.

Give the doctor your complete medical history including:

- What you do for physical activity and what you eat for nutrition
- How old you were when you began to menstruate and whether you usually have regular periods
- If you are sexually active, use birth control pills or have ever been pregnant
- If you have ever had stress fractures or other injuries
- Any changes (up or down) in your weight
- Any medications you are taking or symptoms of other medical problems

- Family history of diseases (i.e., thyroid disease, osteoporosis)
- Factors that cause stress in your life

The doctor will give you complete physical and pelvic examinations and may use laboratory tests to check for pregnancy, thyroid disease, and other medical conditions. In some cases you may also get a bone density test.

Treatment for the female athletic triad often requires help from a team of medical professionals including your doctor, a nutritionist, and a psychological counselor.

Chapter 10

Sleep

Chapter Contents

Section 10.1

Women and Sleep

Reprinted with permission from "Women and Sleep," a brochure from the National Sleep Foundation, www.sleepfoundation.org. © 2001 National Sleep Foundation. Updated August 2003.

Women's Unique Sleep Experiences

Sleep is a basic human need, as important for good health as diet and exercise. When we sleep, our bodies rest but our brains are active. Sleep lays the groundwork for a productive day ahead.

Although most people need eight hours of sleep each night, the National Sleep Foundation (NSF) 1998 Women and Sleep Poll found that the average woman aged 30 to 60 sleeps only six hours and forty-one minutes during the workweek. Research has shown that a lack of enough restful sleep results in daytime sleepiness, increased accidents, problems concentrating, poor performance on the job and in school, and possibly, increased sickness and weight gain.

Getting the right amount of sleep is vital, but just as important is the quality of your sleep. Conditions unique to women, like the menstrual cycle, pregnancy and menopause, can affect how well a woman sleeps. This is because the changing levels of hormones that a woman experiences throughout the month, like estrogen and progesterone, have an impact on sleep. Understanding the effects of these hormones, environmental factors, and lifestyle habits can help women enjoy a good night's sleep.

Understanding Your Monthly Cycle

Changes in women's bodies occur at different times in the menstrual cycle and may affect sleep. For example, the NSF poll found that 50% of menstruating women reported bloating that disturbed their sleep. On average, these women reported disrupted sleep for two to three days each menstrual cycle. These changes can be linked to the rise and fall of hormone levels in the body. The hormone progesterone, which rises after ovulation (when an ovary releases an egg), may cause some women to feel more sleepy or fatigued. However, poor quality sleep is more likely at the beginning of the menstrual cycle when bleeding starts.

Hormones, of course, are not the only factors that influence sleep. Stress, illness, diet, lifestyle and the sleep environment all play a part. Women's sleep experiences vary greatly during the menstrual cycle and certain types of sleep problems are associated with each phase of the cycle:

Before Ovulation (days 1-12): Typically, the period (bleeding or menstruation) occurs for about five days. After the period ends, an egg ripens in the ovary. During menstrual bleeding, women tend to get less restful sleep than at other times. 36% of women polled by NSF said their sleep was most disturbed during the first few days of their menstrual periods.

Ovulation (days 13-14): An egg is released. If the egg is fertilized, pregnancy occurs. Otherwise the cycle continues and a menstrual period results in about 14 days.

After Ovulation (days 15-28): If pregnancy doesn't occur, the lining of the uterine wall begins to break down; it is shed during the menstrual period. Progesterone levels start off high at the beginning of this phase, reaching their peak level around days 19-21. Then levels begin to decrease toward the end of the phase. Women may find it more difficult to fall asleep. This may be related to the rapidly falling levels of progesterone.

Premenstrual syndrome (PMS) symptoms may occur during the later portion of this phase (starting about days 22-28). These include bloating, headaches, moodiness, irritability and abdominal cramps. The most common sleep-related problems reported by women with PMS are: insomnia (difficulty falling asleep, staying asleep, waking up too early or waking unrefreshed), hypersomnia (sleeping too much), and daytime sleepiness.

A healthy sleeper spends about 15-20% of his or her sleep time in deep sleep. Research suggests that women with PMS experience less deep sleep (about 5% of their total sleep) all month long.

Tips That May Help Sleep

If you have difficulty with your sleep for any reason, here are some tips that may help you get a better night's sleep:

- Exercise regularly, but finish your workout at least three hours before bedtime. Exercise may relieve some PMS symptoms and increase the amount of deep sleep.

- Avoid foods and drinks high in sugar (including honey, syrup), and caffeine (coffee, colas, tea, chocolate), as well as salty foods and alcohol before bedtime. Caffeine and alcohol disturb sleep.

- Try to have a standard bedtime routine and keep regular sleep times. Make sure your bedroom is dark, cool and quiet and that your pillows, sleep surface, and coverings provide you with comfort.

- Consult your healthcare professional, if needed.

Pregnancy: Sleeping for Two

Pregnancy is an exciting and physically demanding time. Physical symptoms (body aches, nausea, leg cramps, fetus movements, and heartburn), as well as emotional changes (depression, anxiety, worry) can interfere with sleep. In the NSF poll, 78% of women reported more disturbed sleep during pregnancy than at other times. Sleep related problems also become more prevalent as the pregnancy progresses.

First Trimester (Months 1-3)

High levels of progesterone are produced, increasing feelings of sleepiness. Also, the number of times a woman wakes up during the night to urinate increases. Disturbed sleep patterns may begin. Interrupted sleep can cause daytime sleepiness. Women tend to sleep more during this time than before they were pregnant, or later in pregnancy.

Second Trimester (Months 4-6)

Progesterone levels still rise, but slowly. This allows for better sleep than during the first trimester. The growing fetus reduces pressure on the bladder by moving above it, decreasing the need for frequent bathroom visits. Sleep quality is still worse than it was before pregnancy.

Third Trimester (Months 7-9)

Women experience the most pregnancy-related sleep problems now. They may often feel physically uncomfortable. Heartburn, leg cramps and sinus congestion are common reasons for disturbed sleep, as is an increased need to go to the bathroom. (The fetus puts pressure on the bladder again.) One recent study reported that by the end of pregnancy, 97% of women were waking during the night.

Snoring and Severe Daytime Sleepiness

Pregnant women who have never snored before may begin doing so. About 30% of pregnant women snore because of increased swelling in their nasal passages. This may partially block the airways. Snoring can also lead to high blood pressure, which can put both the mother and fetus at risk. If the blockage is severe, sleep apnea may result, characterized by loud snoring and periods of stopped breathing during sleep. The lack of oxygen disrupts sleep and may affect the unborn fetus. If loud snoring and severe daytime sleepiness (another symptom of sleep apnea and other sleep disorders) occur, consult your physician.

Restless Legs and Poor Sleep

More women (28%) than men (21%) report restless legs syndrome (RLS) symptoms in the NSF's 1998 Omnibus Sleep in America Poll and up to 15 percent of pregnant women develop RLS during the third trimester.

RLS symptoms—crawling or moving feelings in the foot, calf or upper leg—momentarily disrupt sleep. Moving the legs can stop these symptoms temporarily, but the irritation returns when the limb is still. Fortunately, RLS symptoms usually end after delivery of the baby. However, women who are not pregnant can also suffer from RLS. Medications used to treat RLS may cause harm to the fetus and should be discussed with a doctor.

Sleep Tips for Pregnant Women

- In the third trimester, sleep on your left side to allow for the best blood flow to the fetus and to your uterus and kidneys. Avoid lying flat on your back for a long period of time.

- Drink lots of fluids during the day, but cut down before bedtime.

- To prevent heartburn, do not eat large amounts of spicy, acidic (such as tomato products), or fried foods. If heartburn is a problem, sleep with your head elevated on pillows.

- Exercise regularly to help you stay healthy, improve your circulation, and reduce leg cramps.

- Try frequent bland snacks (like crackers) throughout the day. This helps avoid nausea by keeping your stomach full.

- Special pregnancy pillows and mattresses may help you sleep better. Or use regular pillows to support your body.

- Naps may help. The NSF poll found that 51% of pregnant or recently pregnant women reported at least one weekday nap; 60% reported at least one weekend nap.

- Talk to your doctor if insomnia persists.

Once her baby is born, a mother's sleep is frequently interrupted, particularly if she is nursing. Mothers who nurse and those with babies that wake frequently during the night should try to nap when their babies do. Sharing baby care to the extent possible, especially during the night, is important for the mother's health, safety, performance and vitality. After-birth blues (postpartum depression) may also be related to sleep problems. This is usually a temporary condition treatable with professional help.

Understanding Menopause

Menopausal symptoms vary from woman to woman. However, women report the most sleeping problems during menopause. Snoring, for example, has been found to be more common and severe in postmenopausal women.

When a woman approaches natural menopause, her ovaries gradually (over several years) decrease production of estrogen and progesterone. If a woman has her ovaries surgically removed (oophorectomy), periods end immediately, and menopausal symptoms become more severe.

Changing and decreasing levels of estrogen cause many menopausal symptoms including hot flashes, which are unexpected feelings of heat all over the body. They are usually accompanied by sweating. In the NSF poll, 36% of menopausal and post-menopausal women reported hot flashes during sleep. On average, they occurred three days per week and interfered with sleep five days per month. Hot flashes persist for an average of five years. While total sleep time may not suffer, sleep quality does. Hot flashes may interrupt sleep; frequent awakenings cause next-day fatigue.

Treatment with estrogen (Estrogen Replacement Therapy, ERT) or with estrogen and progesterone (Hormone Replacement Therapy, HRT) may relieve menopausal symptoms. The effects of HRT and ERT vary among women depending on the form taken (pill, patch, gel, cream or injection) and the number of years used. [Note: Taking HRT with estrogen and progesterone has also been associated with an increased risk of certain diseases, such as breast cancer, and may not be recommended. Talk to your doctor about HRT.]

Many other products target problems associated with menopause. These include nutritional products and medications such as calcium supplements, vitamin D, and bisphosphonates for the prevention or treatment of osteoporosis (thinning and weakening of the bones); estrogen creams and rings for vaginal dryness; and sleep-promoting drugs for insomnia. All forms of estrogen that enter the blood stream reduce hot flashes.

An alternative treatment for menopausal symptoms may come from soy products (tofu, soybeans, soy milk). They contain phytoestrogen, a plant hormone similar to estrogen.

A few small studies indicate that soy can help lessen hot flashes. Phytoestrogens are also available in over-the-counter nutritional supplements (ginseng, extract of red clover). These supplements are not regulated by the Food and Drug Administration (FDA); their proper doses, long-terms effects and risks are not yet known.

Deciding what, if any, product to use and, if so, for how long, are questions a woman should discuss with her doctor. The answer will depend on personal and family medical history.

Most Common Sleep Problems in Women

Nearly 40 million American men and women suffer from sleep disorders. However, sleep problems affect more women than men. New research exploring women's sleep experiences may lead to specially tailored treatments.

Insomnia

Insomnia is the most common sleep problem. Women are more likely than men to report insomnia. In fact, according to the NSF poll, 53% of women aged 30 to 60 experience difficulty sleeping often or always: 60% of women aged 30 to 39, 47% aged 40 to 49, and 50% aged 50 to 60. Yet only 41% of all the women surveyed think they've had insomnia in the past year. Fortunately, there are a number of approaches

109

to improving sleep, including those you can do yourself such as exercise, establishing regular bedtimes and wake times, dietary changes (less or no caffeine and alcohol), and improving your sleep environment.

If insomnia persists, and lifestyle, behavioral or diet changes do not help, a doctor may prescribe a sleep-promoting medication (hypnotic). In some instances, there may be an underlying and treatable cause, such as depression (women are twice as likely to report depression as men), stress, anxiety or pain. Doctors may prescribe antidepressants (for depression), anxiolytics (anti-anxiety drugs), pain medications, and/or hypnotic medications to improve sleep.

Sleep Apnea

An estimated 12 million plus Americans have sleep apnea including one in four women over 65. While apnea is more common in men, it increases in women after age 50. Sleep apnea is a serious sleep disorder that is characterized by snoring, interrupted breathing during sleep or excessive daytime sleepiness. Recent studies have also found that sleep apnea is associated with increased blood pressure, a risk for cardiovascular disease and stroke. If any of these symptoms appear, it is important to address them with your doctor. A number of effective treatment approaches are available.

Narcolepsy

Feeling sleepy during the day or at times you expect to be awake may indicate a need for more sleep or the presence of a serious but treatable disorder such as those already mentioned or narcolepsy, a chronic neurological disorder that affects approximately one in 2000 people. Narcolepsy symptoms frequently appear in teen years. In addition to excessive daytime sleepiness, people with narcolepsy have sudden sleep attacks (an overwhelming urge to sleep), suddenly lose muscle tone or strength (cataplexy), and may have disturbed nighttime sleep. Recent scientific breakthroughs have led to new understanding of the cause of this condition and new treatments have given doctors more ways to help manage its symptoms.

Nocturnal Sleep-Related Eating Disorder

Persons with nocturnal sleep-related eating disorder (NS-RED), an uncommon condition, eat food during the night while they appear asleep. Since parts of the brain that control memory are asleep, people with NS-RED cannot remember nighttime eating. One study indicates that over 66 percent of sufferers are women. NS-RED can occur during sleepwalking. It can be caused by medications (e.g., some drugs prescribed for depression or insomnia) or by sleep disorders (sleep apnea, restless legs syndrome) that cause awakenings and trigger sleep-eating.

Pain and Sleep

More women (58%) suffer from nighttime pain than men (48%), according to a 1996 NSF Gallup Poll. Pain conditions like migraine, tension headaches, chronic fatigue syndrome and fibromyalgia are all more common among women. Pain may make it harder to fall asleep or lead to nighttime or early morning awakenings. Relaxation techniques, biofeedback, cognitive therapy, and over-the-counter and prescription medications may help. Treatment may target the pain, the sleeping difficulty, or both.

Shift Work

Shift workers—about one in five Americans—work non-traditional hours (not the typical hours of 9 a.m. to 5 p.m.). Difficulty falling asleep is a common effect. However, female shift workers also suffer irregular menstrual cycles, difficulty getting pregnant, higher rates of miscarriages, premature births and low birth-weight babies more than regular day working women, according to several large studies. Changes in exposure to light and lost sleep caused by shift work may have biological or hormonal effects that are not yet entirely understood. Still, most shift-working women do have normal, healthy babies. Women shift workers should consult their doctors if experiencing menstrual difficulties, infertility, or pregnancy.

Travel and Sleep

When traveling to a different time zone, the body takes time to adjust. This causes the physical experience known as jet lag. Helpful tips include avoiding caffeine and alcohol, changing your sleep and wake time before your trip, (to gradually get closer to your new schedule), and exposing yourself to sunlight or bright light upon arrival (in accordance with your new wake up time) may help you overcome jet lag more quickly.

When to See a Doctor

Many sleep problems can be improved by changing your sleep habits, reducing stress, improving your diet, or exercising. If sleep problems persist, it is advised to seek professional help. Your doctor will determine the cause of your sleep problem and may refer you to a sleep disorders center. These centers are staffed with sleep specialists who will ask you questions about your sleep problems and may monitor your sleep overnight.

Section 10.2

Sleep Disorders

Excerpted from "Sleep Disorders," U.S. Department of Health and Human Services, National Women's Health Information Center (NWHIC), August 2002. Available online at http://www.4woman.gov; accessed July 2003.

How much sleep does a person need?

There is no hard and fast answer to this question. The amount of sleep a person needs depends on many things, including age. Most adults need at least 7 to 8 hours of sleep per night, although some people may need as many as 10 hours. Children and adolescents need about 9 hours of sleep, while young infants may need around 16 hours per day. Women in the first 3 months of pregnancy often need a few more hours of sleep than normal, and sleep quality is decreased. When people sleep too little over a period of a few days, they build up a sleep debt, like being overdrawn at a bank.

This debt needs to be repaid sooner or later. A person's body is not able to get used to less sleep than they need. Aging does not seem to change the amount of sleep a person needs, although older people tend to sleep more lightly and for shorter periods of time. About half of the people over 65 have frequent sleeping problems, such as insomnia, and deep sleep stages that are shortened or completely stopped. These changes in sleep may be a normal part of aging, or can be caused by medications or treatments for other health problems.

How can I tell if I have a sleep problem or a sleep disorder?

Because so many people burn the candle at both ends and have large sleep debts, sleep problems are common. Side effects from medications or treatments and stress and worry can also cause sleep problems. For women, hormone changes during pregnancy, menopause, and the menstrual cycle can cause sleep problems.

Sleep experts say that if you feel sleepy during the day, even when doing something boring, you haven't had enough sleep. If you usually fall asleep within 5 minutes of lying down, you probably have a severe sleep debt, maybe even a sleep disorder. Very short periods of sleep throughout the day (sometimes you may not even know that you are sleeping) are also another sign of a sleep disorder. Talk with your health care provider if you are having a problem with sleep or think that you may have a sleep disorder.

What can I do to get a good night's sleep?

Good sleep habits can help you get a good night's sleep. Here are some tips:

- Try to go to bed at the same time every night and get up at the same time every morning. Try not to take naps during the day because naps may make you less sleepy at night.

- Try to avoid caffeine, nicotine, and alcohol late in the day. Caffeine and nicotine are stimulants and can keep you from falling asleep.

- Alcohol can make you wake up later in the night.

- Get regular exercise. Try not to exercise close to bedtime because it may stimulate you and make it hard to fall asleep. Experts suggest not exercising for 3 hours before the time you go to sleep.

- Don't eat a big meal late in the day, although a light snack before bedtime may help you sleep.

- Make your sleeping place comfortable. Be sure that it is dark, quiet, and not too warm or too cold. If light is a problem, try a sleeping mask. If noise is a problem, try earplugs, a fan, or a white noise machine to cover up the sounds.

- Create a routine to help you relax and wind down before sleep, such as reading a book or taking a bath. Watching the news just

113

before bed may keep some people awake, especially if the news is upsetting.

- Try not to use your bed for anything other than sleeping and sex.

- If you can't fall asleep and don't feel sleepy, get up and do something else until you feel sleepy. Just make sure that you don't do anything stimulating.

- If you have trouble lying awake worrying about things, try making a to-do list before you go to bed. This may help you to let go of those worries overnight.

See your health care provider if you think you have a sleep problem or a sleep disorder.

Chapter 11

Smoking

Chapter Contents

Section 11.1

Smoking Is a Woman's Issue

U.S. Department of Health and Human Services, Office of Disease Prevention and Health Promotion, 2001. Available online at http://odphp. osophs.dhhs.gov/pubs/prevrpt/01summer/Summer2001PR.htm; accessed August 2003.

This year alone, lung cancer will kill nearly 68,000 U.S. women— far more deaths than from breast cancer. Many thousands more women will die prematurely from smoking-related diseases, such as heart and respiratory conditions.

Mortality statistics like these support the grim conclusion that smoking-related disease among women is a full-blown epidemic. Smoking is the leading known cause of preventable death and disease among women.

Recent studies have linked smoking or secondhand smoke in some way to breast cancer, depression, attention deficit/hyperactivity disorder, sudden infant death syndrome, infertility, and various respiratory diseases, especially asthma in certain racial and ethnic populations.

Women who smoke experience gender-specific health consequences, including increased risk of various adverse reproductive outcomes. Smoking during pregnancy has adverse health effects. Infants born to women exposed to secondhand tobacco smoke during pregnancy face risks, including decreased birth weight.

Section 11.2

Smoking and Pregnancy

Cigarette smoking during pregnancy can cause serious health problems to an unborn child. Smoking during pregnancy has been linked to premature labor, breathing problems and fatal illness among infants.

An estimated 440,000 Americans die each year from diseases caused by smoking. Smoking is responsible for an estimated one in five U.S. deaths and costs the U.S. at least $150 billion each year in health care costs and lost productivity.

- Smoking during pregnancy is estimated to account for 20 to 30 percent of low-birth weight babies, up to 14 percent of preterm deliveries, and some 10 percent of all infant deaths. The odds of developing asthma are twice as high among children whose mothers smoke more than 10 cigarettes a day. Between 400,000 and 1 million asthmatic children have their condition worsened by exposure to secondhand smoke.

- Maternal smoking during and after pregnancy has been linked to asthma among infants and young children.

- In 1999, 12.3 percent of mothers were reported to have smoked during pregnancy, a 30 percent decline from the 1990 level.

- Smokers inhale nicotine and carbon monoxide, which reach the baby through the placenta and prevent the fetus from getting the nutrients and oxygen needed to grow. Secondhand smoke also adds a risk to pregnancy. Breast milk often contains whatever is in the woman's body. If the woman smokes, the baby ingests the nicotine in her breast milk.

- Reducing frequency of smoking may not benefit the baby. A pregnant woman who reduces her smoking pattern or switches

117

to lower tar cigarettes may inhale more deeply or take more puffs to get the same amount of nicotine as before.

- The most effective way to protect the fetus is to quit smoking. If a woman plans to conceive a child in the near future, quitting is essential. A woman who quits within the first three or four months of pregnancy can lower the chances of her baby being born premature or with health problems related to smoking.

- Pregnancy is a great time for a woman to quit. No matter how long she has been smoking, her body benefits from her quitting because it lessens her chances of developing future tobacco-related health problems, such as lung and heart disease, and cancer.

Additional American Lung Association Resources

Call your local American Lung Association at 1-800-LUNG-USA (1-800-586-4872) to find out more about how to stop smoking for good. The Lung Association is offering a new way to stop smoking through its Freedom From Smoking® online smoking cessation clinic. The program is based on the Lung Association's Freedom From Smoking® program, which has already helped thousands of smokers quit smoking for good. The Freedom From Smoking® online smoking cessation clinic can be accessed day or night, seven days a week, on any schedule a smoker chooses.

Visit www.ffsonline.org and stop smoking today!

Section 11.3

Kicking the Smoking Habit

Excerpted from the National Institutes of Health, National Heart, Lung, and Blood Institute's brochure "The Healthy Heart Handbook for Women," NIH No. 03-2720. Revised February 2003. Available online at http://www.nhlbi.nih.gov; accessed August 2003.

The good news is that quitting smoking greatly reduces your risk of heart disease and other serious disorders. Just 1 year after you stop smoking, your heart disease risk will drop by more than half. Within several years, it will approach the heart disease risk of someone who has never smoked. No matter how long you have been smoking, quitting will lessen your chances of developing heart disease.

Getting Ready to Quit

- Get motivated. Take some time to think about all the benefits of being smoke free. Besides the health benefits of quitting, what else do you have to gain? Money saved from not buying cigarettes? Loved ones no longer exposed to secondhand smoke? A better appearance? No more standing outside in the cold or rain for a smoke? Write down all of the reasons you want to stop smoking.

- Sign on the dotted line. Write a brief contract that states your intention to stop smoking, your quitting date, and some ways you plan to reward yourself for becoming an ex-smoker. Have someone sign it with you.

- Line up support. Ask the person who cosigns your contract—or another friend or family member—to give you special support in your efforts to quit. Plan to get in touch with your support person regularly to share your progress and to get encouragement. If possible, quit with a friend or spouse.

Breaking the Habit

- Know yourself. To quit successfully, you need to know your personal smoking triggers. These are the situations and feelings

119

that usually bring on the urge to light up. Some common triggers are drinking coffee, having an alcoholic drink, talking on the phone, watching someone else smoke, and experiencing stress.

- Make a list of your own personal triggers. Especially during the first weeks after quitting, try to avoid as many triggers as you can.

- Find new habits. Replace your triggers with new activities that you don't associate with smoking. For example, if you have always had a cigarette with a cup of coffee, switch to tea for a while. If stress is a trigger for you, try a relaxation exercise such as deep breathing to calm yourself. (Take a slow, deep breath, count to five, and release it. Repeat 10 times.)

- Keep busy. Get involved in activities that require you to use your hands, such as needlework, jigsaw puzzles, or fix-up projects around your house or apartment. When you feel the urge to put something in your mouth, try some vegetable sticks, apple slices, or sugarless gum. Some people find it helpful to inhale on a straw or chew on a toothpick until the urge passes.

- Keep moving. Walk, garden, bike, or do some yoga stretches. Physical activity will make you feel better and help prevent weight gain.

- Know what to expect. During the first weeks after quitting, you may experience temporary withdrawal symptoms, such as headaches, irritability, tiredness, and trouble concentrating. While these feelings are not pleasant, it is important to know that they are signs that your body is recovering from smoking. Most symptoms end within 2 to 4 weeks.

- Ask for help. Several free or low-cost programs are available to help people stop smoking. They include programs offered by local chapters of the American Lung Association and the American Cancer Society. Other low-cost programs can be found through hospitals, health maintenance organizations (HMOs), workplaces, and community groups. Some programs offer special support groups for women.

- Be good to yourself. Get plenty of rest, drink lots of water, and eat three healthy meals each day. If you are not as productive or cheerful as usual during the first weeks after quitting, be gentle with yourself. Give yourself a chance to adjust to your new nonsmoking lifestyle. Congratulate yourself for making a major, positive change in your life.

Chapter 12

Women's Safety and Health Issues at Work

- Women currently comprise 46% of the 137 million workers in the United States, with their share of the labor force projected to reach 48% by 2008.

- In 1999, 75% (46 million) of employed women worked full-time, while 25% (16 million) worked part-time.

- In 1999, 3.7 million women held multiple jobs.

- Sixty percent of women age 16 and over were either employed or looking for work in 1999.

- Of employed women, 40% held technical, sales, and administrative support positions; 32% worked in managerial and professional specialties; and 17% worked in service occupations in 1999.

Musculoskeletal Disorders

Sprains and strains, carpal tunnel syndrome, tendonitis, and other musculoskeletal disorders account for more than half (52%) of the injuries and illnesses suffered by female workers, as compared to 45% for male workers.

Further research is needed to determine the factors that place women at greater risk for musculoskeletal disorders. Research will

Centers for Disease Control and Prevention, National Institute for Occupational Safety and Health, 2001. Available online at http://www.cdc.gov/niosh; accessed May 2003.

examine if physical differences between men and women, or differences in the jobs they hold, contribute to this increased risk for women.

NIOSH is conducting research on musculoskeletal disorders among women in the telecommunication, health care, service, and data entry industries. In a study relating to musculoskeletal disorders, NIOSH worked with the Internal Revenue Service (IRS) to examine interventions for reducing discomfort among IRS data transcribers—an occupation comprised primarily of female workers. They found that periodic rest breaks throughout the work shift reduced musculoskeletal discomfort, while allowing workers to maintain job performance.

Job Stress

Stress at work is a growing problem for all workers, including women. In one survey 60% of employed women cited stress as their number one problem at work. Furthermore, levels of stress-related illness are nearly twice as high for women as for men.

Many job conditions contribute to stress among women. Such job conditions include heavy workload demands; little control over work; role ambiguity and conflict; job insecurity; poor relationships with coworkers and supervisors; and work that is narrow, repetitive, and monotonous. Other factors, such as sexual harassment and work and family balance issues, may also be stressors for women in the workplace.

Job stress has been linked with cardiovascular disease, musculoskeletal disorders, depression, and burnout. NIOSH is conducting studies to identify workplace factors that are particularly stressful to women, and potential prevention measures.

Reproductive Hazards

Three-quarters of women of reproductive age are in the workforce. Over half of the children born in the United States are born to working mothers. NIOSH conducts both basic research and population-based studies to learn whether women may be at risk for reproductive health hazards related to their work environment.

The following are examples of NIOSH research on reproductive hazards: NIOSH found no association between video display terminals (VDTs) and miscarriages, low birth-weights in newborns, or preterm deliveries.

NIOSH is working with the Federal Aviation Administration (FAA) to determine if exposure to cosmic ionizing radiation or circadian rhythm disruption increases the risk for adverse reproductive outcomes among female flight attendants.

NIOSH and the University of Cincinnati are assessing the effects of jet fuel exposure on the reproductive health of female Air Force personnel.

Violence in the Workplace

Homicide: Homicide is the leading cause of injury death for women in the workplace. Homicide accounts for 40% of all workplace deaths among female workers. Workplace homicides are primarily robbery-related, and often occur in grocery/convenience stores, eating and drinking establishments, and gasoline service stations.

Over 25% of female victims of workplace homicide are assaulted by people they know (coworkers, customers, spouses, or friends). Domestic violence incidents that spill into the workplace account for 16% of female victims of job-related homicides.

Nonfatal Assault: Female workers are also at risk for nonfatal violence. Women were the victims in nearly two-thirds of the injuries resulting from workplace assaults. Most of these assaults (70%) were directed at women employed in service occupations, such as health care, while an additional 20% of these incidents occurred in retail locations, such as restaurants and grocery stores.

Women in Non-Traditional Employment

Women in non-traditional employment may face health and safety risks due to the equipment and clothing provided to them at their workplace. Personal protective equipment (PPE) and clothing (PPC) are often designed for average-sized men. The protective function of PPE/PPC (such as respirators, work gloves, and work boots) may be reduced when they do not fit female workers properly.

Women who work in nontraditional employment settings may also face specific types of stressors. For instance, they may be exposed to sexual harassment and gender-based discrimination.

Cancer

An estimated 180,000 new cases of breast cancer and 12,000 new cases of cervical cancer will be diagnosed in 2000. Workplace exposures to hazardous substances may play a role in the development of these types of cancer. NIOSH is studying several hazardous substances to determine whether there is a link to cancers that affect women, such as cervical and breast cancer.

Health Care Workers

Ninety-two percent of the 4.3 million nurses and nursing aides in the U.S. are female. In addition to being at risk for incidents of musculoskeletal disorders, workplace violence, and exposure to hazardous substances, health care workers face other hazards including latex allergy and needlestick injuries. NIOSH has established a new initiative to study the health and safety of health care workers.

Needlestick Injuries: Between 600,000-800,000 needlestick injuries occur annually in health care settings, mostly involving nurses. These injuries pose both physical and emotional threats to health care workers, as serious infections from bloodborne pathogens (such as hepatitis B virus, hepatitis C virus, and human immunodeficiency virus [HIV]) may result.

Latex Allergy: Health care workers may have an increased risk for developing latex allergy due to their use of latex gloves. Among health care workers who experience frequent latex exposure, 8-12% develop sensitivity to latex. Latex sensitivity may lead to symptoms of latex allergy, such as skin rashes; hives; nasal, eye, or sinus symptoms; asthma; and (rarely) shock.

Chapter 13

Factors Affecting the Health of Women of Color

Health Facts about Women of Color

- The acquisition of quality care and the resulting health outcomes for women of color are shaped by various sociocultural-economic factors. These include the physical and social environments (especially for American Indians/Alaska Natives, Latinos, and blacks), linguistic isolation (especially Asian Americans, Latinos, and Native Hawaiians or Other Pacific Islanders), and racism (especially blacks and Asian Americans).

- Although women of color generally have shorter life expectancies than white women, selected populations of Asian women (Japanese, Filipino, and Chinese in both Hawaii and California) and Hispanic women (in California and Puerto Rico) report the longest life expectancies among women, equaling or exceeding that of white women.

- American Indian/Alaska Native and black American women report the shortest life expectancies.

"Health Facts about Women of Color" from the National Institutes of Health, *Women of Color Health Data Book*, 2002. Available online at http://www.nih.gov; accessed August 2003. "Health Problems in African American Women," "Health Problems in Asian American/Pacific Islander and Native Hawaiian Women," and "Health Problems in Hispanic American/Latina Women" excerpted from the publications by the U.S. Department of Health and Human Services, National Women's Health Information Center (NWHIC), May 2003. Available online at http://www.4woman.gov; accessed August 2003.

- Despite declining death rates from heart disease over the past 50 years, diseases of the heart remain the major cause of death for all females, except Asian and Pacific Islander females, for whom they are the second major cause of death.

- In addition to heart disease, other prominent causes of death for women of color are: cancers (especially for blacks), diabetes mellitus (all women of color), cerebrovascular diseases (especially American Indians/Alaska Natives), unintentional injuries, and HIV/AIDS (especially black women).

- Obesity, a problem for many women of color, is related in part to sedentary lifestyles and diets of poverty (high in fat and low in fruits and vegetables) and contributes to the development of both diabetes and heart disease. American Indian, Native Hawaiian, American Samoan, and black women are the most likely to be overweight or obese.

- Cigarette smoking among black females of all ages has declined since the late 1980s, although smoking has increased slightly among younger Hispanic and Asian American women over this period. Between 1997 and 1999, American Indian/Alaska Native women (32 percent) reported the highest smoking rate, followed by black women (21 percent) and Latinas (13 percent).

- Most new cases of AIDS (acquired immunodeficiency syndrome) among women are reported among African American and Hispanic women. Eighty percent of the new cases reported among women in 2000 were among these two subpopulations that together constitute only 25 percent of all women.

- The incidence of low- and very-low-birthweight infants varies considerably by the race/ethnicity of the mothers of the infants. For example, in 1999, non-Hispanic black mothers were most likely to give birth to low-birthweight infants (13 percent of live births to these mothers), while Chinese mothers were least likely to do so (5 percent).

- Many women of color do not avail themselves of preventive health tests such as Pap smears and breast exams on a regular basis due to a variety of factors (availability of insurance coverage, accessibility of facilities, cultural beliefs, and lack of information). For example, one study found that two thirds of Asian immigrants in California had never had a Pap smear, and 70 percent had never had a mammogram.

- People of color were disproportionately represented among the nearly 43 million people without health insurance in 1999. Among the low-income people within each racial/ethnic group, the most likely to be uninsured were Hispanics (44 percent), Asians and Pacific Islanders (42 percent), and blacks (28 percent).

- Although the measured incidence of depression and other mental health problems varies by study and among subpopulations of women of color, a majority of Hispanic, African American, and Asian women in one study reported an unmet need for mental health care in the past year.

- Collecting data about women of color is problematic, with undercounting, failing to collect data for the subpopulations within each group, and misidentifying women of color being some of the major issues.

- A greater number of community-based medical facilities with culturally sensitive health care providers are needed to serve women of color.

Health Problems in African American Women

What health problems affect a lot of African American women?

- Overweight and Obesity: Fifty percent of adult African American women are obese.

- Diabetes: Overall, African Americans are twice as likely to have diabetes than Whites. Type 2 diabetes is becoming more common in African American children under 20 years old. African Americans experience higher rates of at least three of diabetes' most serious complications: eye disease, amputation and kidney failure.

- High Blood Pressure: The number of African Americans with high blood pressure is high: one out of three African Americans have it.

- Kidney Disease: Diabetes is the leading cause of kidney failure in African Americans. African Americans tend to have kidney failure at an earlier age than Whites.

- HIV/AIDS: HIV is the leading cause of death for African American women between the ages of 25 and 44.

- Lupus: It is more common in African American women and other minorities than in White women. The Centers for Disease Control and Prevention (CDC) reports that between 1979 and 1998, 70% more African American women (between 45 and 65 years old) died from systemic lupus erythematosus (SLE).

- Breast Cancer: Except for African Americans 20-24 years old, African American women are more likely than White women to get breast cancer before age 40. However, they are less likely than White women to get breast cancer after age 40. African American women are more likely than White women to die from breast cancer. Researchers are trying to find out why this happens. Some reasons may be that tumors are found at a later (more advanced) stage so there are less treatment options, or patients don't follow-up after getting abnormal test results. Other reasons might include being overweight or not being able to get a mammography.

- Other Cancers: New cases of certain cancers occur more often in African American women, including colorectal cancer, pancreatic cancer, and lung cancer. The death rate from colorectal cancer and pancreatic cancer is higher among African American women than other racial groups. Overall, African American women are more likely to die from cancer than persons of any other racial and ethnic group. There is not enough information to figure out why African Americans bear this cancer burden. Some reasons may be poor access to health care, poverty, tumors found at a later (more advanced) stage, different belief systems, fear of talking about cancer, and lack of trust of the medical system.

- Pregnancy-Related Death: African American women die in childbirth more frequently than other American women. They have a higher chance of having pregnancy-related high blood pressure (preeclampsia) and seizures from high blood pressure (eclampsia).

- Heart Disease: African American women are more likely to die from heart disease than other groups of women. In addition, studies have shown that African Americans don't receive the same care for heart disease as Whites because they don't receive the same procedures and treatments.

- Stroke: African Americans are twice as likely to die from a stroke or its complications than any other racial or ethnic group in the U.S.

- High Cholesterol: High cholesterol is a health problem for African American women. However, African American women have lower cholesterol levels than White women.

- Sexually Transmitted Diseases (STDs): Overall, African Americans have higher rates of STDs than Whites for chlamydia, gonorrhea, syphilis, herpes, and hepatitis B.

- Asthma: Asthma is a growing concern in this country, especially for African Americans. African Americans go into the hospital more than Whites because of asthma and are more likely to die from asthma.

- Uterine Fibroids: While no one knows for sure what will increase a woman's chances of getting fibroids, researchers have found that African American women are 2 to 3 times more likely to get them than women of other racial groups. African American women also tend to get fibroids at a younger age than do other women with fibroids.

- Sickle Cell Anemia: Every year, about 1 in 500 African Americans are born with sickle cell anemia. This means that they got the sickle gene from both parents. People who have only one gene are carriers of the sickle cell, but won't get sickle cell anemia themselves. They can pass the gene to their children. It is estimated that one in 12 African Americans have one sickle cell gene.

- Osteoporosis: While White and Asian women have the highest rates of osteoporosis, African American women are at risk as well. As African American women get older, their risk of developing osteoporosis more closely resembles the risk of White women. Lupus and sickle cell anemia, which are more common in African American women, increase the risk for osteoporosis.

- Tuberculosis (TB): Among all women with TB, 81% of TB cases affect minority women. African American women have the highest number of TB cases, compared to all other women.

- Infant Deaths: African American women have the highest number of infant deaths in the U.S.

Health Problems in Asian American/Pacific Islander and Native Hawaiian Women

What health problems affect a lot of Asian American/ Pacific Islander and Native Hawaiian women?

- Obesity and overweight: Being overweight is a problem for Pacific Islanders. Native Hawaiians and Samoans are among the most obese people in the world.

- Diabetes: Data on how many cases of diabetes are in the Asian American/Pacific Islander and Native Hawaiian population are limited. Some groups within these populations are at increased risk for diabetes. For example, data collected from 1996 to 2000 suggest that Native Hawaiians are 2.5 times more likely to have diagnosed diabetes than White residents of Hawaii of similar age. Guam's death rate from diabetes is five times higher than that of the U.S. mainland. And it is one of the leading causes of death in American Samoa. People with diabetes have a higher chance of having problems with their skin, mouth, kidneys, heart, nerves, eyes, and feet.

- Heart Disease: Heart disease is the main cause of death for American women. Overall, Asian/Pacific Islander and Native Hawaiian women have much lower rates of heart disease than women of other minority groups, but it is still the leading cause of death within their own group. Heart disease risk and death rates are higher among Native Hawaiians and some Asian Americans (Asian Indians) partly because of higher rates of obesity, diabetes, and high blood pressure.

- Stroke: Among Asian Americans/Pacific Islanders, the risk of stroke is higher at ages 35 to 64 than for Whites.

- High Cholesterol: Among Asian American/Pacific Islander women, high cholesterol rates are highest in Japanese women. Asian American/Pacific Islander women also have low cholesterol screening rates.

- High Blood Pressure: Among Asian American/Pacific Islander women, high blood pressure is more of a problem for Filipino women. And all Asian American/Pacific Islander women have much lower blood pressure screening rates than other minority women.

- Hepatitis B: Your risk of getting the virus is higher if you were born in Southeast Asia or the Pacific Islands. Compared to the U.S. average this disease is 25 to 75 times more common among Samoans and immigrants from Cambodia, Laos, Vietnam, and China.

- Tuberculosis: Among all women with TB, 81% of TB cases affect minority women. Of these cases, 26% are among Asian American/Pacific Islander women (second only to African American women, who make up 30% of TB cases among minority women).

- Cervical Cancer: New cases of cervical cancer among Vietnamese women are nearly 5 times those of White women. And, on average, Asian American/Pacific Islander women have much lower rates of Pap test screening than other groups.

- Breast Cancer: Breast cancer is less common in Asian American/Pacific Islander and Native Hawaiian women than it is in White or African American women. But, more Asian American/Pacific Islander and Native Hawaiian women have breast cancer than do women of Hispanic or American Indian/Alaska Native descent. Also, the number of Asian American/Pacific Islander women who have been diagnosed with breast cancer has increased. Chinese American and Japanese American women have higher rates of breast cancer than women of their same age in China and Japan. At first, it was believed a Western diet (higher in fat) could explain this difference, but this has not been proven. Among all other populations in the United States, Asian American/Pacific Islander women have the lowest death rate from breast cancer. But, among certain Pacific Islanders, death rates from breast cancer are much higher than among other ethnic groups. For example, Native Hawaiians have the highest death rate from breast cancer than for any racial/ethnic group in the Unites States. Breast cancer also is the leading cause of death among Filipino women. We do not know why the rates vary between these groups. But, among all ethnic groups in this country, Asian American/Pacific Islander and Native Hawaiian women are the least likely to have ever had a mammogram.

- Suicide: Asian American women have the highest suicide rate among women 65 or older. And suicide rates are higher than the national average for Native Hawaiians. One possible reason for the higher rate of suicide among Asian American/Pacific Islander and Native Hawaiian women is that seeking mental health support is not socially acceptable in those cultures. And many of them wait to seek treatment until symptoms of mental health problems, such as depression, reach crisis levels. Nearly one out of two Asian American/Pacific Islanders will have problems using mental health treatment because they do not speak English or cannot find services that meet their language needs.

• Osteoporosis: While all women are at risk for getting osteoporosis, Asian American women have a higher risk because of their lower bone mass and density and smaller body frames. They also have a lower intake of calcium compared to other groups of women. As many as 90% of Asian Americans are lactose intolerant or cannot easily digest dairy products.

Health Problems in Hispanic American/Latina Women

What health problems affect a lot of Hispanic American/ Latina women?

• Obesity and overweight: Obesity is 1.5 times more common in Mexican American women (reaching 52%) than in the general, female population.

• Diabetes: Diabetes, including gestational diabetes that occurs during pregnancy, is more common in Hispanic American/ Latinos than in Whites. Mexican Americans, the largest Hispanic/ Latino subgroup, are two times more likely to have diabetes than Whites. Also, residents of Puerto Rico are two times more likely to have diagnosed diabetes than U.S. Whites. Within the Hispanic American/Latino population, diabetes is more prevalent in women than it is in men. Hispanic Americans/Latinos have a 2 times higher rate of retinopathy (eye disease) and kidney disease (including end-stage kidney failure). And Hispanic American/Latina women with diabetes are 7.6 times more likely to develop peripheral vascular disease (problems with blood flow in the veins) than non-diabetic women, and three to four times more likely to have heart disease or a stroke. Mexican American women, especially when they are overweight, have higher rates of gestational diabetes than non Hispanic White women.

- High Cholesterol: Among Mexican American women ages 20 to 74, almost half have borderline-high risk total cholesterol levels. Low-density lipoprotein (LDL) or bad cholesterol levels of 130 mg/dL or higher are related to a higher risk of coronary heart disease. And 41.6% of Mexican American women have an LDL cholesterol level in that range.

- Heart Disease: Heart disease risk and death rates are higher among Mexican Americans partly because of higher rates of obesity and diabetes.

- Stroke: Among Hispanic Americans/Latinos, the risk of stroke is 1.3 times higher at ages 35 to 64 than for non-Hispanics.

- HIV/AIDS: Even though males account for the largest proportion (81%) of AIDS cases reported among Hispanic Americans/ Latinos in the United States, the number of cases among females is rising. Females represent 19% of all AIDS cases among Hispanic Americans/Latinos, but account for 23% of cases reported in 2000 alone. And the rate of HIV infection is seven times higher in Hispanic American/Latina women than in White women. For the largest proportion (47%) of adult and adolescent Hispanic American/Latina women with AIDS, heterosexual contact (mostly with injection drug users) is the cause for their disease. Injection drug use accounts for an additional 40% of AIDS cases among Hispanic American/Latina women.

- Depression: The rate of depression in Hispanic American/Latina women remains about twice that of men. And major depression (also known as clinical depression, in which symptoms last for at least 2 weeks but usually for several months or longer) and dysthymia (a type of depression that lasts for at least two years) may be diagnosed slightly more frequently in Hispanic American/Latino women than in White women. Possible differences in how symptoms appear may affect the way depression is recognized and diagnosed among minorities. For example, African Americans are more likely than Hispanics to report symptoms of depression that affect their whole body, such as appetite change and body aches and pains.

- Other Cancers: Hispanic Americans/Latinos have a lower rate of new cancer cases and lower death rates for all cancers combined, but a higher burden of cancers of the stomach, liver, and cervix than Whites. There are gaps in access to and use of cancer screening programs among Hispanic Americans/Latinos. Death rates from cancers of the breast and cervix, all of which can be found early by screening, decreased less among Hispanic Americans/Latinas than among non-Hispanics.

- Breast Cancer: Breast cancer is the most commonly diagnosed cancer and the leading cause of cancer death among Hispanic American/Latina women. Although breast cancer is diagnosed about 30% less often among women of Hispanic origin, it is more often diagnosed at a later stage (when the disease is more advanced) than when found in non-Hispanic women, even when access to health care is adequate. Lower rates of using screening tests like mammography among Hispanic American/Latina women is thought to add to this later diagnosis.

- Cervical Cancer: Study results show that the number of new cases of invasive cervical cancer among Hispanic American/Latina women (age 30 years and older) is about twice that for non Hispanic women. But Hispanic American/Latina women in the Southwest and Midwest have similar rates to non-Hispanics. Overall, the death rate from cervical cancer is 40% higher among Hispanic American/Latina women than non-Hispanic women. Although invasive cervical cancer can be prevented by regular screening, Hispanic American/Latina women have a low rate of Pap testing.

- Smoking and Lung Cancer: Lung cancer is the second cause of cancer deaths among Hispanic American/Latina women (behind breast cancer). And the death rates for lung cancer in these women have increased every year. Among Hispanic American/Latino high school students, 31.5% of females smoke cigarettes.

- Illicit Drug Use: Illicit drugs are illegal drugs, like heroin, marijuana, ecstasy, cocaine, PCP, and LSD. Subgroups of Hispanic Americans/Latinos vary in their rates of substance abuse, alcohol dependence, and need for illicit drug abuse treatment. But overall, compared to the total U.S. population, Mexicans and Puerto Ricans have high rates of illicit drug use, heavy alcohol use, alcohol dependence, and need for drug abuse treatment.

Chapter 14

Women with Disabilities

Chapter Contents

Section 14.1

Special Health Issues for Women with Disabilities

"Special Summary of Health Care Needs of Women with Disabilities." Excerpted with permission from: Nosek MA, Howland CA, Rintala DH, Young ME, and Chanpong GF. National Study of Women with Physical Disabilities: Final Report. Houston: Center for Research on Women with Disabilities, 1997. © Baylor College of Medicine. Despite the date of this document, the topics addressed will still be of interest to women with disabilities.

In 1992, the Center for Research on Women with Disabilities was awarded a three-year grant by the National Center for Medical Rehabilitation Research within the National Institutes of Health to examine and conduct research on issues of concern to women with disabilities and disseminate the findings nationally.

Our study examined a broad range of issues facing women with physical disabilities. It consisted of two phases. Phase I was a qualitative interview study of 31 women with physical disabilities which helped us understand all the various aspects of sexuality from the point of view of the woman with a disability. The themes were identified in these interviews fell into six basic domains: 1) sense of self, 2) relationship issues, 3) information about sexuality, 4) sexual functioning, 5) abuse, and 6) general and reproductive health. With the assistance of national and local advisors, including consumers, researchers, medical professionals, social workers, and educators, the research team developed a questionnaire that represented all the primary themes from the qualitative study and issues raised in the literature. In Phase II, we identified 1,150 women with physical disabilities around the country who volunteered to participate in the study or who were recruited through independent living centers in each federal region. We sent each of them two copies of this questionnaire, one for her to complete and one for her to give to an able-bodied female friend to complete. We received responses from 45% of this sample or a total of 946 women, 504 of whom had physical disabilities and 442 who did not have disabilities.

We collected an enormous volume of information in this study. The survey included 311 questions with more than a thousand variables, yielding more than a million bits of data. For the last few years, we've been analyzing these data in each of the six domains we identified early in the study. Thanks to supplemental funding through the Centers for Disease Control and Prevention, we were able to spend an additional year conducting further analysis of our data on health issues for women with physical disabilities.

The findings of this study will, we hope, lay the foundation for further research on issues of concern to women with disabilities, and empower advocates to press for change in service systems so that they can more effectively assist women with disabilities to achieve independence, equality, and quality of life.

Women with disabilities have limited opportunities to establish romantic relationships.

- Compared to women without disabilities, women with disabilities were less satisfied with how often they date and perceived more constraints on attracting dating partners.

- Even when women with disabilities were outgoing with strong social skills and many friends, their friendships were less likely to evolve into romantic relationships than for able-bodied women.

- The large majority (87%) of the women with disabilities had had at least one serious romantic relationship or marriage. Fifty-two percent were involved in a serious relationship at the time of the study versus 64% of the women without disabilities.

- Among the women with disabilities who were not married or in a serious relationship at the time of the study, 42% said it was because no one had asked them. Only 27% of women without disabilities listed that as a reason for not being in a relationship.

- More than half of the women with disabilities believed that disability was not a major cause of the ending of a marriage or other serious relationship.

- Only 38% of the women with disabilities in this sample had borne children compared to 51% of women without disabilities.

- Women with disabilities were significantly more likely than those without disabilities to stay in a bad marriage for fear of losing custody of their children.

Self-esteem in women with physical disabilities is more strongly influenced by social and environmental factors than by the fact of having a disability.

- More than three-quarters of the women with disabilities had high self-esteem and a positive body image. Whether the woman had a severe disability or a mild disability, incurred disability earlier or later in life, or had ever been in special education didn't make much difference in self-esteem.

- Women who were working, who were in a serious romantic relationship, or who had never experienced physical or sexual abuse reported high self-esteem, whether or not they had a disability. Among women who were not working, not in a serious romantic relationship, or who had experienced physical or sexual abuse, the women with disabilities had much lower self-esteem than the women without disabilities.

- Abuse is a very serious problem for women with disabilities. They have even fewer options for escaping or resolving the abuse than women in general.

- The same percentage (62%) of women with and without disabilities had experienced emotional, physical, or sexual abuse, but women with disabilities experienced abuse for longer periods of time.

- In addition to the types of abuse experienced by all women, women with disabilities were sometimes abused by withholding needed orthotic equipment (wheelchairs, braces), medications, transportation, or essential assistance with personal tasks, such as dressing or getting out of bed.

- Women with disabilities face serious barriers to accessing existing programs to help women remove violence from their lives.

Women with physical disabilities have as much sexual desire as women in general; however, they do not have as much opportunity for sexual activity.

- Ninety-four percent of women with disabilities had had sexual activity with a partner in their lifetime. Forty-nine percent were sexually active at the time of the study, compared to 61% of women without disabilities.

- Forty-nine percent of the women with disabilities believed that they did not have adequate information about how their disability affects their sexual functioning.

- Women with disabilities reported significantly lower levels of sexual activity, sexual response, and satisfaction with their sex lives.

- Level of sexual activity was not significantly related to severity of disability.

Women with physical disabilities encounter serious barriers to receiving general and reproductive health care.

- Thirty-one percent of the women with physical disabilities who participated in this study were refused care by physicians because of their disability.

- Women with physical disabilities reported considerable difficulty locating physicians who were knowledgeable about their disability to help them manage their pregnancy.

- More women with physical disabilities reported chronic urinary tract infections, heart disease, depression, and osteoporosis, at younger ages than the comparison group of women without disabilities.

- There was a much higher rate of use of public health clinics, specialists, and emergency departments among women with disabilities compared to women without disabilities.

Section 14.2

Health Care Utilization among Women with Disabilities

"Health Care Utilization." Excerpted with permission from: Nosek MA, Howland CA, Rintala DH, Young ME, and Chanpong GF. National Study of Women with Physical Disabilities: Final Report. Houston: Center for Research on Women with Disabilities, 1997. © Baylor College of Medicine. Despite the date of this document, the topics addressed will still be of interest to women with disabilities.

According to the literature, women and persons with disabilities consume a larger share of health care services than the general population. We wanted to know more about the experience of women with disabilities in accessing health care services. In the interviews that began this study, we found our participants very eager to talk about these experiences; indeed, many used the opportunity to vent some very long held frustrations and deep negative feelings.

They complained bitterly about inaccessibility in health care settings, lack of knowledge among health care providers about their disability, and a perception that they were not getting the same quality of health care, particularly reproductive health care, as women in general. In the national survey, we focused our questions on the types of health care providers used within the past year, as well as the types of health care facilities used. We analyzed differences in utilization patterns between women with and without disabilities.

We also asked some general questions about how well their physicians were able to deal with their disability as it might affect an ordinary health problem.

Results

Women with physical disabilities who participated in this study were more likely to have used every major category of health care provider within the past 12 months than women without disabilities. Significantly more women with disabilities had seen general practitioners, rehabilitation specialists, obstetricians/gynecologists, and other specialists.

Ninety-one percent of women with disabilities had seen specialists of some type within the past year. Women with disabilities who lived alone were five times more likely to see specialists during the past year. Women who worked full- or part-time were less likely to see specialists. There was a slight trend for women with lower levels of functional impairment and women who work to be less likely to see specialists.

Age, household income, duration of disability, self-esteem, perceived control of life, urban or rural residence, or education level did not increase the odds of seeing specialists. It is interesting to note that 24% of women with disabilities and 20% of women without disabilities used alternative health care providers, such as curanderos, homeopathists, and acupuncturists.

Women with physical disabilities were also more likely to have used every major category of health care facility within the past 12 months than women without disabilities. Significantly more women with disabilities used public health clinics, rehabilitation hospitals, and emergency rooms. We were curious about the high rate of emergency room use, and tried to identify factors that were associated with it. Various disability and socioeconomic factors did not seem to be related; however, we found that women who perceived more control over their lives were less likely to use emergency rooms. Although more women with disabilities (54%) reported seeing private physicians than women without disabilities (45%), this difference was not significant.

Five items in the national survey asked specifically about the ability of health care providers and facilities to accommodate disability-related needs. These items were grounded in statements made by women with disabilities who participated in the qualitative interviews that preceded the national survey. Thirty-nine percent reported that their physicians do not speak directly to them if a family member or other person accompanies them. Thirty-one percent have had a physician refuse to see them because of their disability. Twenty-six percent believed their physicians were not well-informed about how their disability affects their reproductive health. Thirty-six percent had difficulty finding a physician who was willing or able to manage their pregnancy. More than half of women with spinal cord injury had this problem. Fifty-six percent reported that the hospital could not accommodate their disability-related needs when they gave birth.

Conclusion

Serious barriers exist that reduce the quality of health care available to women with physical disabilities. Architectural barriers in physicians' offices and hospitals still exist, despite the requirements of the Americans with Disabilities Act. There are invisible barriers as well, such as policies that deny service to women who cannot independently mount an examination table, and the refusal of physicians to see women solely on the basis of their disability, also in violation of the Americans with Disabilities Act. Advocacy is needed to inform persons in charge of medical facilities and clinical practices about their obligation to comply with legal requirements for physical and policy accessibility.

Our finding that women with disabilities make significantly greater use of services from specialists and emergency rooms has strong implications. With the advent of managed care, there are more stringent regulations on the use of specialists. For women whose health depends on timely access to physicians who have the specialized knowledge they need, these regulations could seriously affect their ability to maintain good health and prevent minor conditions from escalating into major ones that require more involved and more expensive treatment. Many of the complications of immobility and disability-related diagnoses are not taught in primary care training programs. A specialist may be the most appropriate primary care provider for some women with disabilities.

This may also be an insight into the disproportionately high use of emergency rooms we found among women with disabilities. The many barriers to accessing health care, both within medical systems and in the community (such as lack of accessible transportation and attendant services) contribute to delayed treatment. When knowledgeable providers are not available or when systems barriers prevent them from delivering services in a timely manner, otherwise controllable health problems become ones that can only be handled in an emergency room. When we see the use of emergency room services declining, we will know that health care systems have made progress in removing some of these barriers to quality health care service.

Part Two

Gynecological Concerns

Chapter 15

Menstruation and the Menstrual Cycle

Menstruation is a woman's monthly bleeding. It is also called menses, menstrual period, or period. When a woman has her period, she is menstruating. The menstrual blood is partly blood and partly tissue from the inside of the uterus (womb). It flows from the uterus through the small opening in the cervix, and passes out of the body through the vagina. Most menstrual periods last from three to five days.

What is the menstrual cycle?

Menstruation is part of the menstrual cycle, which helps a woman's body prepare for the possibility of pregnancy each month. A cycle starts on the first day of a period. The average menstrual cycle is 28 days long. However, a cycle can range anywhere from 23 days to 35 days.

The parts of the body involved in the menstrual cycle include the brain, pituitary gland, uterus and cervix, ovaries, fallopian tubes, and vagina. Body chemicals called hormones rise and fall during the month and make the menstrual cycle happen. The ovaries make two important female hormones, estrogen and progesterone. Other hormones involved in the menstrual cycle include follicle-stimulating

Excerpted from "Menstruation and the Menstrual Cycle," U.S. Department of Health and Human Services, National Women's Health Information Center (NWHIC), November 2002. Available online at http://www.4woman.gov; accessed July 2003.

hormone (FSH) and luteinizing hormone (LH), made by the pituitary gland.

What happens during the menstrual cycle?

In the first half of the menstrual cycle, levels of estrogen rise and make the lining of the uterus grow and thicken. In response to follicle-stimulating hormone, an egg (ovum) in one of the ovaries starts to mature. At about day 14 of a typical 28-day cycle, in response to a surge of luteinizing hormone, the egg leaves the ovary. This is called ovulation.

In the second half of the menstrual cycle, the egg begins to travel through the fallopian tube to the uterus. Progesterone levels rise and help prepare the uterine lining for pregnancy. If the egg becomes fertilized by a sperm cell and attaches itself to the uterine wall, the woman becomes pregnant. If the egg is not fertilized, it either dissolves or is absorbed into the body. If pregnancy does not occur, estrogen and progesterone levels drop, and the thickened lining of the uterus is shed during the menstrual period.

What is a typical menstrual period like?

During the menstrual period, the thickened uterine lining and extra blood are shed through the vaginal canal. A woman's period may not be the same every month, and it may not be the same as other women's periods. Periods can be light, moderate, or heavy, and the length of the period also varies. While most menstrual periods last from three to five days, anywhere from two to seven days is considered normal. For the first few years after menstruation begins, periods may be very irregular. They may also become irregular in women approaching menopause. Sometimes birth control pills are prescribed to help with irregular periods or other problems with the menstrual cycle.

Sanitary pads or tampons, which are made of cotton or another absorbent material, are worn to absorb the blood flow. Sanitary pads are placed inside the panties; tampons are inserted into the vagina.

At what age does a girl get her first period?

Menarche is another name for the beginning of menstruation. In the United States, the average age a girl starts menstruating is 12. However, this does not mean that all girls start at the same age. A girl can begin menstruating anytime between the ages of 8 and 16.

Menstruation will not occur until all parts of a girl's reproductive system have matured and are working together.

How long does a woman have periods?

Women usually continue having periods until menopause. Menopause occurs around the age of 51, on average. Menopause means that a woman is no longer ovulating (producing eggs) and therefore can no longer become pregnant. Like menstruation, menopause can vary from woman to woman and may take several years to occur. Some women have early menopause because of surgery or other treatment, illness, or other reasons.

When should I see a health care provider about my period?

You should consult your health care provider for the following:

- If you have not started menstruating by the age of 16.
- If your period has suddenly stopped.
- If you are bleeding for more days than usual.
- If you are bleeding excessively.
- If you suddenly feel sick after using tampons.
- If you bleed between periods (more than just a few drops).
- If you have severe pain during your period.

Chapter 16

Menstrual Hygiene Products

Having a menstrual period is a normal and regular event in a woman's life. The average woman will have menstrual periods from about ages 12 to 51. However, many women do not like talking about products they use while having their periods.

This chapter explains the types of menstrual hygiene products available. It may help you select the products that are best for you.

Sanitary Pads

Types of Pads

Pads are worn inside your underwear to collect menstrual flow. They come in different sizes, thicknesses, and styles. The choice is based on your comfort and the amount of your flow.

Regular maxi. Regular maxi pads are the traditional rectangular-shaped sanitary pads. They are about a half-inch thick. You should choose a maxi pad for medium- to heavy-flow days.

Thin maxi. Thin maxi pads are not as thick as regular maxi pads. Thin maxi pads are for lighter-flow days. Ultra thin maxi pads are also available.

American College of Obstetricians and Gynecologists. *Menstrual Hygiene Products.* (Patient Education Pamphlet No. AP116). Washington, DC. © ACOG 1997. Reviewed by David A. Cooke, M.D. on June 30, 2003.

Long. Long or super pads are 1 to 4 inches longer than regular maxi pads. Long pads are often used for extra protection during the night or for heavy-flow days.

Options

Some pads have tabs that wrap around and attach to the underside of your underwear with an adhesive. This feature is called wings.

Winged pads are usually the same size as regular pads. Deodorant pads are also available. These pads contain perfume. Some women notice that the perfume irritates the skin. If you are concerned about the smell of menstrual blood, you can control any smell by changing the pad often.

Things to Consider

Absorbency and a comfortable fit are the main features women look for when buying menstrual products. Because the amount of menstrual flow is not the same every day, to find the best absorbency you may want to use several different types of pads during your period.

Panty Liners

Panty liners or panty shields are shorter and thinner than maxi pads. They are made to use on light-flow days or along with tampons. Women sometimes wear panty liners to collect everyday (nonmenstrual) vaginal secretions. This shouldn't be necessary. Some vaginal discharge is normal. Cotton underwear will help absorb these normal secretions.

Tampons

Types of Tampons

Unlike pads, tampons include a rating on the package for their absorbency. The absorbency of the tampon you use should vary based on the amount of your flow. For heavy-flow days, you may need super or super plus. As your menstrual flow gets lighter, you may want to use regular or junior tampons or sanitary pads.

You can tell how absorbent a tampon is by how often you need to change it. You should need to change a tampon after four to six hours of use.

Tampons come with a variety of applicators. The basic choices are plastic with a covered tip, cardboard with an exposed tip, and cardboard with a covered tip.

Things to Consider

A tampon is comfortable to wear—once inserted, you shouldn't feel it. If you can feel the tampon in place, it may be too long or be placed improperly.

Tampons are a good choice for active women. They can be worn while swimming and don't interfere with physical exercise.

Tampons should be inserted carefully to avoid irritation.

Tampons may be more difficult to remove on light-flow days because they absorb vaginal secretions along with menstrual fluid.

A rare, but serious, condition called toxic shock syndrome (TSS) can be related to tampon use. The risk of TSS increases with higher-absorbency tampons. To lower your risk of TSS, choose a tampon with the lowest absorbency to meet your needs.

Menstruation is a normal, healthy process. Practicing good hygiene is as important during menstruation as it is at any other time of the month. The wide variety of menstrual products available makes it easier to ensure menstruation doesn't affect your daily activities.

Chapter 17

Tampon Safety and Toxic Shock Syndrome

According to the grapevine in 12-year-old Jerri's North Carolina school, tampons not only cause AIDS, but also can be lost in a woman's body, never to be seen again.

If you're hooked into the Internet, you may notice that tampon tales such as these get more creative as they're passed around. The latest stories claim tampons are tainted with cancer-causing toxins and that rayon tampons are especially dangerous. Another Internet rumor suggests that manufacturers add asbestos to tampons to promote excessive bleeding and boost sales.

"It can be hard to tell what stuff is true," says Jerri.

The truth is that tampons can't get lost forever in a woman's body. Rayon tampons are as safe as cotton ones. And asbestos has never had anything to do with fibers that make up tampons.

"The only way asbestos could be connected to tampons would be through tampering," says Mel Stratmeyer, Ph.D., chief of the Food and Drug Administration's health sciences branch. "And we haven't received any reports of such tampering."

FDA regulates tampons as medical devices, and "we ensure that tampon design and materials are safe through a solid, scientifically valid premarket review process," says Colin Pollard, chief of FDA's obstetrics and gynecology devices branch. Tampon manufacturers

---

Excerpted from "Tampon Safety: TSS Now Rare, but Women Still Should Take Care," U.S. Food and Drug Administration, *FDA Consumer*, March-April 2000. By Michelle Meadows.

153

conduct a battery of safety studies, and tampons must pass through FDA review and clearance before they can be marketed.

FDA also regulates the absorbency ratings for tampons. While high levels of absorbency were initially linked to an infection called toxic shock syndrome (TSS), FDA recently proposed a rule to provide an absorbency term for 15- to 18-gram tampons (ultra absorbency) that may help women manage heavier menstrual flows.

"Tampons with this absorbency are available in other countries with very low rates of toxic shock syndrome," explains Kimber Richter, M.D., deputy director of FDA's office of device evaluation. TSS is the only disease with a proven association to tampon use, according to FDA and the national Centers for Disease Control and Prevention.

Tampons and TSS

Any fear still surrounding tampon use likely dates from a time when TSS was first identified. About half of all cases occur in women using tampons, although the exact link between TSS and tampons remains unclear.

Tampons enjoyed a quiet history from 1933—when the first ones hit the market—until about 1980. That's when CDC noticed a sharp rise in the number of cases of TSS, a serious and sometimes fatal disease caused by toxin-producing strains of the *Staphylococcus aureus* bacterium. Experts believe the bacterium releases one or more toxins into the bloodstream.

Between October 1979 and May 1980, 55 TSS cases and seven deaths were reported. Most were among women who experienced onset of illness within a week following their periods. The TSS epidemic reached its peak in 1980 with a total of 813 cases of menstrual-related TSS, including 38 deaths, according to CDC. CDC carried out national and state-based studies to pinpoint TSS risk factors and used its national surveillance system to track trends. Research suggested one factor was the use of very highly absorbent tampons made from new materials.

Studies showed that women who used Proctor & Gamble's Rely tampons were at substantially greater risk for TSS than other tampon users. This brand consisted of polyester foam and a special type of highly absorbent cellulose, a combination no longer used in tampons. "TSS was not limited to Rely, but it did play a major role," says Pollard. Proctor & Gamble voluntarily withdrew that tampon from the market in 1980, and competing manufacturers of tampons made from other superabsorbent materials began removing them as well.

TSS Cases Drop Dramatically

Compared with the 813 menstrual TSS cases in 1980, there were only three confirmed cases in 1998 and six in 1997. "Although there is some underreporting of cases, this is a real decline," says Rana Hajjeh, M.D., a medical epidemiologist with CDC's division of bacterial and mycotic diseases. She attributes the drop in TSS rates to the removal of Rely from the market and advances in the way FDA regulates tampon materials and absorbency. Women also are much better educated about TSS prevention, she says.

Today, tampon manufacturers in this country produce tampons made of rayon, cotton, or a blend of the two. Cotton is commonly referred to as natural, while rayon is considered synthetic. But consumers shouldn't assume that synthetic means bad and natural means safer, says Jay Gooch, Ph.D., a toxicologist and senior scientist at Proctor & Gamble. Rayon is made from cellulose fibers derived from wood pulp. "Technically speaking, rayon is synthetic, but it's more like natural cellulose than it is different," Gooch says. "There is a lot of confusion out there about what rayon is and a lot of unsupported allegations about the safety of the two fibers." Previous CDC studies have found no increased risk with rayon versus cotton for the same absorbency and brand of tampon.

TSS Warning Signs

Symptoms of toxic shock syndrome can be hard to recognize because they mimic the flu. If you experience sudden high fever, vomiting, diarrhea, dizziness, fainting, or a rash that looks like a sunburn during your period or a few days after, contact your doctor right away. Also, if you're wearing a tampon, remove it immediately. One or two weeks after initial symptoms begin, flaking and peeling of the skin occurs, mainly on the palms and soles. If your doctor determines that your symptoms are TSS, you will probably be sent to a hospital for treatment. With proper treatment, patients usually get well in two to three weeks.

Women under 30, especially teenagers, are at a higher risk for TSS, because some females that age may not yet have antibodies to the toxin. Using any kind of tampon—cotton or rayon of any absorbency— puts a woman at greater risk for TSS than using menstrual pads.

Tips to Avoid Tampon Trouble

The strategy had worked for years, says Tracy, 28. She always inserted a small tampon on the morning she expected her period. But a few years ago, her period started one day late. "By the time it came, I had forgotten about the first tampon," she says. "The bleeding was so heavy that I figured I must not have had one in. So I put another one in."

All day she changed her tampon every few hours like she normally does. Then on one trip to the bathroom that night, she noticed a second string. When she finally removed the first tampon, the mild cramps she had experienced all day worsened. The pain became so intense she couldn't walk. Severe cramps and heavy bleeding ultimately landed her in the emergency room.

Putting in a tampon and forgetting about it is rare, but it does happen, says Gerald Joseph, M.D., former chairman of the department of obstetrics and gynecology at the Ochsner Medical Foundation. Joseph says he sees such cases—mostly among women under 30—a few times each year. Joanne, 44, says she forgot once and didn't realize the tampon was still there until six days later when she went to her doctor complaining of foul odor and vaginal discharge.

FDA recommends the following tips to help avoid tampon problems:

• Follow package directions for insertion.

• Choose the lowest absorbency for your flow.

• Change your tampon at least every 4 to 8 hours.

• Consider alternating pads with tampons.

• Know the warning signs of toxic shock syndrome.

• Don't use tampons between periods.

Michelle Meadows is a writer in Laurel, Maryland.

Chapter 18

Premenstrual Syndrome

What is premenstrual syndrome (PMS)?

Premenstrual syndrome (PMS) is a group of symptoms related to the menstrual cycle. PMS symptoms occur in the week or two weeks before your period (menstruation or monthly bleeding). The symptoms usually go away after your period starts. PMS may interfere with your normal activities at home, school, or work. Menopause, when monthly periods stop, brings an end to PMS.

The causes of PMS are not yet clear. Some women may be more sensitive than others to changing hormone levels during the menstrual cycle. Stress does not seem to cause PMS, but may make it worse. PMS can affect menstruating women of any age.

PMS often includes both physical and emotional symptoms. Diagnosis of PMS is usually based on your symptoms, when they occur, and how much they affect your life.

What are the symptoms of PMS?

PMS often includes both physical and emotional symptoms. Common symptoms are: breast swelling and tenderness; fatigue and trouble sleeping; upset stomach, bloating, constipation, or diarrhea; headache; appetite changes or food cravings; joint or muscle pain;

Excerpted from "Premenstrual Syndrome," U.S. Department of Health and Human Services, National Women's Health Information Center (NWHIC), July 2002. Available online at http://www.4woman.gov; accessed July 2003.

tension, irritability, mood swings, or crying spells; anxiety or depression; and trouble concentrating or remembering.

Symptoms vary from one woman to another. If you think you have PMS, try keeping track of your symptoms for several menstrual cycles. You can use a calendar to note which symptoms you are having on which days of your cycle, and how bad the symptoms are. If you seek medical care for your PMS, having this kind of record is helpful.

How common is PMS?

Estimates of the percentage of women affected by PMS vary widely. According to the American College of Obstetricians and Gynecologists, up to 40 percent of menstruating women report some symptoms of PMS. Most of these women have symptoms that are fairly mild and do not need treatment. Some women (perhaps five to ten percent of menstruating women) have a more severe form of PMS.

What treatment is available for PMS?

A combination of lifestyle changes and other treatment may be needed. If your PMS is not so bad that you need medical help, a healthier lifestyle may help you feel better and cope with symptoms.

- Adopt a healthier way of life. Exercise regularly, get enough sleep, choose healthy foods, don't smoke, and find ways to manage stress in your life.

- Try avoiding excess salt, sugary foods, caffeine, and alcohol, especially when you are having PMS symptoms.

- Be sure that you are getting enough vitamins and minerals. Take a multivitamin every day that includes 400 micrograms of folic acid. A calcium supplement with vitamin D can help keep bones strong and may help with PMS symptoms.

- In more severe cases, drugs such as diuretics, ibuprofen, birth control pills, or antidepressants may be used.

Although PMS does not seem to be related to abnormal hormone levels, some women respond to hormonal treatment. For example, one approach has been to use drugs such as birth control pills to stop ovulation from occurring. There is evidence that a brain chemical, serotonin, plays a role in severe forms of PMS. Antidepressants that alter serotonin in the body have been shown to help many women with severe PMS.

Chapter 19

Menstrual Problems

Chapter Contents

Section 19.1

Menstrual Disorders Overview

Some women sail through their monthly periods with little or no concern. With few symptoms to worry about, other than the menstrual flow itself, their periods are like clockwork, starting and stopping at nearly the same time every month. For other women, however, the menstrual cycle introduces a host of physical and emotional symptoms that cause discomfort or worry. Menstrual cycle disorders include abnormal uterine bleeding, fibroids, premenstrual syndrome, and premenstrual dysphoric disorder, among other conditions.

Most menstrual cycle disorders are benign, but that doesn't mean that they aren't overwhelming or shouldn't be evaluated. There are many treatment options to correct menstrual cycle disorders. The first and most important step is to discuss your symptoms with your health care professional so he or she can accurately diagnose your condition and help you choose the best way to make your menstrual cycle tolerable.

Abnormal Uterine Bleeding

Heavy menstrual bleeding is a common problem for many women. One in five women bleed so heavily that they sometimes have to put their normal lives on hold just to deal with the heavy blood flow. The general term for this condition is called abnormal uterine bleeding (AUB). It is used to describe menstrual periods that are too heavy (menorrhagia), too long (hypermenorrhea) and bleeding that occurs between periods (metrorrhagia). AUB may also be used to describe missed periods (amenorrhea).

How heavy is heavy? In general, AUB describes menstrual bleeding heavy enough to interfere with normal activities. Blood loss during a normal menstrual period is about 2.5 ounces, but if you have AUB, you may bleed as much as 10 to 25 times that amount each month. It's a distressing and, sometimes, painful problem.

Irregular periods can be common at various stages of your life—during your teen years when you first begin to menstruate, and as you near menopause, around the age of 50, for example. In the three to five years just prior to menopause, your periods may suddenly become lighter or heavier because you are ovulating less often. If you are past menopause and you aren't taking any hormones, any uterine bleeding you experience is considered abnormal and should be evaluated immediately by a health care professional.

The best way to determine if your periods are normal is to determine how predictable the time between your periods is. A woman having periods every 21 to 35 days lasting three to four days does not have AUB. A woman having periods every 21 to 35 days lasting three days some months and 10 days other months is likely not to be ovulating regularly and may have AUB.

Types of AUB

There are three types of abnormal uterine bleeding: dysfunctional, structural, and bleeding secondary to underlying disorders, such as von Willebrand disease and hemophilia, for example.

Dysfunctional uterine bleeding can be caused by hormonal imbalances. As many as 75 percent of women with excessive menstrual bleeding have a hormone-related disorder that is responsible for their AUB condition. Hormonal imbalances occur when your body produces too much or not enough of certain hormones. These imbalances also be associated with: weight loss or gain; a heavy exercise regimen; stress; illness; and use of some medications.

Nearly one half of women with AUB and almost all of women with dysfunctional uterine bleeding are not ovulating regularly. Ovulation, which is the release of the egg from the ovary, is accompanied by production of progesterone, the hormone that is most important in keeping periods regular.

Women who fail to ovulate for many months or years can end up with endometrial hyperplasia—a condition where the lining of your uterus grows excessively. It happens because the delicate balance between the hormones of progesterone and estrogen in your body is disrupted. If left untreated for a long time, the condition can become cancerous.

Chronic failure to ovulate may cause the ovaries to produce excessive levels of androgens (a reproductive hormone found in small amounts in women and in greater amounts in men). This condition may cause cysts to develop on your ovaries and is known as polycystic ovarian disease. The symptoms of polycystic ovarian disease include: irregular uterine bleeding; irregular periods from an early age; infertility; acne; excessive facial hair or hair on your abdomen or chest; and obesity.

Other hormonal causes of dysfunctional uterine bleeding include thyroid or adrenal gland imbalance. Heavy bleeding may be caused by medical conditions, such as:

- blood clotting disorders such as Von Willebrand disease, ITP [immune thrombocytopenic purpura], or hemophilia

- liver or kidney disease

- leukemia

- medications, such as anticoagulant drugs and some synthetic hormones

- the Copper-T IUD, which may also cause heavy periods

- normal pregnancy

- miscarriage

- ectopic pregnancy, which occurs when a fertilized egg begins to grow outside your uterus, typically in your fallopian tubes

- chronic medical problems, such as diabetes, lupus, or sarcoidosis

Structural causes of excessive bleeding include: polyps; scar tissue; infection; pre-cancerous conditions; and uterine fibroids.

Fibroids don't always cause excessive bleeding. In fact, about half of all women who have fibroids don't have any symptoms at all.

Amenorrhea—No Bleeding

Some women don't have heavy menstrual bleeding—they have the opposite problem: no menstrual periods at all. This condition, called amenorrhea, or the absence of menstruation, is normal before puberty, after menopause, and during pregnancy. If you don't have a monthly period and don't fit into one of these categories, then you need to discuss your condition with your health care professional.

Primary amenorrhea is diagnosed if you reach the age of 18 and haven't yet begun to menstruate. It's usually caused by some problem in your endocrine system, which regulates your hormones. This medical condition can be caused by a number of things, such as a problem with your ovaries, your nervous system, your adrenal glands, or an abnormally functioning pituitary gland that affects how you mature at puberty. Birth defects that prevent some of your reproductive anatomy from developing normally (Turner syndrome, for example) are other causes of primary amenorrhea.

Secondary amenorrhea is diagnosed if you've had regular periods, but then they suddenly stop for at least three months or longer. This condition can be precipitated by other problems that affect estrogen levels, including stress, weight loss, exercise or illness; or problems affecting the pituitary (elevated levels of the hormone prolactin), thyroid (hyperthyroidism or hypothyroidism) or adrenal glands (Cushing disease, for example). Secondary amenorrhea can also occur if you've had an ovarian tumor or have had your ovaries surgically removed. Celiac disease, which causes abnormalities in the digestive tract, is also associated with late puberty, early menopause, and amenorrhea.

Menstrual Cramps, PMS, and PMDD

Most women have experienced menstrual cramps before or during their period at some point in their lives. For some, it's part of the regular monthly routine. But if your cramps are especially painful and persistent, you should consult your health care professional.

Pain from menstrual cramps is a result of contractions of your uterus, which are caused by prostaglandins. Prostaglandins circulate in your bloodstream and they can cause diarrhea because they also speed up contractions in your intestines. They can also lower your blood pressure by relaxing blood vessels. If you're having severe menstrual pain, you might also find you have some diarrhea or an occasional feeling of faintness where you suddenly become pale and sweaty.

Premenstrual syndrome, or PMS, is a term commonly used to describe a wide variety of severe physical and psychological symptoms associated with the menstrual cycle. Approximately 30 to 40 percent of all women experience symptoms severe enough to disrupt their lifestyles. PMS symptoms are more severe and disruptive than the premenstrual symptoms that as many as 75 percent of all women experience.

There are more than 150 documented symptoms of PMS; the most common is depression. Symptoms develop about seven to 10 days before each period, and disappear once your period begins or soon after. Some of the physical symptoms associated with PMS are: bloating; swollen, painful breasts; fatigue; constipation; headaches; and clumsiness.

Some of the emotional symptoms associated with PMS are: anger; anxiety or confusion; mood swings and tension; crying and depression; and an inability to concentrate.

No one knows what causes PMS. However, researchers now know that PMS is not a simple result of an imbalance of estrogen and progesterone—commonly referred to as female hormones, or any other single hormonal factor.

A complex interaction of neurotransmitters (such as dopamine, norepinephrine, and serotonin) as well as other brain chemicals are now suspected of having a more direct relationship in triggering PMS. But exactly how these brain chemicals change with or affect the menstrual cycle remains unclear. Estrogen excesses, progesterone deficiencies, vitamin B6 deficiencies, low levels of serotonin (a brain chemical that affects mood), an excess of prolactin (a protein hormone that induces lactation), and altered glucose metabolism are among the many different theories that attempt to explain PMS, but none has been proven.

Features of PMS that distinguish it from other menstrual cycle symptoms are: symptoms tend to increase in severity as the cycle progresses; symptoms are relieved when menstrual flow begins or shortly after; and symptoms are present for at least three consecutive menstrual cycles

Symptoms of PMS may worsen with age and increase in severity following each pregnancy. Women who experience PMS may have an increased sensitivity to alcohol at specific times during their cycle. They often have a sister or mother who also suffers from PMS, suggesting a genetic component exists for the disorder.

Premenstrual dysphoric disorder (PMDD) is different from the more common PMS—it's far more severe. Women who experience PMDD (about five to seven percent of all women) say that it significantly interferes with lives. Experts equate the difference between PMS and PMDD to the difference between a mild tension headache and a migraine.

The most common symptoms of PMDD are heightened irritability, anxiety, and mood swings. Women who have a history of major depression, postpartum depression, or mood disorders are at higher risk for PMDD than other women. Although some symptoms of PMDD and major depression overlap, they are different. PMDD-related symptoms (both emotional and physical) are cyclical. When a woman starts her period, the symptoms subside within a few days. Depression-related symptoms, however, are not associated with the menstrual cycle. Without treatment, depressive mood disorders can persist or weeks, months, or years.

Section 19.2

Amenorrhea

What is amenorrhea?

Amenorrhea is when a woman does not get her monthly period. Women normally do not menstruate before puberty, during pregnancy, and after menopause. If amenorrhea happens at other times, it may be the symptom of a treatable medical condition.

There are two types of amenorrhea: primary amenorrhea and secondary amenorrhea. Primary amenorrhea is when a young woman never gets her first period. Secondary amenorrhea is when a woman who has had normal menstrual cycles stops getting her monthly period.

What causes amenorrhea?

Amenorrhea can be caused by any number of changes in the organs, glands, and hormones involved in menstruation.

Primary amenorrhea. Possible causes include:

- Failure of the ovaries (female sex organs that hold eggs)

- Problems in the nervous system or the pituitary gland (a gland in the brain that makes a hormone involved in menstruation)

- Poorly formed reproductive organs

In many cases, the cause of primary amenorrhea is not known.

Secondary amenorrhea. Common causes of secondary amenorrhea are: pregnancy; breast feeding; stopping of the use of birth control pills; menopause; and some birth control methods, such as Depo Provera.

Other causes of secondary amenorrhea include: stress; poor nutrition; depression; certain drugs; extreme weight loss; overexercising;

ongoing illness; sudden weight gain or being very overweight (obesity); problems with hormone-making glands, including the thyroid (rare); and tumors on the ovaries (rare).

A woman who has had her uterus or ovaries removed will also stop menstruating.

How can I know if I have amenorrhea?

If you miss your period, contact your health care provider. First, he or she will want to know if your period has stopped because of a normal condition such as pregnancy or menopause. (Most women go through menopause in their early fifties.) You will be given a physical and pelvic exam. You will also be asked to describe your symptoms and medical history. A sample of blood and urine may be taken for testing.

In some cases, finding the cause of amenorrhea can be difficult. You can help your health care provider by keeping a record of changes in your menstrual cycle. Note how long your periods last and when you had your last period. Also report any drugs you are taking and changes in your diet and/or exercise program. You should also report any emotional problems you are having, including stress.

How is amenorrhea treated?

Amenorrhea from normal causes, such as pregnancy, does not need to be treated. In other cases, treatments will depend on the cause. Treatments include:

- Dieting and exercising to lose weight (for amenorrhea caused by obesity)
- Dieting to gain weight (for amenorrhea caused by extreme weight loss). Amenorrhea may be the symptom of anorexia nervosa, a serious eating disorder. If you or someone you care about has this condition, get help right away.
- Learning ways to manage stress
- Changing exercise levels
- Hormones ordered by a health care provider
- Surgery (rarely)

When should I see my health care provider?

See your health care provider if you:

- Miss a period
- Have trouble with your balance, coordination, or vision
- Begin producing breast milk though you have not given birth
- Have extra growth of body hair
- Are over 16 years old and haven't had your first period

How can I prevent secondary amenorrhea?

The best way to prevent secondary amenorrhea is to maintain a healthy lifestyle. Stay at a healthy weight, learn ways to cope with stress and emotional problems and get a pelvic exam and Pap test once a year.

Where can I learn more?

Call the American College of Obstetricians and Gynecologists, (202) 863-2518.

Section 19.3

Dysmenorrhea

What is dysmenorrhea?

Dysmenorrhea is the medical term for menstrual cramps. There are two types of dysmenorrhea: primary dysmenorrhea and secondary dysmenorrhea. Primary dysmenorrhea is common menstrual cramps. Cramps usually begin one to two years after a woman starts getting her period. Pain is usually felt in the lower abdomen or back and can be mild to severe. Common menstrual cramps usually become less painful as a woman ages and may stop entirely if the woman has a baby.

Secondary dysmenorrhea is pain caused by a disorder in the woman's reproductive organs. Pain from secondary dysmenorrhea usually begins earlier in the menstrual cycle and lasts longer than common menstrual cramps.

What are the symptoms of menstrual cramps?

- Aching pain in the abdomen (Pain can be severe at times.)
- Feeling of pressure in the abdomen
- Pain in the hips, lower back, and inner thighs

When cramps are severe, symptoms may include:

- Upset stomach, sometimes with vomiting
- Loose stool

What causes common menstrual cramps?

Menstrual cramps are caused by contractions in the uterus, a muscle. The uterus, the hollow pear-shaped organ where a baby grows, contracts throughout a woman's menstrual cycle. During menstruation, the uterus contracts more strongly. If the uterus contracts too strongly, it can press against nearby blood vessels, cutting off the supply of oxygen to the muscle tissue of the uterus. Pain results when part of the muscle briefly loses its supply of oxygen.

How can I relieve mild menstrual cramps?

To relieve mild menstrual cramps:

- Take aspirin or another pain reliever such as acetaminophen or ibuprofen. (Note: For best relief, you must take ibuprofen as soon as bleeding or cramping starts.)

- Place a heating pad or hot water bottle on your lower back or abdomen.

You should also:

- Rest when needed.
- Avoid foods that contain caffeine.
- Avoid smoking and drinking alcohol.
- Massage your lower back and abdomen.

Women who exercise regularly often have less menstrual pain. To help prevent cramps, make exercise a part of your weekly routine.

If these steps do not relieve pain, your health care provider can order medications for you, including:

- Ibuprofen (higher dose than is available over-the-counter)
- Oral contraceptives (women on birth control pills have less menstrual pain)

What causes menstrual cramps from secondary dysmenorrhea?

Menstrual pain from secondary dysmenorrhea is caused by a disease in the woman's reproductive organs. Conditions that can cause secondary dysmenorrhea include:

- Endometriosis—A condition in which the tissue lining the uterus (the endometrium) is found outside of the uterus.

169

- Pelvic inflammatory disease (PID)—An infection caused by bacteria (a type of germ) that starts in the uterus and can spread to other reproductive organs.

- Cervical stenosis—Narrowing of the opening to the uterus.

- Tumors (also called fibroids)—Growths on the inner wall of the uterus.

How can I know if my cramps are normal?

If you have severe or unusual menstrual cramps or cramps that last for more than two or three days, contact your health care provider.

Both primary and secondary menstrual cramps can be treated, so it's important to get checked.

First, you will be asked to describe your symptoms and menstrual cycles. Your health care provider will also perform a pelvic exam. During this exam, your doctor inserts a speculum (an instrument that lets the clinician see inside the vagina) and examines your vagina, cervix and uterus. The doctor will feel for any lumps or changes, and a small sample of vaginal fluid may be taken for testing.

If secondary dysmenorrhea is suspected, further tests may be needed. If a medical problem is found, your health care provider will discuss treatments.

If you use tampons and develop the following symptoms, get medical help right away:

- Fever over 102 degrees Fahrenheit
- Vomiting
- Diarrhea
- Dizziness, fainting, or near fainting
- A rash that looks like a sunburn

These are symptoms of toxic shock syndrome, a life-threatening illness.

Where can I learn more?

Call the American College of Obstetricians and Gynecologists at (202) 863-2518.

Chapter 20

Pelvic Pain

Many women have pain in their pelvic region at some point in their lives. Each woman responds to pain in her own way. Some women are bothered by pain more than others. You should discuss any pain with your doctor, but even more so if it disrupts your daily life, if it worsens over time, or if you've noticed a recent increase in pain.

Finding the cause of pelvic pain can be a long process. Often there is more than one reason for the pain, and its exact source can be hard to pin down.

Causes of Pelvic Pain

Acute Pain

Acute (sharp) pain starts over a short time (a few minutes to a few days). It often has one cause.

Infection. Pelvic pain can be caused by an infection or inflammation.

Pelvic inflammatory disease (PID) is a broad term used to describe infection of the uterus, fallopian tubes, and ovaries. Most cases of PID are thought to come from sexually transmitted diseases (STDs).

Vaginal infection (vaginitis) can sometimes be painful, mainly during and after sex.

American College of Obstetricians and Gynecologists. *Pelvic Pain.* (Patient Education Pamphlet No. AP099). Washington, DC. © ACOG 1999.

Infections of the urethra, bladder, or kidneys (urinary tract infections) may cause pain, too.

Ovarian Cysts. Sometimes a cyst may form on an ovary. A cyst is a sac filled with fluid. It is somewhat like a blister. Some cysts on the ovaries form as a result of the normal process of ovulation (release of an egg from the ovary). Often a cyst begins fairly quickly but goes away within a day or two. Some cysts can last a long time. These cysts are often felt as a dull ache or heaviness.

Ectopic Pregnancy. A tubal or ectopic pregnancy is one that starts outside the uterus, often in one of the fallopian tubes. This happens most often in women who have some damage to their tubes. The pain often starts on one side of the abdomen after a missed period.

Chronic Pain

Chronic pain can be either intermittent (it can come and go) or constant (it is there most of the time). Intermittent chronic pain often has a distinct cause.

Dysmenorrhea. Dysmenorrhea is a case of long-term, intermittent chronic pain. Although some mild pain is common during a woman's menstrual period, some women have severe pain with their periods.

Endometriosis and Adenomyosis. Sometimes menstrual cramps can be a sign of disease. If they get worse over the years or stay strong beyond the first one or two days of flow, they may be due to a disease such as endometriosis or adenomyosis.

The cause of endometriosis and the reasons for pain during the menstrual cycle are not known for sure.

Adenomyosis occurs when the endometrium buries itself in the muscle wall of the uterus. This can cause menstrual cramps.

Ovulation Pain. Pain that is felt around the time of ovulation is sometimes called mittelschmerz (German for "middle pain").

Constant Chronic Pain

Some women may feel pain almost every day. This may mean that a problem has gotten worse. Or it could mean that a person has become less able to cope with pain.

Other Causes of Pain

Adhesions or scar tissue can form as a result of the healing process.

Fibroids may grow on the inside of the uterus, on its outer surface, or within the wall of the uterus. It is not known for certain what causes fibroids.

Other causes of lower abdominal and pelvic pain include:

- Diverticulitis (inflammation of a pouch bulging from the wall of the colon)
- Irritable bowel syndrome (a condition that may cause alternating bouts of diarrhea and constipation and often seems to be related to stress)
- Kidney or bladder stones
- Appendicitis
- Muscle spasms or strain

Diagnosis

Because there are so many causes of pelvic pain, your doctor may use many tests to rule out likely causes of your pain.

Physical Factors

The evaluation begins with an exam. Cultures and blood tests are sometimes needed to look for infection.

Other studies are sometimes useful to find the cause of pain.

Treatment

Acute pain or intermittent chronic pain often involves treatment of one specific condition. Treatment of constant chronic pain is not like that.

Medications

If you have had a problem such as a urinary tract infection or vaginitis before and it has come back, your doctor may prescribe medication over the phone.

Drugs that reduce inflammation, such as ibuprofen, can be used to lessen the pain of dysmenorrhea.

For other problems, treatment with hormones may help. Combination oral contraceptives (birth control pills) can be used to relieve pain from menstrual cramps.

Antidepressants have been used in some patients with pelvic pain when other treatments have not worked.

Most people try to use as little pain medication as they can. When treating chronic pain, it is better to use a nonnarcotic pain medication as part of a routine. Pain medication may only take the edge off the pain. It may not get rid of it. It is best to avoid strong narcotic medication.

Surgery

Certain problems may be treated with surgery. The type of surgery depends on your exact problem.

Other Treatments

Heat therapy, muscle relaxants, nerve block, and relaxation exercises may all help to treat other causes of pelvic pain.

Finally

Because pelvic pain has a number of causes, finding the source of your pain can be a long and involved process. This may frustrate you, but try not to give up. Even when there is no one cause found for pelvic pain, there are treatments that may help.

Chapter 21

Uterine, Cervical, and Ovarian Disorders

Chapter Contents

Section 21.1

Common Uterine Conditions

Excerpted from "Common Uterine Conditions: Options for Treatment," by the Agency for Healthcare Research and Quality, December 1997. Available online at http://www.ahrq.gov; reviewed and revised by David A. Cooke, M.D. on June 30, 2003.

Endometrial Hyperplasia

Hyperplasia is a condition in which the lining of the uterus becomes too thick, which results in abnormal bleeding. Hyperplasia is thought to be caused by too much estrogen.

Depending on your age and how long you have had hyperplasia, your doctor may want to do a biopsy before beginning treatment to rule out cancer. Treatment options include:

- Hormone treatment with birth control pills or progesterone helps some women who have hyperplasia.

- Hysterectomy is often recommended to treat hyperplasia. Because some types of hyperplasia can lead to cancer, your doctor will watch your condition carefully if you choose not to have a hysterectomy.

Uterine Prolapse

If you have uterine prolapse, it means that your uterus has tilted or slipped. Sometimes it slips so far down that it reaches into the vagina. This happens when the ligaments that hold the uterus to the wall of the pelvis become too weak to hold the uterus in its place. Uterine prolapse can cause feelings of pressure and discomfort. Urine may leak.

Treatment choices depend on how weak the ligaments have become, your age, health, and whether you want to become pregnant. Options that do not involve an operation include:

- Exercises (called Kegel exercises) can help to strengthen the muscles of the pelvis. How to do Kegel exercises: Tighten your pelvic muscles as if you are trying to hold back urine. Hold the muscles tight for a few seconds and then release them. Repeat this exercise up to 10 times. Repeat the Kegel exercises up to four times each day.

- Taking estrogen to limit further weakening of the muscles and tissues that support the uterus. Taking estrogen can improve this condition, but because of recent studies showing multiple risks associated with estrogen use, you should carefully discuss the risks and benefits of this kind of therapy with your doctor.

- Inserting a pessary—which is a rubber, diaphragm-like device—around the cervix to help prop up the uterus. The pessary does have drawbacks. It may dislodge or cause irritation, it may interfere with intercourse, and it must be removed regularly for cleaning.

- Watchful waiting.

Surgical treatments include:

- Tightening the weakened muscles without taking out the uterus. This is usually done through the vagina, but it also can be done through the abdomen. Although this is a type of surgery, it is not as extensive as a hysterectomy.

- Hysterectomy. Doctors usually recommend this operation if symptoms are bothersome or if the uterus has dropped so far that it is coming through the vagina.

Very Heavy Menstrual Bleeding

As you get closer to menopause, it may be hard to tell when your period is going to start. The time between your periods may be longer or shorter than usual. When it does start, bleeding may be very heavy and last for several weeks.

You may have dysfunctional uterine bleeding or DUB. DUB most often affects women over 45. Usually it is caused by an imbalance in the chemicals in the body (hormones) that control the menstrual cycle.

Younger women also may have heavy bleeding. Usually it is because of an irregular menstrual cycle. A woman may go for several months without a period, but the lining of her uterus continues to build up. When finally her body sheds the uterine lining, she may have very heavy bleeding.

The symptoms can be very upsetting and may make you feel limited in the things you can do. Sometimes, the symptoms are a sign of a more serious problem.

Your doctor will probably do a blood test. Depending on the results, your medical history, and your age, the doctor may recommend that you have a biopsy to rule out endometrial hyperplasia. Treatment options include:

- Birth control pills or other medicines may be helpful.

- Another choice is watchful waiting.

- A surgical procedure called endometrial ablation may help to relieve very heavy menstrual bleeding. Endometrial ablation causes sterility (inability to become pregnant), but it does not trigger menopause. The long-term effects of endometrial ablation are unknown.

- Hysterectomy is an option in some women who have very heavy bleeding, particularly in older women, or if there are other conditions present that are improved by hysterectomy.

Do you have a bleeding disorder?

If you have very heavy periods (lasting more than 7 days or soaking more than one pad or tampon every 2 to 3 hours), frequent or long-lasting nosebleeds, easy bruising, or prolonged oozing of blood after dental work, you may have a bleeding disorder such as von Willebrand Disease. This is not the same as very heavy menstrual bleeding, but it can be an underlying cause.

Section 21.2

What Is a Retroverted Uterus?

A retroverted uterus is the medical term used to describe a uterus that is tipped or tilted backward away from the belly. The condition is also referred to as a tipped uterus or tilted uterus. All three terms are interchangeable. The uterus is normally suspended in a straight up and down position or slightly forward toward the belly. A retroverted uterus is usually congenital or something you are born with, but can be caused by labor while giving birth.

In most cases, a retroverted uterus does not cause any problems.

However, some women with a retroverted uterus experience pain during sexual intercourse. This happens when the penis hits the cervix or uterus during sex. This condition is known as collision dyspareunia. Women may also suffer pain during menstruation or experience infertility because of a retroverted uterus.

A retroverted uterus can be repositioned through:

- Exercises—Although doctors differ in their opinion on effectiveness, a knee-chest exercise may be prescribed to reposition a retroverted uterus temporarily. Note that the doctor will only recommend exercise therapy if he or she can reposition the uterus manually in the office. The knee-chest exercise will not be effective if the uterus has become fixed in the retroverted position because of endometriosis, fibroid tumors, pelvic infection, or other cause.

- Pessary—A pessary is a plastic or silicone device that is placed in the vagina to reposition a tipped uterus. It can be used on a temporary or permanent basis, though long-term use has been linked to inflammation, ulceration, and other complications.

- Surgery—The minimally invasive UPLIFT uterine suspension procedure can provide lasting pain relief in most cases of collision dyspareunia. Uterine suspension can also relieve dysmenorrhea

179

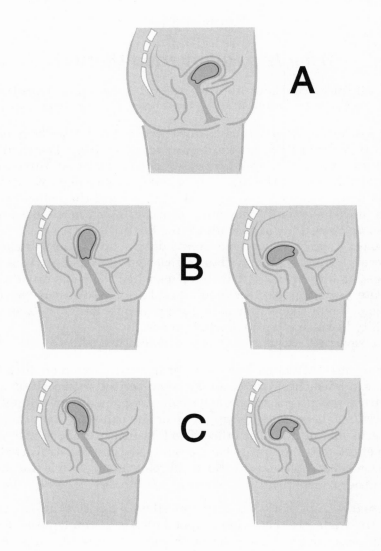

Figure 21.1. *What is a retroverted uterus? Figure 21.2a shows a normal or forward (anteverted) resting position of the uterus. Figure 21.2b shows a retroverted uterus (backward facing). Figure 21.2c shows a retroflexed uterus (backward facing with a crimp).*

in a significant number of women who have painful periods and have no other identifiable pathologies other than a retroverted uterus. The UPLIFT procedure can be performed on an outpatient basis, has a short recovery time and has demonstrated a success rate of over 85% in reducing or eliminating the pain associated with a retroverted uterus.

How do I know if I have a retroverted uterus?

Your physician can perform a simple physical exam to find out. This can be done during a routine pelvic exam as shown in Figure 21.2. If you suspect that you have a retroverted uterus, please discuss it with your physician.

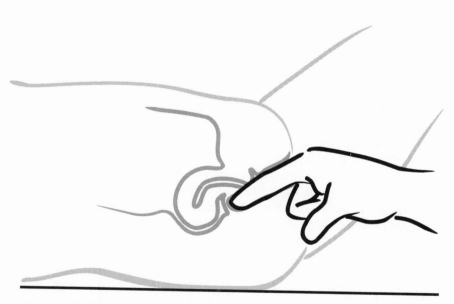

Figure 21.2. *Retroverted or tipped uterus.*

Section 21.3

Adenomyosis

Reprinted with permission of Brigham and Women's Hospital, Center for Uterine Fibroids. © 1998 Brigham and Women's Hospital, Center for Uterine Fibroids. Available online at http://www.fibroids.net/html/ adenomyosis.htm. Reviewed by David A. Cooke, M.D. on June 30, 2003.

What Is Adenomyosis?

Adenomyosis is a benign disease of the uterus in which components normally limited to the endometrium (the thin innermost uterine layer) are found within the myometrium (the middle muscular layer of the uterus). The exact prevalence of adenomyosis is not known because the diagnosis can be made only by microscopic examination of uterine specimens obtained during surgery or, less often, during biopsy. Some studies estimate that 20% of women have adenomyosis; however, with careful microscopic analysis of multiple myometrial samples from an individual uterine specimen, the prevalence increases to as high as 65%.

The cause of adenomyosis is also unknown. The most widely accepted theory of adenomyosis development postulates that the barrier between the endometrium and myometrium, which normally prevents invasion of endometrial glands and stroma into the myometrium, is compromised, allowing invasion to occur. This process is thought to occur only in the presence of estrogen, however, little scientific evidence exists to support this hypothesis.

Adenomyosis most commonly affects women between the ages of 40 and 50 years and is associated with a past history of childbirth. Approximately 80% of women with this disorder have given birth. However, the incidence of adenomyosis does not correlate with increasing number of pregnancies.

Adenomyosis is also associated with other uterine disorders. More than 80% of women with adenomyosis have another pathologic process in the uterus; 50% of patients have associated fibroids (benign smooth muscle tumors of the uterus), approximately 11% have endometriosis (endometrial tissue outside of the uterus, most commonly in the ovaries), and 7% have endometrial polyps (benign outgrowths of endometrial tissue). The symptoms of these associated conditions often obscure the diagnosis of adenomyosis.

A typical uterus with adenomyosis is boggy [does not contract] and uniformly enlarged. Approximately 80% of uteri with adenomyosis weigh more than 80 grams (a normal uterus weighs approximately 50 grams), but it is unusual for a uterus in which adenomyosis is the only pathologic process to exceed 200 grams.

Symptoms of Adenomyosis

Symptoms of adenomyosis include abnormal uterine bleeding and pelvic pain. Approximately 60% of women with adenomyosis experience abnormal uterine bleeding, which usually manifests as either hypermenorrhea (prolonged and/or profuse uterine bleeding, also called menorrhagia) or metrorragia (irregular, acyclic bleeding). Dysmenorrhea (pelvic pain during menstruation) is the second most common symptom in patients with adenomyosis, occurring in 25% of cases.

A review of the literature demonstrates that only 15% of cases of adenomyosis are correctly diagnosed before surgery. The reason for this low percentage of preoperative diagnosis is two-fold; first, many patients with adenomyosis are asymptomatic in the absence of other uterine pathology, and second, the presence of adenomyosis is often overshadowed by associated pathology (e.g., leiomyomas, endometriosis).

D&C (dilation and curettage) does not aid in diagnosis. (In this procedure, the cervix is gradually dilated to allow removal of the uterine lining.) Pelvic ultrasonography may be suggestive but is not definitive. The usefulness of other imaging studies such as MRI (magnetic resonance imaging) is currently undetermined.

Treatment

Areas of adenomyosis do not lend themselves to local surgical excision. The only definitive treatment for adenomyosis, therefore, is total hysterectomy (surgical removal of the entire uterus). Synthetic steroid hormones such as progestins are not helpful and may actually increase the level of pelvic pain in some patients. GnRH (gonadotropin releasing hormone) agonists have been used in a few cases, resulting in a transient decrease in uterine size, in amenorrhea (cessation of menstrual cycling), and even in the ability to conceive. Unfortunately, regrowth of the adenomyosis and recurrence of symptoms are usually documented within six months of cessation of therapy.

Section 21.4

Intrauterine Adhesions

Reprinted with permission of the American Society for Reproductive Medicine, http://www.asrm.org. © 1996. Reviewed by David A. Cooke, M.D. on June 30, 2003.

Trauma to and/or infection of the uterine lining (endometrium) may lead to the formation of intrauterine adhesions or destruction of the endometrial lining. Intrauterine adhesions are defined as scar tissue inside the uterine cavity.

Causes

The principle cause of intrauterine adhesions is trauma to the uterine cavity. This may occur following dilation and curettage (D&C), an outpatient surgical procedure during which the cervix is dilated and the tissue contents of the uterus are emptied. D&C may be performed for excess uterine bleeding after childbirth, pregnancy termination, or other gynecological conditions. Less commonly, prolonged use of an intrauterine device (IUD), infections of the endometrium (endometritis), and surgical procedures involving the uterus (such as removal of fibroids) may also lead to the development of intrauterine adhesions.

Symptoms

Women with intrauterine adhesions may have no obvious problems. Many patients, however, may experience menstrual dysfunction in the form of absent, light, or infrequent menstruation. Also, they may be unable to achieve pregnancy, or experience recurrent miscarriages. Less commonly, pelvic pain or dysmenorrhea (painful menstrual periods) may be present.

Diagnosis

Hysterosalpingography (HSG), an x-ray procedure, is a common method used to diagnose intrauterine adhesions. During an HSG, a solution is injected into the uterus to illustrate the inner shape of the uterus and determine if the fallopian tubes are open. Hysteroscopy is also used to diagnose intrauterine adhesions. This is a procedure in which a thin, telescope-like instrument is inserted through the cervix to allow direct visualization of the uterine cavity. Although HSG is a useful screening test, hysteroscopy is the most accurate method of evaluating intrauterine adhesions. Both HSG and hysteroscopy can be performed in an office setting without general anesthesia.

Treatment

Surgical removal of intrauterine adhesions with hysteroscopic guidance is generally recommended. Following removal of the adhesions, many surgeons recommend temporarily placing a device, such as a plastic catheter, inside the uterus in an effort to keep the walls of the uterus apart and prevent adhesions from reforming. Hormonal treatment with estrogens and progestins, and non-steroidal anti-inflammatory medications, are frequently prescribed after surgery to lessen the chance of adhesion reformation.

Reproductive Outcome

Reproductive outcome appears to correlate with the type and extent of the adhesions. After treatment, patients with mild to moderate adhesions have full-term pregnancy rates of approximately 70 to 80 percent, and menstrual dysfunction is frequently alleviated. Alternatively, patients with severe adhesions or extensive destruction of the endometrial lining may only have full-term pregnancy rates in the 20 to 40 percent range after treatment. Women with extensive damage to the endometrium unresponsive to conventional therapy by hysteroscopy may be offered gestational surrogacy.

Section 21.5

Endometriosis

Excerpted from "Endometriosis," a booklet produced by the National Institutes of Health, National Institute of Child Health and Human Development, NIH Pub. No. 02-2413, September 2002. Available online at http://www.nichd.nih.gov; accessed July 2003.

Endometriosis is one of the most common gynecological diseases, affecting more than 5.5 million women in North America alone. The two most common symptoms of endometriosis are pain and infertility. Some women have pain before and during their periods, as well as during or after sex.

This pain can be so intense that it affects a woman's quality of life, from her relationships, to her day-to-day activities. Some women don't have any symptoms from endometriosis. Others may not find out they have the disease until they have trouble getting pregnant.

What is endometriosis?

Endometriosis occurs when tissue like that which lines the inside of uterus grows outside the uterus, usually on the surfaces of organs in the pelvic and abdominal areas, in places that it is not supposed to grow.

The word endometriosis comes from the word endometrium—endo means inside and metrium means mother. Health care providers call the tissue that lines the inside of the uterus (where a mother carries her baby) the endometrium.

Health care providers may call areas of endometriosis by different names, such as implants, lesions, or nodules.

Most endometriosis is found in the pelvic cavity: on or under the ovaries; behind the uterus; on the tissues that hold the uterus in place; and on the bowels or bladder. In extremely rare cases, endometriosis areas can grow in the lungs or other parts of the body.

What are the symptoms of endometriosis?

One of the most common symptoms of endometriosis is pain, mostly in the abdomen, lower back, and pelvic areas. The amount of pain a woman feels is not linked to how much endometriosis she has. Some women have no pain even though their endometriosis is extensive, meaning that the affected areas are large, or that there is scarring. Some women, on the other hand, have severe pain even though they have only a few small areas of endometriosis.

General symptoms of endometriosis can include (but are not limited to):

- Extremely painful (or disabling) menstrual cramps; pain may get worse over time
- Chronic pelvic pain (includes lower back pain and pelvic pain)
- Pain during or after sex
- Intestinal pain
- Painful bowel movements or painful urination during menstrual periods
- Heavy menstrual periods
- Premenstrual spotting or bleeding between periods
- Infertility

In addition, women who are diagnosed with endometriosis may have gastrointestinal symptoms that resemble a bowel disorder, as well as fatigue.

Does having endometriosis mean I'll be infertile or unable to have children?

About 30 percent to 40 percent of women with endometriosis are infertile, making it one of the top three causes of female infertility. Some women don't find out that they have endometriosis until they have trouble getting pregnant.

If you have endometriosis and want to get pregnant, your health care provider may suggest that you have unprotected sex for six months to a year before you have any treatment for the endometriosis.

The relationship between endometriosis and infertility is an active area of research. Some studies suggest that the condition may change the uterus so it does not accept an embryo. Other work explores whether endometriosis changes the egg, or whether endometriosis gets in the way of moving a fertilized egg to the uterus.

How do I know that I have endometriosis?

Currently, health care providers use a number of tests for endometriosis. Sometimes, they will use imaging tests to produce a picture of the inside of the body, which allows them to locate larger endometriosis areas, such as nodules or cysts. The two most common imaging tests are ultrasound, a machine that uses sound waves to make the picture, and magnetic resonance imaging (MRI), a machine that uses magnets and radio waves to make the picture.

The only way to know for sure that you have the condition is by having surgery. The most common type of surgery is called laparoscopy. In this procedure, the surgeon inflates the abdomen slightly with a harmless gas. After making a small cut in the abdomen, the surgeon uses a small viewing instrument with a light, called a laparoscope, to look at the reproductive organs, intestines, and other surfaces to see if there is any endometriosis. He or she can make a diagnosis based on the characteristic appearance of endometriosis. This diagnosis can then be confirmed by doing a biopsy, which involves taking a small tissue sample and studying it under a microscope.

Your health care provider will only do a laparoscopy after learning your full medical history and giving you a complete physical and pelvic exam. This information, in addition to the results of an ultrasound or MRI, will help you and your health care provider make more informed decisions about treatment.

Are there treatments for endometriosis?

Currently, we have no cure for endometriosis. Even having a hysterectomy or removing the ovaries does not guarantee that the endometriosis areas and/or the symptoms of endometriosis will not come back. There are a number of treatments for both pain and infertility related to endometriosis, however. They include:

- Pain medication—Works well if your pain or other symptoms are mild. These medications range from over-the-counter remedies to strong prescription drugs.

- Hormone therapy—Is effective if your areas are small and/ or you have minimal pain. Hormones can come in pill form, by shot or injection, or in a nasal spray. Common hormones used to treat endometriosis pain are progesterone, birth control pills, Danocrine, and gonadotropin-releasing hormone (GnRH).

- Surgical treatment—Is usually the best choice if your endo-metriosis is extensive, or if you have more severe pain. Surgical treatments range from minor to major surgical procedures.

Section 21.6

Uterine Fibroids

Excerpted from "Fast Facts about Uterine Fibroids," a booklet produced by the National Institutes of Health, National Institute of Child Health and Human Development, NIH Pub. No. 02-7103, June 2002. Available online at http://www.nichd.nih.gov; accessed July 2003.

What are uterine fibroids?

Uterine fibroids are tumors or lumps made of muscle cells and other tissue that grow within the wall of the uterus.

Fibroids may grow as a single tumor or in clusters. A single fibroid can be less than one inch in size or can grow to eight inches across or more. A bunch or cluster of fibroids can also vary in size.

Where do uterine fibroids grow?

Most fibroids grow within the wall of the uterus. Health care providers put fibroids into three groups based on where they grow. Submucosal fibroids grow just underneath the uterine lining. Intramural fibroids grow in between the muscles of the uterus. Subserosal fibroids grow on the outside of the uterus. Additionally, some fibroids grow on stalks (also called peduncles) that grow out from the surface of the uterus, or into the cavity of the uterus.

What are the symptoms of uterine fibroids?

Many women don't feel any symptoms with uterine fibroids. But fibroids can cause the following symptoms:

- Heavy bleeding or painful periods
- Bleeding between periods

- Feeling full in the lower abdomen—sometimes called pelvic pressure

- Urinating often (results from a fibroid pressing on the bladder)

- Pain during sex

- Lower back pain

- Reproductive problems, such as infertility, multiple miscarriages, and early onset of labor during pregnancy

Does having uterine fibroids mean that a woman will be infertile or unable to have children?

In some cases, fibroids can prevent a woman from getting pregnant through natural methods. However, advances in treatments for fibroids and infertility have greatly improved the chances for a woman to get pregnant, even if she has uterine fibroids.

Researchers are still looking into what role, if any, uterine fibroids play in infertility. Currently, though, there are few answers. One study's results suggest that only submucosal fibroids have a negative impact on fertility, but these results are not yet confirmed. The relationship between fibroids and infertility remains a very active research area.

How do I know that I have uterine fibroids?

Unless you start to have symptoms, you probably won't know that you have uterine fibroids.

Sometimes, health care providers find fibroids during a routine gynecological exam.

- During this exam, the health care provider checks out the size of your uterus by putting two fingers of one hand into the vagina, while applying light pressure to your abdomen with the other hand.

- If you have fibroids, your uterus may feel larger-than normal; or, if you have fibroids, your uterus may extend into places it should not.

If your health care provider thinks that you have fibroids, he or she may use imaging technology—machines that create a picture of the inside of your body without surgery—to confirm the diagnosis. Some common types of imaging technology include:

- Ultrasound, which uses sound waves to form the picture;

- Magnetic resonance imaging or MRI, which uses magnets and radio waves to build the picture;

- X-rays, which use a form of electromagnetic radiation to see into the body; and

- CT or cat scan, which takes x-rays of the body from many angles to provide a more complete image. Sometimes, health care providers use a combination of these technologies.

Sometimes, however, the only way to confirm the presence of uterine fibroids is through surgery.

- Laparoscopy—In this procedure, the surgeon makes a small cut into the abdomen, after inflating it with a harmless gas; then, using a small viewing instrument with a light in it, the doctor can look for fibroids.

- Your health care provider may suggest a procedure called a hysteroscopy, which involves inserting a camera on a long tube through the vagina directly into the uterus to see the fibroids.

Keep in mind that because these are surgical procedures, you will need time to recover from them. However, the amount of recovery time you'll need may vary.

What are the treatments for uterine fibroids?

If a woman has uterine fibroids, but shows no symptoms or has no problems, she may not need any treatment. The provider will check the fibroids at a woman's routine gynecological exam to see if they have grown.

If a woman has pain now and then or feels mild symptoms, her health care provider may suggest pain medication, ranging from over-the-counter remedies to strong prescription drugs.

If a woman has many symptoms or feels pain often, she may benefit from medical therapy—that is, therapy using certain medications rather than surgery. Keep in mind that many medications have side effects, some of them serious.

If a woman has moderate symptoms of fibroids, surgery may be the best form of treatment.

- Myomectomy removes only the fibroids and leaves the healthy areas of the uterus in place. This procedure can preserve a woman's ability to have children.

- Hysterectomy is used when a woman's fibroids are large, or has heavy bleeding, and she is either near or past menopause, or doesn't want children. Hysterectomy is the only sure way to cure uterine fibroids. In general, recovery time from a hysterectomy is one to two months.

- Health care providers now have hysterectomy options that differ in how invasive they are. Abdominal hysterectomy is a procedure that involves a cut into the abdomen to remove the uterus. Vaginal hysterectomy is less invasive because the doctor reaches the uterus through the vagina, instead of making a cut into the abdomen. This procedure may not be an option if the fibroids are very large.

Section 21.7

Ovarian Cysts

U.S. Department of Health and Human Services, National Women's Health Information Center (NWHIC), April 2001. Available online at http://www.4woman.gov; accessed July 2003.

What are ovarian cysts?

The ovaries produce the eggs in the female reproductive system. Eggs grow, develop, and mature in the ovaries and then are released during ovulation, part of the monthly menstrual cycle that occurs during the childbearing years. Ovarian cysts are fluid-filled sacs that form on the ovaries when the follicles (sacs) on the ovary that contain the egg mature, but do not release the egg into the fallopian tube where it would be fertilized. A woman can develop one cyst or many cysts. Ovarian cysts can vary in size—from as small as a pea to as big as a grapefruit. Most cysts are small and do not cause symptoms. Some cysts might cause a dull ache in the abdomen because they are twisted, bleeding, or have burst; others might cause pain during sexual intercourse. Most cysts are benign (not cancerous). A few cysts, though, may turn out to be malignant (cancerous). For this reason, your doctor should check all cysts. If ovarian cysts are found early, many of the problems they cause can be treated. There are different types of ovarian cysts:

Functional cysts: These cysts are completely normal and form during ovulation. The follicles (sacs) on the ovary that contain the egg often do not mature, and become cysts. These cysts usually disappear during menstruation, before another menstrual cycle begins. If not, they will shrink in about one to three months. Your doctor may want to check in a few months to make sure the cyst has gotten smaller. Only women who are ovulating form functional cysts. If you are in menopause or past menopause and not having periods, you should not have functional cysts.

Endometriomas: These cysts develop in women who have endometriosis, a condition in which tissue from the lining of the uterus (endometrium) grows in other areas, such as on the fallopian tubes, the ovaries, and on other organs outside of the uterus in the stomach. These may be filled with a thick, brown blood and so also are called chocolate cysts. Because uterine tissue is sensitive to hormones, it bleeds monthly, which may cause it to form a growing cyst on the ovary. These cysts can be painful during sexual intercourse and during menstruation.

Benign cystic tumors (cystadenomas): These tumors are non-cancerous and are often filled with a fatty liquid. They develop from cells on the outer surface of the ovary. Some of these tumors, called dermoid cysts, are lined with structures such as hair, or pieces of bone. They are often small and may not cause symptoms. They can, however, become large and uncomfortable.

Multiple Cysts: Women who do not ovulate regularly can develop multiple cysts. This is a disorder in which the ovaries are enlarged and contain many small cysts. This can be caused by a condition called polycystic ovary syndrome (PCOS). Symptoms of PCOS include irregular menstrual periods, infertility, and increased body hair.

When are women most likely to have ovarian cysts?

Ovarian cysts are very common during the childbearing years. Most often, cysts in women of this age group are not cancerous. Women who are past menopause (ages 50 to 70), however, and have ovarian cysts, have a higher risk of having ovarian cancer. If you are over 50 and have an ovarian cyst, your doctor will probably want to do surgery to remove it. However, if you think you might have a cyst, at any age, you should tell your health care provider.

How are ovarian cysts diagnosed and treated?

Ovarian cysts usually are found during routine pelvic examinations. During this examination, your doctor is able to feel the swelling of the cyst on your ovary. Once a cyst is found, the doctor may perform an ultrasound, or a screening to see if the cyst is hollow or solid, determine its size and exact location, and see if it contains fluid or abnormal structures that help show its type. The doctor may decide to wait and see if the cyst will shrink on its own in a few months. If you frequently develop cysts, your doctor may prescribe birth control pills to prevent you from ovulating. This will prevent follicles from developing and new cysts from forming. Your doctor might talk with you about birth control pills, and if they are right for you.

If the cyst does not go away after several menstrual periods, if it has gotten larger or more painful, or it does not appear to be a functional cyst, your doctor may want to perform other tests or procedures to look at and remove the cyst. To detect your risk for ovarian cancer, your doctor may want to do a blood test to measure a substance in the blood called CA-125. The amount of this protein is increased in the blood of women with ovarian cancer. However, some ovarian cancers do not produce enough CA-125 to be detected by the test, and there are other non-cancerous diseases that also increase the levels of CA-125. For these reasons, the CA-125 test is recommended mostly for women who are at high risk for the disease.

If the cyst is small and looks benign on the ultrasound, your doctor may perform a laparoscopy. This procedure is done under general anesthesia on an outpatient basis and allows the doctor to closely examine all of your reproductive organs. A very small incision is made above or below the navel, and a small instrument that acts like a telescope is inserted into the abdomen. If the cyst is small and looks benign, it can be removed after the doctor makes very small incisions in the pubic hairline.

If the cyst is too large to remove this way, the doctor may perform a procedure called a laparotomy. This procedure involves making bigger incisions in the stomach to remove the cyst. While you are under general anesthesia, the doctor is able to have the cyst tested to find out if the tissue is cancerous. If it is cancerous, the doctor will then be able to remove other tissue that could be affected, like the ovary, fallopian tubes, uterus, or lymph nodes. Before any surgery, your doctor will talk to you about what will happen during the surgery, the risks, and how long it will take you to recover. It is important to remember that most cysts are not cancerous and relatively harmless if treated properly.

Section 21.8

Polycystic Ovary Syndrome

Excerpted from the publication by the U.S. Department of Health and Human Services, National Women's Health Information Center (NWHIC), April 2001. Available online at http://www.4woman.gov; accessed July 2003.

The ovaries are the organs that produce the eggs in the female reproductive system. Polycystic ovary syndrome (PCOS) is a syndrome in which the ovaries are enlarged and have several fluid-filled sacs or cysts. These cysts may look like a string of pearls or a pearl necklace. A woman can develop one cyst or many cysts. Polycystic ovaries are usually 1.5 to 3 times larger than normal. Women with PCOS may experience a number of other symptoms as well. PCOS is a leading cause of infertility and is the most common reproductive syndrome in women of childbearing age. An estimated five to 10% of women of childbearing age have PCOS (ages 20 to 40). At least 30% of women have some symptoms of PCOS.

What causes ovarian cysts?

Eggs grow, develop, and mature in the ovaries and then are released during ovulation, part of the monthly menstrual cycle that occurs during the childbearing years. Ovarian cysts are fluid-filled sacs that form on the ovaries when the follicles (sacs) on the ovary that contain the egg mature, but do not release the egg into the fallopian tube where it would be fertilized.

195

What are the other symptoms of PCOS?

Some of the other symptoms of PCOS include:

- Infrequent menstrual periods, no menstrual periods, and/or irregular bleeding

- Infrequent or no ovulation

- Increased serum levels of male hormones, such as testosterone

- Inability to get pregnant within six to 12 months of unprotected sexual intercourse (infertility)

- Pelvic pain that lasts longer than six months

- Weight gain or obesity

- Diabetes, overproduction of insulin, and inefficient use of insulin in the body

- Abnormal lipid levels (such as high or low cholesterol levels, and high triglycerides)

- High blood pressure (over 140/90)

- Excess growth of hair on the face, chest, stomach, thumbs, or toes

- Male-pattern baldness or thinning hair

- Acne, oily skin, or dandruff

- Patches of thickened and dark brown or black skin on the neck, groin, underarms, or skin folds

- Skin tags, or tiny excess flaps of skin in the armpits or neck area

How is PCOS diagnosed?

Diagnosing PCOS involves several steps. Your doctor will take a detailed medical history about your menstrual cycle and reproductive history, including information about methods of birth control and pregnancies. You also will receive a pelvic and physical exam. During a pelvic exam, the doctor is able to feel the swelling of the cysts on your ovary. Once cysts are found, the doctor may perform a vaginal ultrasound, or a screening to examine the cysts and the endometrium (lining of the uterus). If your doctor suspects you have PCOS, he or she may recommend having blood tests to measure hormone levels.

Women with PCOS can have high levels of hormones, such as test-osterone. Your doctor also may test your insulin and glucose levels, to look for diabetes or insulin resistance (inefficient use of insulin in the body). Many women with PCOS have these conditions.

Lastly, your doctor may test your levels of cholesterol and triglyc-erides since they often are abnormal in women with PCOS. Once your doctor makes a diagnosis, you will work together to decide how to best treat and manage your condition.

Does PCOS put women at risk for other conditions?

Women with PCOS can be at an increased risk for developing sev-eral other conditions.

Irregular menstrual periods and the absence of ovulation cause women to produce estrogen, but not progesterone. Without progest-erone, which causes the endometrium to shed each month as a men-strual period, the endometrium may grow too much and undergo cell changes. This is a precancerous condition called endometrial hyper-plasia. If the thickened endometrium is not treated, over a long pe-riod of time it may turn into endometrial cancer. PCOS also is linked to other diseases that occur later in life, such as insulin resistance, Type II diabetes, high cholesterol, hardening of the arteries (athero-sclerosis), high blood pressure, and heart disease.

Depression or mood swings also are common in women with PCOS. Although more research is needed to find out about this link, there are studies linking depression to diabetes. Therefore, in PCOS, depres-sion may be related to insulin resistance. It also could be a result of the hormonal imbalances and the cosmetic symptoms of the condition. Acne, hair loss, and other symptoms of PCOS can lead to poor self-esteem. Infertility and miscarriages also can be very stressful. Medi-cations that restore the balance to hormone levels or antidepressants can help these feelings.

How is PCOS treated?

Because there is no cure for PCOS, it needs to be managed to pre-vent further problems. There are many medications to control the symptoms of PCOS. Doctors most commonly prescribe the birth con-trol pill for this purpose. Birth control pills regulate menstruation, reduce androgen levels, and help to clear acne. Your doctor will talk to you about whether the birth control pill is right for you and which kind to take. Other drugs can help with cosmetic problems. There also are drugs available to control blood pressure and cholesterol. Progestins and insulin-sensitizing medications can be taken to induce a menstrual period and restore normal cycles. Eating a balanced diet low in carbohydrates and maintaining a healthy weight can help lessen the symptoms of PCOS. Regular exercise helps weight loss and also aids the body in reducing blood glucose levels and using insulin more efficiently.

Although it is not recommended as the first course of treatment, surgery called ovarian drilling is available to treat PCOS. This involves laparoscopy, which is done under general anesthesia on an outpatient basis. A very small incision is made above or below the navel, and a small instrument that acts like a telescope is inserted into the abdomen. During laparoscopy, the doctor then can make punctures in the ovary with a small needle carrying an electric current to destroy a small portion of the ovary. The success rate is less than 50% and there is a risk of developing adhesions or scar tissue on the ovary.

Chapter 22

Vaginal and Vulvar Disorders

Chapter Contents

Section 22.1

Vaginal Infections and Vaginitis

Excerpted from "Vaginal Infections and Vaginitis," U.S. Department
of Health and Human Services, National Women's Health Information
Center (NWHIC), October 2000.

What is vaginitis?

Vaginal infections are often accompanied by vaginitis, which is an
inflammation of the vagina characterized by discharge, irritation, and/
or itching. The cause of vaginitis cannot be adequately determined
solely on the basis of symptoms or a physical examination. Laboratory tests allowing microscopic evaluation of vaginal fluid are required
for a correct diagnosis. A variety of effective drugs are available for
treating vaginal infections and accompanying vaginitis.

What is bacterial vaginosis?

Bacterial vaginosis (BV) is the most common cause of vaginitis
symptoms among women of childbearing age. BV (previously called
nonspecific vaginitis) can be transmitted through sexual activity although the organisms responsible also have been found in young
women who are not sexually active. BV is due to a change in the balance among different types of bacteria in the vagina. Additionally,
intrauterine devices (IUDs) increase the risk of acquiring bacterial
vaginosis.

What is trichomoniasis?

Trichomoniasis, sometimes referred to as trich, is a common STD
that affects 2 to 3 million Americans yearly. It is caused by a single-
celled protozoan parasite called *Trichomonas vaginalis*. Trichomoniasis is primarily an infection of the urogenital tract: the urethra is the
most common site of infection in men, and the vagina is the most common site of infection in women.

What is a vaginal yeast infection?

Vulvovaginal candidiasis (VVC), sometimes referred to as candidal vaginitis, monilial infection, or vaginal yeast infection, is a common cause of vaginal irritation. It has been estimated that approximately 75 percent of all women will experience at least one episode of VVC during their lifetime. There is no direct evidence that VVC is transmitted by sexual intercourse.

Section 22.2

Bacterial Vaginosis (BV)

Excerpted from "Bacterial Vaginosis," National Center for HIV, STD and TB Prevention, Division of Sexually Transmitted Diseases, September 2000.

What is bacterial vaginosis?

Bacterial vaginosis (BV) is the most common vaginal infection in women of childbearing age, and it is sometimes accompanied by discharge, odor, pain, itching, or burning.

Women with BV often have an abnormal vaginal discharge with an unpleasant odor. Some women report a strong fish-like odor, especially after intercourse. The discharge is usually white or gray; it can be thin. Women with BV may also have burning during urination or itching around the outside of the vagina, or both. Some women with BV report no signs or symptoms at all.

Who is at risk for bacterial vaginosis?

Any woman can get BV. However, some activities or behaviors can upset the normal balance of bacteria in the vagina and put women at increased risk: having a new sex partner or multiple sex partners; douching; or using an intrauterine device (IUD) for contraception. Pregnant women are at increased risk for complications of BV.

What is the treatment for bacterial vaginosis?

BV is treatable with antimicrobial medicines prescribed by a health care provider. Two different medicines are recommended as treatment for BV: metronidazole or clindamycin. Either can be used with non-pregnant or with pregnant women, but the recommended dosages differ. Women with BV who are HIV-positive should receive the same treatment as those who are HIV-negative. BV can recur after treatment.

Section 22.3

Genital Candidiasis (Yeast Infections)

"Genital Candidiasis—General Information," Centers for Disease Control and Prevention, National Center for Infectious Diseases, Division of Bacterial and Mycotic Diseases, December 2002.

What is genital candidiasis/VVC?

Candidiasis, also known as a yeast infection or VVC, is a common fungal infection that occurs when there is overgrowth of the fungus called *Candida*. *Candida* is always present in the body in small amounts. However, when an imbalance occurs, such as when the normal acidity of the vagina changes or when hormonal balance changes, *Candida* can multiply. When that happens, symptoms of candidiasis appear.

Women with VVC usually experience genital itching or burning, with or without a cottage cheese-like vaginal discharge. Males with genital candidiasis may experience an itchy rash on the penis.

How common is genital candidiasis/VVC, and who can get it?

Nearly 75% of all adult women have had at least one genital yeast infection in their lifetime. On rare occasions, men may also experience genital candidiasis. VVC occurs more frequently and more severely in people with weakened immune systems. There are some other conditions that may put a woman at risk for genital candidiasis: pregnancy; diabetes mellitus; use of broad-spectrum antibiotics; and use of corticosteroid medications

How is genital candidiasis/VVC transmitted?

Most cases of *Candida* infection are caused by the person's own *Candida* organisms. *Candida* yeasts usually live in the mouth, gastrointestinal tract, and vagina without causing symptoms. Symptoms develop only when *Candida* becomes overgrown in these sites. Rarely, *Candida* can be passed from person to person, such as through sexual intercourse.

How is genital candidiasis/VVC treated?

Antifungal drugs which are taken orally, applied directly to the affected area, or used vaginally are the drugs of choice for vaginal yeast infections. Although these drugs usually work to cure the infection (80%-90% success rate), infections that do not respond to treatment are becoming more common, especially in HIV-infected women receiving long-term antifungal therapy. Prolonged and frequent use of these treatments can lessen their effectiveness.

Section 22.4

Vulvar Problems

American College of Obstetricians and Gynecologists. *Vulvar Problems.* (Patient Education Pamphlet No. AP088). Washington, DC. © ACOG 2001.

Certain health problems can affect the vulva (the outer part of the female genital area). Some problems are minor. Others are more serious. Finding and treating changes early can help prevent more serious problems. You can help find problems by doing a vulvar self-exam.

How to Find Vulvar Problems

Just as you would examine your breasts or skin for changes, you should examine your vulva. A good way to screen for vulvar problems is to do a vulvar self-exam once a month.

Why Do a Self-Exam?

The vulvar self-exam will help you to be aware of any changes in the vulvar area that could signal a problem.

What Am I Looking For?

When you examine your vulva, you should look for:

- Redness
- Swelling
- Dark or light spots
- Blisters
- Bumps
- Any other changes

Tell your doctor if you see any changes or have symptoms that don't go away. Symptoms include:

- Itching
- Bleeding
- Discomfort
- Burning

If a problem does occur, you are more likely to find it at an early stage if you have examined yourself regularly.

Types of Vulvar Problems

Contact dermatitis. Contact dermatitis is caused by irritation of the skin of the vulva. It is not always easy to find the cause.

The main symptoms of contact dermatitis are redness and itching.

Yeast infections. Yeast infections are the most common type of vulvar infections.

Sexually transmitted diseases. Sexually transmitted diseases (STDs) can affect the vulva.

- *Genital warts.* Genital warts (condyloma), like warts on other parts of the body, are caused by human papillomavirus (HPV). They often are spread through sexual contact.

- *Genital herpes.* Genital herpes infection is caused by herpes simplex virus. It can be spread through sexual contact.

Problems in other areas. Problems that affect other parts of the body also may affect the vulva. Psoriasis, for instance, is a skin disease that can appear on the vulva as red, thick, scaly patches that may itch.

Vulvodynia. Vulvodynia means vulvar pain. The symptoms of vulvodynia include burning, stinging, irritation or rawness.

Vulvar dystrophy. A vulvar dystrophy is abnormal skin on the vulva. The skin can be too thin (lichen sclerosus), too thick (hyperplasia), or a mixture of both.

Vulvar intraepithelial neoplasia. Vulvar intraepithelial neoplasia (VIN) is a type of precancer. Precancer means it may turn into cancer if it is not found and treated early.

Invasive cancer. Invasive cancer of the vulva occurs most often in areas of the vulva where there is chronic inflammation or VIN. Symptoms include itching, discomfort, and bleeding.

Melanoma. Melanoma is a form of skin cancer. During a vulvar self-exam, look for changing moles or dark spots on your skin that have edges that are not even.

Finally

The vulvar self-exam can help alert you to vulvar problems. Talk to your doctor about any changes or symptoms you notice.

Section 22.5

Vaginitis

What is vaginitis?

It is any irritation in the vagina. It often causes an abnormal discharge.

How common is vaginitis?

Vaginitis is one of the most common reasons women seek health care. You will most likely have it some time in your life. You may have it more than once. It usually is not serious. But it can be annoying and uncomfortable.

How can I tell if I have vaginitis?

You will have a vaginal irritation or an abnormal vaginal discharge. The discharge may have an unpleasant odor. You may notice the odor more right after vaginal intercourse. You also may have vaginal itching or burning. And you may feel as if you need to urinate more often than usual.

What are normal vaginal fluids like?

They are either thick and whitish or slippery and clear. It depends on where you are in your menstrual cycle. There is little odor and no itching or burning. Regular bathing keeps the fluids from getting stale or uncomfortable.

The fluids come from the walls of your vagina. They also come from your cervix at certain times in your cycle. They leave the body through the vagina.

How much fluid you produce depends on the hormones that guide your menstrual cycle. Usually there is more fluid just before you ovulate, when you are pregnant, or when you are sexually excited.

You will have less fluid just before your period and while you breastfeed.

What are vaginal fluids for?

- They wash the vagina clean.
- They lubricate it during sexual intercourse.
- They nourish acid-producing bacteria that fight infections.

What are abnormal vaginal fluids like?

Watch for changes in color, quantity, or texture of the fluid; unpleasant odors; bleeding, spotting, or bloody discoloration; or itching and/or burning of the vagina or vulva.

What causes abnormal vaginal discharges?

They are caused by vaginal infections or irritation (vaginitis), cervical infections or irritation (cervicitis), or sexually transmitted infections.

What causes vaginitis?

Vaginitis is caused by infections, lack of the hormone estrogen, irritants, or allergies. The infections that cause vaginitis are candidiasis, bacterial vaginosis, and trichomoniasis.

What is atrophic vaginitis?

Atrophic vaginitis is a vaginal irritation without a discharge. It is caused by the lack of estrogen due to childbirth—especially if it is followed by breastfeeding, menopause, removal of the ovaries, or radiation treatments. Atrophic vaginitis occasionally occurs in girls before their first period.

Lack of estrogen dries and thins vaginal tissue. It may also cause spotting. Estrogen creams and oral tablets can help restore lubrication and decrease soreness and irritation.

What irritants can cause vaginitis?

Objects and chemicals left in the vagina may cause irritations that lead to vaginitis. Do not leave tampons, toilet tissue, contraceptives, or other objects in the vagina longer than necessary.

What can stimulate allergies that can cause vaginitis?

Some women are allergic to substances put in the vagina, including chemicals, medicines, latex condoms, diaphragms and cervical caps, and spermicides.

What is cervicitis?

It is an irritation of the cervix. It can be caused by infections like gonorrhea, chlamydia, or herpes. Less commonly it occurs in women who are sensitive to certain chemicals, including those in spermicides, latex, and tampons. There may be an abnormal discharge from the cervix. It can look and feel just like a vaginal discharge. That's why cervicitis is often confused with vaginitis.

What is vulvitis?

It is an irritation of the vulva—the soft folds of skin outside the vagina. It may result from a yeast infection or the discharge caused by vaginitis.

The vulva and vagina may also be irritated by:

- scented or colored toilet paper
- perfumed soaps or bubble baths
- shampoos and hair conditioners
- laundry detergents (especially enzyme-activated cold-water formulas)
- feminine hygiene sprays
- spermicides
- douches that are too strong or used too often
- hot tub and swimming pool water
- wearing tight pants, underwear, or pantyhose without a cotton crotch
- wearing wet bathing suits for long periods of time

- rubbing against a bicycle seat
- horseback riding

Section 22.6

Vulvodynia

This fact sheet is reprinted with permission from The Interstitial Cystitis Association. © 1999. For more information, call 800-HELP-ICA (800-435-7422), or visit www.ichelp.org.

What Is Vulvodynia?

The term vulvodynia is derived from "vulva" and the Greek word "odynia" meaning pain. There are four basic types of vulvodynia, and they are not always easy to distinguish from each other: vulvar vestibulitis, dysesthetic vulvodynia, cyclic vulvovaginitis (yeast-related), and vulvar dermatoses. Many doctors are still not familiar with vulvodynia and, as a result, patients are frequently misdiagnosed or go undiagnosed altogether. The pain of vulvodynia isn't always accompanied by visible skin changes and sometimes patients are told, "It's all in your head." But the condition is very real.

The Vulva

The vulva is considered to be the visible parts of the female genitals. The parts most often affected by vulvodynia include the inner labia, the clitoral glans, the paraurethral (Skene) glands located on each side of the urethral opening, the vulvovaginal (Bartholin) glands located on each side of the vaginal opening, the membranes surrounding the vaginal opening (called the introitus), small minor vestibular glands around the vaginal opening, and the hymen.

Four Types of Vulvodynia

The four types of vulvodynia are described. Careful diagnostic evaluation is important in order to distinguish these conditions from each other and from others with similar symptoms and to choose the most effective treatment.

- Vulvar vestibulitis—Inflammation around the vestibule, or opening to the vagina. This condition may occur alone or in combination with other types of vulvar pain. Symptoms of vulvar vestibulitis include sensations of burning, dry, raw, or tight skin, and may range from mild to severe. Pain is usually caused by external touch, or by pressure caused by intercourse, tampon insertion, tight pants, bicycling, or horseback riding. A few patients, however, may have symptoms without touching or pressure. Some patients with vulvar vestibulitis only have discomfort with intercourse. Others are uncomfortable on a daily basis and find it difficult to sit or walk. Some women cannot tolerate intercourse, but others can, although there is usually some degree of discomfort. Women with severe, enduring pain may develop vaginismus, a spasm of the pelvic floor muscles that makes intercourse or tampon insertion difficult or impossible.

- Dysesthetic vulvodynia—Vulvar pain caused by irritated or inflamed nerves. Pain may encompass the inner labia, or may extend beyond the vulva to the anus or groin area, or down the inner thighs. Some women experience sharp pains or deep aching. This type is most common in postmenopausal women and women with fibromyalgia and may also be seen with interstitial cystitis.

- Cyclic vulvovaginitis—The yeast *Candida* normally inhabits the mouth, vagina, intestinal tract, and skin. If *Candida* overgrows in the vagina or on the vulva, it can cause itching, burning, inflammation, and swelling. *Candida* may affect the vulva without causing any obvious vaginal discharge. Skin may tear or split from swelling. The cause of chronic *Candida* infection is unknown, but various theories have suggested an allergy to yeast or fermented products, immune suppression, or some type of autoimmune response to yeast. Symptoms may flare around the time of menses.

- Vulvar or mucous dermatoses—Skin disorders that occur on the vulva's membranes may cause chronic itching or burning. When scratched, these areas become inflamed, more irritated and hypersensitive, and can be caused, or made worse, by overuse of topical medications or frequent douching. This category includes several skin eruptions characterized by the term lichen, which merely describes a tough, scaly, or peeling appearance. The most common is lichen simplex, but lichen sclerosis and lichen planus are two other skin problems that affect the vulva.

Who Gets Vulvodynia?

For reasons that are unclear, approximately 70% of women with vulvodynia are white with fair complexions. Most patients are of childbearing age, but young girls and postmenopausal women can get the condition as well. Vulvar vestibulitis and dysesthetic vulvodynia are the most common forms of vulvodynia that occur in IC [interstitial cystitis] patients. A study published in the journal *Urology* (May 1997) revealed that 10% of women with interstitial cystitis also have symptoms of vulvodynia.

What Causes Vulvodynia?

The precise cause of vulvodynia is unknown. Various theories suggest infection (viral, fungal, or bacterial); an allergic response to environmental irritants; an autoimmune response to the body's own chemistry; increased or high concentration of oxalate crystals in the urine; irritation of the muscles that support the bladder, uterus, and rectum (called the pelvic floor muscles); or irritation of the nerves that innervate the vulva. There is no evidence that vulvodynia is a sexually transmitted disease—except for *Candida*, which can be passed from partner to partner during sexual activity.

How Is Vulvodynia Diagnosed?

The hallmark of vulvar vestibulitis is an exquisite sensitivity of the tiny gland openings at the entrance to the vagina when touched with a cotton-tipped applicator. This is called the touch test. In addition, about two thirds of patients with vulvar vestibulitis have visible, tiny red spots at these points. Others may have inflamed surface blood vessels that the doctor can see with the aid of a magnifying instrument called a colposcope.

In dysesthetic vulvodynia there may or may not be visible skin irritation and generalized sensations of irritation or burning, not related to touch or pressure. If skin rashes are present, their cause should be investigated.

Even when *Candida* is suspected of causing chronic vulvar irritation, it cannot always be seen on cultures. It is thought that some women with a history of *Candida* infections may develop a hypersensitivity to very low concentrations of *Candida*.

Vulvar dermatoses are skin disorders, but it is important to rule out overuse of medications (especially topical steroids), or infectious causes (such as herpes, human papillomavirus, and allergic reactions). Skin lesions need to be evaluated and classified in order to choose the most effective treatment, so a biopsy may be helpful in this category.

Treatments

Like other chronic conditions, vulvodynia can have periods of flare and remission. At present, there are treatments that offer partial or complete relief, including:

- Oral medications. Antihistamines or sedatives such as Atarax and Vistaril inhibit mast cells from releasing substances that can irritate mucous membranes. Medications that may control dysesthetic vulvodynia caused by nerve irritation include tricyclic antidepressants such as Elavil and Tofranil and anticonvulsants such as Tegretol and Neurontin.

- Biofeedback programs or Kegel exercises done at home can strengthen the pelvic muscles. These exercises may also relieve vaginismus muscle spasms. Biofeedback equipment can ensure that you are doing the exercises correctly and can monitor progress.

- Interferon, an antiviral drug injected into the affected area, works best in patients who also have human papillomavirus.

- Anti-*Candida* creams such as clotrimazole or azole. For stubborn cases, low dose, suppressive therapy of Diflucan once or twice a week may be required for several months.

- Low-oxalate diet and supplements of calcium citrate. Oxalate crystals, which are normal byproducts of the body's metabolism, are excreted in the urine. Oxalates are very acidic and can irritate the mucous membranes of the vulva when overproduced. One theory maintains that an oxalate insult to the skin over a long period of time is the cause of vulvar pain. Calcium citrate alkalizes the urine and suppresses the secretion of oxalates. A low-carbohydrate, low-oxalate diet may also be helpful. Foods that are high in oxalates include all beans, beer, beets, berries, celery, chard, chocolate, eggplant, some grapes, green peppers, peanuts, rutabagas, spinach, squash, and tofu, to name a few.

- Surgery removes the hypersensitive tissue of the vestibule and hymen. It works best for women with pure vulvar vestibulitis, who experience pain only upon touch (tampon insertion, intercourse). Often considered as a last resort, surgery has a high success rate for appropriate candidates.

Self-Help Tips

Medical treatments for vulvodynia may not always work, or if they do, they may take a while to take effect. In the meantime, there are a number of self-help remedies that patients and their doctors have found that provide some relief or may prevent flare-ups or worsening of symptoms. These include:

- Wear only cotton underwear and loose clothing. Try stockings and thigh highs instead of pantyhose.

- During sex, avoid the use of lubricants that contain preservatives and chemicals. Pure almond oil or vegetable oil or commercial lubricants with glycerine (such as Astroglide) are usually tolerated the best. Apply at the initiation of sexual activity, since being touched is often as painful as intercourse itself.

- Use only white or unbleached toilet tissue and 100% cotton fiber sanitary products.

- Try baking soda soap for washing clothes. Wash new underwear before wearing and always rinse thoroughly after hand washing to remove soap residue. Avoid fabric softener liquids or dryer sheets.

- Avoid the use of perfumed creams and soaps, Vaseline, oils, lanolin, bubble bath, bath oils or feminine deodorant products.

- Use a bidet (a low basin with a spray device used for washing the genitals) if one is available.

- Baking soda douches may temporarily soothe inflamed areas, or rinsing the vulva with clear water from a squeeze bottle after urinating may help ease burning.

- Wash hair in the sink to avoid getting shampoo on the vulvar area in the shower.

- Place a compress of Aveeno (a powdered oatmeal bath treatment) over the vulva three to four times a day. Put two tablespoons of Aveeno in one quart of water. Mix in a jar and refrigerate. Patients report that this is especially helpful after intercourse or when symptoms are in a state of flare.

- Avoid contraceptive devices and creams that can irritate sensitive tissues.

- Don't sit or remain in a wet bathing suit.

- Avoid constipation or a full bladder, since any fullness may put pressure on the vulva. Exercise and lots of fiber from whole grains, fruits, and vegetables are the key to regularity. If this isn't enough, daily use of a psyllium product such as Metamucil will help.

- A prescription of 5% lidocaine (Xylocaine) topical ointment applied to the vestibule 10 to 15 minutes before intercourse may make sex more comfortable for some women. Check with your doctor for a prescription and instructions on use. Ointments may be tolerated better than creams because they don't contain any preservatives.

- Discharge from vaginal yeast or bacterial infections can irritate vulvar tissues. If you suspect such an infection, see your doctor promptly for diagnosis and treatment.

Always check with your doctor before initiating any home remedy or treatment.

Finding Help

Vulvodynia is often misdiagnosed or undiagnosed and consequently is mistreated or untreated. There is an urgent need for education and awareness about this condition among both patients and doctors.

Chapter 23

Gynecological Surgeries and Procedures

Chapter Contents

Section 23.1

Laparoscopy

American College of Obstetricians and Gynecologists. *Laparoscopy*. (Patient Education Pamphlet No. AP061). Washington, DC. © ACOG 1998. Reviewed by David A. Cooke, M.D. on July 25, 2003.

To diagnose certain problems, a doctor needs to look directly into the abdomen and at the reproductive organs. This can be done with laparoscopy.

The word laparoscopy comes from the Greek words that mean "look into the abdomen." A laparoscope is a small telescope that is inserted into the abdomen through a small incision (cut). It brings light into the abdomen so the doctor can see inside.

Uses of Laparoscopy

There are several reasons why laparoscopy may be recommended. Laparoscopy may be used if you have problems with infertility or if you want to be sterilized. It is also used to check for ectopic pregnancy, causes of pelvic pain, and masses.

Diagnosis and Surgery

Laparoscopy is often used to diagnose causes of abdominal pain. If the doctor finds that he or she can treat the condition during the procedure, diagnostic laparoscopy can turn into operative laparoscopy. This procedure is used to treat many health problems.

- Endometriosis. Tissue like endometrium (the lining of the uterus) sometimes grows in places outside of the uterus. One way to be certain that endometriosis is present is by laparoscopy.

- Adhesions. Sometimes tissues in the abdomen stick together and form scar tissue called adhesions. Adhesions can cause pain. They often can be separated during laparoscopy.

- Fibroids. Fibroids are growths that form on the inside, outside, or within the wall of the uterus. Laparoscopy can diagnose some fibroids.

- Ovarian cysts. Ovaries sometimes develop cysts (fluid-filled sacs). These cysts may be harmless, causing only mild pain.

- Hysterectomy. The laparoscope can be used to assist in a vaginal hysterectomy (removal of the uterus through the vagina). The laparoscope is used to help the doctor see inside the abdomen during part of the surgery.

Infertility and Sterilization

Women who have trouble getting pregnant may have laparoscopy to find problems like endometriosis or cysts.

Laparoscopy is also used for sterilization. In this operation, the doctor uses the laparoscope as a guide to block the fallopian tubes by cutting, clipping, or burning them.

Ectopic Pregnancy

When a woman has pain in her lower abdomen during early pregnancy, the doctor may suspect an ectopic pregnancy. An ectopic pregnancy is one that may be located in the tube instead of the uterus. It may rupture the tube and cause abdominal bleeding that may require emergency surgery.

Benefits of Laparoscopy

In the past, most surgery involving reproductive organs was done by laparotomy. Now, many of these same procedures are done through the laparoscope. There are many benefits to laparoscopy—a shorter hospital stay, smaller incisions, and a shorter recovery.

The Procedure

The anesthesia used depends on the type of procedure, your doctor's advice, and your personal choice. General anesthesia is usually used so that you will not be awake.

After the anesthesia is given, a small cut is made below or inside the navel. A gas, such as carbon dioxide or nitrous oxide, is usually put into the abdomen. The gas swells the abdomen so the pelvic reproductive organs can be seen more clearly.

The laparoscope is placed through the cut. Another cut is often made above the pubic region. Through this cut, an instrument is used to move the organs into view.

Other surgical instruments can be inserted through the scope or through another small cut. After the procedure, the instruments are removed and the gas released. The cuts are then closed, usually with stitches that dissolve. In a few hours you can go home. You should plan to have someone take you home and stay with you, at least for awhile.

Possible Problems

Although problems seldom occur with laparoscopy, there can be some complications. You may have some bleeding, reactions to the anesthesia, or injury to other organs.

Recovery

The recovery time from laparoscopy is much shorter than that from regular surgery. It is safe to resume normal activities as soon as you feel up to it, usually within a few days. If you are sexually active, talk with your doctor about when you can have sex again.

Finally

Laparoscopy can be useful in diagnosing and treating many gynecologic problems. It has taken the place of surgery in some cases and offers the benefits of fewer problems and shorter recovery.

Section 23.2

Dilation and Curettage (D&C)

D&C—also known as dilatation (dil-ah tay´-shun) and curettage
(koo-re tahzh´)—is a minor surgical procedure in which the surgeon
first dilates or opens the woman's cervix and then inserts a thin, spoon
shaped instrument. The instrument is then used to remove a sample
of the internal lining of the uterus, or to remove the portion of the
internal lining that is causing bleeding. Dilatation, therefore, stands
for opening the cervix; curettage means the scraping of the uterine
wall.

This section will explain:

- Why you may need to have a D&C
- How D&C is performed
- What to expect before and after the procedure

D&C is one of the most common surgical procedures. However, as
routine as a D&C is, no two women undergoing a D&C are alike. The
reasons for and the outcome of any D&C depend on your overall
health, your age, the severity of uterine bleeding, and any other abnormalities that may exist in your uterus, such as polyps (typically
harmless, benign growths).

This section is not intended to take the place of your surgeon's
professional opinion. Rather, the information presented here can help
you to begin to understand the basics of this surgical procedure. Read
this material carefully. If you have more questions, discuss them
openly with your doctor.

The Uterus and the Cervix

The uterus is a muscular, pear-shaped organ that has three main
functions:

1. to receive an egg that has been fertilized by sperm in the ovary

2. to nurture and house the fetus (unborn baby) during its development

3. to use its muscular walls to push the baby out when it is ready to be born

Because it is a muscular organ, the uterus has contractions or cramps that occur during the entire monthly cycle, even throughout pregnancy and delivery. The contractions are more intense during your menstrual period but they also occur throughout the month—you may not even feel them. At menstruation, the cervix opens to release blood and to shed the lining of the uterus, called the endometrium (en-doh me ´tree-um).

The cervix is located at the base of the uterus and serves as the valve between the uterus and the vagina. Through the cervical canal, semen enters the uterus, blood flows from the uterus during menstruation, and babies are delivered during birth.

Who Needs to Undergo a D&C?

It is estimated that 70 percent of all women who have a D&C performed are 15 to 44 years old. The procedure is done for two reasons: to diagnose a problem, and to treat a problem. By doing a D&C, your surgeon can evaluate the causes of any abnormal bleeding from your uterus, determine the cause of severe menstrual pain, or gain information about why you are unable to get pregnant. This elective procedure is also commonly performed after a miscarriage (losing the fetus) to empty the uterus of remaining tissue associated with the pregnancy.

- Abnormal uterine bleeding is the most common reason why a D&C is done. However, reproductive-age women may be treated with hormones to attempt to stabilize the uterine lining before an operation is advised. If hormone treatment is unsuccessful, a D&C is done to establish the cause of abnormal bleeding so that a normal bleeding pattern can be restored.

- Polyps are generally harmless (benign) growths that can occur in the cervix or uterus. A cervical polyp can be irritated by sexual intercourse. A uterine polyp can cause abnormal bleeding.

In either case, these conditions can be treated through a D&C, during which the polyp is scraped off. Removed polyps are routinely sent to a lab to make sure they are not cancerous.

- Fibroid tumors are modular benign tumors of the muscular wall of the uterus and are almost never cancerous. If one protrudes into the uterine cavity, however, abnormal bleeding may occur in rare situations. If bleeding is very heavy, a D&C can identify and sometimes scrape away a small tumor of this type, although usually a more extensive operation is required.

- D&C is sometimes done to remedy a condition called endometrial hyperplasia, in which the uterine lining has become too thick.

- Sometimes a woman experiences bleeding after menopause. If vaginal bleeding occurs after a cessation of at least six months, you should see a doctor immediately. He or she may recommend a D&C.

About the Procedure

D&C can be done on an inpatient or outpatient basis, in either a hospital or freestanding surgery center. Prior to the procedure, you may be given a sedative. An IV may be started either before or after you enter the operating room. The vaginal area will be washed.

There are three steps in the D&C procedure:

1. You will be positioned on your back on a gynecological table; your knees will be bent and your feet will be in stirrups. At this time, the surgeon will pass a series of dilators (narrow instruments of increasing thicknesses) into the vagina and the cervix, gradually opening the strongly contracted muscles of the cervix.

2. When the cervix is opened sufficiently, the surgeon will insert a curette (a thin spoon-like instrument) into the uterus to scrape the lining. Tissue and specimens will be removed and examined by the doctor and are sent to a pathology lab for evaluation.

3. A nurse will then put a sanitary napkin in place before you are taken to the recovery room. The operation takes about 10 minutes. You will be in the recovery room for about 30 minutes.

After the Procedure

In most cases, you will be discharged from the surgery center or hospital on the same day that a D&C is done. However, you may be kept longer if you have another medical condition, such as diabetes or heart disease, or if some complication arises from the procedure or the anesthetic used.

The results of the laboratory evaluation of the removed tissue are usually available in several days. At that time, your doctor will recommend treatment for conditions that are identified by the procedure.

You will be encouraged to walk to the bathroom and resume normal nonstrenuous activity as soon as you are comfortable doing so. Expect slight bleeding and staining for anywhere from five to 14 days following a D&C.

You should refrain from sexual intercourse and the use of tampons for at least seven days or until the bleeding has stopped. Use sanitary napkins during this time. Also, douches should be avoided for two weeks after the operation because the operated area may be exposed to bacteria that can cause infection or inflammation.

Following the D&C, you will be given oral medication for any postoperative pain, such as severe cramps. Most pain disappears within 24 hours. You may also be given an antibiotic to prevent infection.

A D&C procedure leaves no scar. If your occupation does not involve heavy physical work, you can plan on returning to your job within two to four days.

Surgery by Surgeons

A fully trained surgeon is a physician who, after medical school, has gone through years of training in an accredited residency program to learn the specialized skills of a surgeon. One good sign of a surgeon's competence is certification by a national surgical board approved by the American Board of Medical Specialties. All such board-certified surgeons have satisfactorily completed an approved residency training program and have passed a rigorous specialty examination.

The letters F.A.C.S. (Fellow of the American College of Surgeons) after a surgeon's name are a further indication of a physician's qualifications. Surgeons who become Fellows of the College have passed a comprehensive evaluation of their education, training, and professional qualifications, and their credentials have been found to be consistent with the standards established and demanded by the College.

Section 23.3

Hysterectomy

Hysterectomy is the surgical removal of the uterus, or womb. This chapter will explain:

- Why you may need to have a hysterectomy
- How hysterectomy is performed
- What to expect before and after the operation

Remember, no two women undergoing a hysterectomy are alike. The reasons for and the outcome of any surgical procedure depend on your age, the severity of your problem, and your general health. This brochure is not intended to take the place of your surgeon's professional opinion. Rather, it is intended to help you understand the basic elements of this surgical procedure. Read this information carefully. If you have questions after reading this material, discuss them openly and honestly with your surgeon.

Why Are Hysterectomies Performed?

Hysterectomy may be performed to treat a variety of gynecological (female reproductive system) problems. It is an elective procedure 90 percent of the time.

Today most hysterectomies are done to treat benign (non-cancerous) fibroid tumors of the uterus. While not life-threatening, these growths cause pelvic pain, excessive bleeding, or pain during sexual intercourse. Fibroid tumors are common and usually do not require surgery. Other forms of treatment which preserve the uterus and childbearing capacity are also available. You should discuss these options with your surgeon.

Endometriosis is a condition in which the tissue lining the uterus becomes displaced and grows in other parts of the abdomen, where it can cause pain. Endometriosis is the second most common reason for a woman to have a hysterectomy. However, the practice of treating endometriosis by performing hysterectomy has been declining in the last decade because other treatments have evolved. You should discuss these other options with your surgeon first to see if another treatment for endometriosis may be effective for you.

Prolapse of the uterus is another reason why some women decide to undergo a hysterectomy. In this condition, the uterus descends or sags into the vagina due to stretching of the ligaments and fibrous tissue that usually hold it in place.

Women with cancer of the uterus or cancer of the cervix require special types of treatment which may include a simple or radical hysterectomy. These women should seek the counsel of a gynecologic oncologist.

Are All Hysterectomies the Same?

You may hear different names used to refer to this type of operation. That is because there are different types of hysterectomies. A total hysterectomy or panhysterectomy applies only to the removal of the uterus and cervix. When the ovaries and fallopian tubes on both sides of the uterus are also removed, the procedure is called a hysterectomy and bilateral salpingo-oophorectomy ("salpingo" is from the Greek word for "tube," while "oophor" is from the Greek word for "bearing eggs," that is, the ovaries). A radical hysterectomy is a much more extensive procedure and is only performed in special situations such as cancer of the uterus or cervix. It includes removal of the uterus, cervix, and surrounding tissue, the upper vagina, and usually the pelvic lymph nodes. A surgeon with special training in gynecologic oncology performs this type of procedure.

Is Hysterectomy Mainly for Older Women?

You may be surprised to know that 42, a relatively young age, is the average age of women undergoing hysterectomy. More than three-fourths of all women who have a hysterectomy are between 20 and 49 years of age.

Is There Any Reason to Avoid or Delay Hysterectomy?

It is not sensible to have a hysterectomy in order to prevent cancer of the cervix or uterus. In this case, the risks of having a major operation outweigh any supposed cancer-protection benefits. Furthermore, hysterectomy is not considered to be the first choice for sterilization in most healthy women. Another procedure, tubal ligation, is a cheaper, easier, and safer method for most women.

Hysterectomy may not be advisable if your problem has not been adequately diagnosed. For instance, if you have pelvic pain that is not specifically caused by the uterus, a hysterectomy may not relieve your pain. The pain may be due to problems in your digestive, urinary, or skeletal systems. In these cases, your doctor will want to do the proper tests and X rays to locate the exact source of your pain. In addition to the tests and X rays indicated, a diagnostic laparoscopy may be helpful in selecting the appropriate treatment.

Similarly, most women with abnormal bleeding, especially menopausal or post-menopausal women, should have an endometrial biopsy (EMB) or a dilatation and curettage (D&C) procedure to rule out uterine cancer before undergoing a hysterectomy. Hysteroscopy (a surgical procedure in which a gynecologist uses a small lighted telescopic instrument to view the inside of the uterus) should not be performed until uterine cancer has been ruled out by D&C or EMB. If cancer is present within the uterus, the hysteroscope has the potential to push it out through the fallopian tubes into the abdominal cavity.

Finally, women who are obese, who have diabetes, high blood pressure, or some other chronic conditions, are at increased risk during any type of operation. For these women, hysterectomy should only be considered if reasonable alternatives have been exhausted.

If you have any questions about hysterectomy, ask your doctor. If it would make you feel more confident about your medical treatment, get a second opinion from another physician who is qualified to diagnose and treat your condition. Unless you have a severe pelvic infection, or uncontrollable bleeding, you do not have to rush into having a hysterectomy. Even with a diagnosis of cancer, a short delay to seek another qualified opinion is usually safe and worthwhile.

How Do I Decide If I Should Have a Hysterectomy?

You will no longer be able to get pregnant after a hysterectomy. Thus, before you choose elective hysterectomy, you must consider both the severity of your problem and your desire to have children in the future.

Although this operation may improve your quality of life by relieving chronic symptoms such as pain or bleeding, some women are willing to tolerate these conditions.

225

Ask yourself:

- Do I want to become pregnant in the future?
- How do I feel about not having a uterus?
- What is my husband's (or partner's) attitude toward this operation?

Ask your surgeon:

- What will happen if I don't have a hysterectomy?
- What are the risks of a hysterectomy in my particular case?
- Is my condition likely to improve on its own, stay the same, or get worse?
- Is a hysterectomy medically necessary or recommended to relieve my particular symptoms?

Before your operation, you will be asked to sign a document giving your "informed consent" to the operation. This form lets you know any risks or possible complications that can be caused by the surgical procedure. Some states have specific laws that pertain to hysterectomies. These laws require surgeons to explain the alternatives and the risks of the procedure and are intended to make sure you understand the potential after-effects of the operation.

How Is Hysterectomy Performed?

The surgeon can remove the uterus through a surgical incision made either inside the vagina or in the abdomen. In both the vaginal and abdominal approaches, the surgeon detaches the uterus from the fallopian tubes and ovaries as well as from the upper vagina.

Abdominal Hysterectomy

When a hysterectomy is performed through an incision in the abdomen, it allows the surgeon to see the pelvic organs easily and gives him or her more operating space than is permitted in a vaginal hysterectomy.

Thus, for large pelvic tumors or suspected cancer, your surgeon may decide to do the procedure abdominally. Patients who have an abdominal hysterectomy require a longer hospital stay than those who have a vaginal hysterectomy. In addition, they may experience greater discomfort immediately following the operation, and will have a visible scar. However, the surgeon often can make a less noticeable horizontal incision, called a bikini-cut, that extends along the top of the pubic hairline.

Vaginal Hysterectomy

The vaginal approach to hysterectomy is ideal when the uterus is not enlarged or when the uterus has dropped as a result of the weakening of surrounding muscles. This approach is technically more difficult than the abdominal procedure because it offers the surgeon less operating space and less opportunity to view the pelvic organs. However, it may be preferred if a patient has a prolapsed uterus, if the patient is obese, or in some cases has early cervical or uterine cancer. A vaginal hysterectomy leaves no external scar.

A variation on vaginal hysterectomy is LAVH (laparoscopic-assisted vaginal hysterectomy). A laparoscope is a device the surgeon can use to examine the inside of the pelvis. LAVH is an alternative for women who have ovarian disease but previously had only one choice: an abdominal hysterectomy that leaves a long incision. With LAVH, much of the procedure is done through tiny incisions using a laparoscope. The rest of the procedure then can be finished vaginally.

Stages of Recovery

After the operation, you will likely remain in the recovery room for one to three hours. You may be given pain medication, and possibly antibiotics to prevent infection.

You will probably be able to walk around your room the day after your operation, depending on the type of procedure you underwent. Most patients go home the third day following an abdominal hysterectomy and by the first or second day after a vaginal hysterectomy or LAVH.

Complete recovery from abdominal hysterectomy usually takes six to eight weeks because the incision is typically five inches long. During your recovery, you can expect a gradual increase in activities. Avoid all lifting during the first two weeks of your recovery period and get plenty of rest. In the weeks following the surgical procedure, you can begin to do light chores, some driving, and even return to work, provided your occupation does not involve too much physical activity.

Around the sixth week following the operation, you can take tub baths and resume sexual activity. Women who have had vaginal hysterectomies generally recover more quickly.

Risks or Complications?

Hysterectomy is regarded as one of the safest operations. Nevertheless, no operation is without risk. Severe complications and even death occasionally occur with this operation.

The uterus is located between the ureters (small tubes which transport urine from the kidneys to the bladder) on each side, the urinary bladder in front, and the rectum behind. All of these structures are subject to injury, especially if the operation is difficult, as can occur with large fibroids, endometriosis, or cancer. Bleeding and infection can also occur, but most infections are now avoided by using antibiotics. Blood clots in the legs (DVT-deep vein thromboses) sometimes occur postoperatively and can break off and travel to the lungs causing a sometimes fatal pulmonary embolism (blood clot). These clots largely can be avoided in high-risk patients by using special stockings during the operation or by using blood thinners.

Long-Term Effects

After having a hysterectomy, you will no longer be able to get pregnant and will no longer have menstrual periods. If you were premenopausal (still menstruating) before the operation and have your fallopian tubes and ovaries removed, you will experience all of the symptoms of menopause as your body gets used to different hormone levels. These symptoms may include hot flashes and perhaps irritability and depression. If the symptoms are severe, your doctor may prescribe hormone replacement medication.

Hysterectomy usually has no physical effect on your ability to experience sexual pleasure or orgasm.

Following hysterectomy, the ovaries will continue to function; however, the actual occurrence of menopause will be difficult to determine since the uterus has been removed and the patient will no longer have periods. As the age of menopause, approximately age 50, is approached, symptoms such as hot flashes may warrant testing to see if hormone replacement therapy is indicated.

If you experience vaginal dryness, it can be remedied by using prescription hormone creams or pills, or water-soluble lubricants that you can purchase at the pharmacy.

A sense of loss following the removal of any organ is normal and takes time for adjustment. While depression following hysterectomy does not happen to everyone, it is more common if the operation was done because of cancer or severe illness, rather than as an elective operation. Additionally, if you are under age 40 or the operation interfered with your plans to have children, depression is more likely to occur. This depression can be temporary, depending on your general outlook on life, and the availability of a good support group of family and friends.

Most women experience an improvement of mood and increased sense of well-being following hysterectomy. For many, relief from fear of pregnancy results in heightened sexual enjoyment following the procedure.

Surgery by Surgeons

A fully trained surgeon is a physician who, after medical school, has gone through years of training in an accredited residency program to learn the specialized skills of a surgeon. One good sign of a surgeon's competence is certification by a national surgical board approved by the American Board of Medical Specialties. All such board-certified surgeons have satisfactorily completed an approved residency training program and have passed a rigorous specialty examination.

The letters F.A.C.S. (Fellow of the American College of Surgeons) after a surgeon's name are a further indication of a physician's qualifications. Surgeons who become Fellows of the College have passed a comprehensive evaluation of their education, training, and professional qualifications, and their credentials have been found to be consistent with the standards established and demanded by the College.

Part Three

Breast Health

Chapter 24

Normal Breast Development and Anatomy

Although the general shape of a breast is circular or tear-drop, breast tissue can be found from the collar bone to the bra line, and from the breast bone to the armpit. That is why it is important for you to examine that entire area during breast self examination, and for the surgeon to make a wide enough incision during a mastectomy.

Breasts are made up of milk-producing glands and milk-carrying ducts, imbedded in fatty tissue and fibrous supportive tissue. The glands are grouped in sections, called lobes. Each lobe has many smaller lobules which end in dozens of tiny grape-like bulbs where milk is produced. That is why breasts usually feel lumpy to the touch. Slender tubes called ducts carry the milk from the lobes to the nipple.

Two muscles, the pectorals major and the pectorals minor, are attached to the ribs under the breast. There are no muscles within the breast itself.

Arteries and veins carry blood to and from the breast, supplying it with nutrients and oxygen. Lymph ducts collect lymph (the fluid that leaks out of the blood vessels and accumulates between cells) and bring it back into the main circulation. Along the way, lymphatic fluid is filtered through small bean-shaped organs called lymph nodes.

Most of the lymphatic fluid from the breast drains toward the armpit area(the maxilla), where it is filtered through the maxillary lymph nodes.

How Breasts Grow and Change

From birth to old age, breasts go through more changes than almost any other organ in the body.

One to two years before menarche (the first menstrual period) breasts begin to grow under the influence of the female hormones estrogen and progesterone.

During reproductive years, variations in the levels of these hormones cause the breasts to go through monthly cycles: milk glands become engorged and the breasts swell, as if getting ready for a pregnancy, then return to their inactive state again.

At menopause, levels of hormones drop, many milk-producing glands shrink and disappear, and some of the breast tissue is replaced with fat.

All these changes sometimes damage the cells' DNA—the genetic material that tells the cell how to divide and grow. This damage may lead to cancer.

Vladimir Lange is a physician and the founder and CEO of Lange Productions, a leading producer of medical communications focusing on breast health and other health topics.

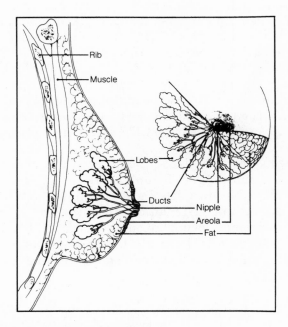

Figure 24.1. *Anatomy of the breast.*

Chapter 25

Breastfeeding

Why should I breastfeed?

Here are just some of the many good reasons why you should breastfeed your baby:

- Breast milk is the most complete form of nutrition for infants. Breast milk has just the right amount of fat, sugar, water, and protein that is needed for a baby's growth and development. Most babies find it easier to digest breast milk than they do formula.

- Breast milk has agents (called antibodies) in it to help protect infants from bacteria and viruses. Breastfed babies are more able to fight off infection and disease, such as diarrhea, ear infections, allergies and asthma. They are sick less often and have fewer visits to health care providers.

- Nursing uses up extra calories, making it easier to lose the pounds of pregnancy. It also helps the uterus to get back to its original size and lessens any bleeding you might have after giving birth.

- Breastfeeding lowers the risk of breast cancer and may lower the risk of ovarian cancer.

Excerpted from the publication by the U.S. Department of Health and Human Services, National Women's Health Information Center (NWHIC); July 2003. Available online at http://www.4woman.gov; accessed August 2003.

- Breastfeeding can help you bond with your baby. Physical contact is important to newborns and can help them feel more secure, and warm and comforted.

How long should I breastfeed?

One of the best things that only you can do is to breastfeed your baby for as long as possible. The longer a mom and baby breastfeeds, the greater the benefits are for both mom and baby.

Babies should be fed with breast milk only—no formula—for the first six months of life. Ideally, though, babies should receive breast milk through the first year of life, or for as long as both you and your baby wish. Solid foods can be added to your baby's diet, while you continue to breastfeed, when your baby is six months old. For at least the first six months, breastfed babies don't need supplements of water, juice, or other fluids. These can interfere with your milk supply if they are introduced during this time.

If I decide to breastfeed, is there a right way to do so?

There are several tips for making breastfeeding a good experience for both you and your baby. However, you can prevent the most common challenges or problems by following the three most important tips about breastfeeding:

- Nurse early and often. Try to breastfeed your baby within the first hour after birth. Newborns need to nurse frequently, at least every two hours, and not on a strict schedule. This stimulates your breasts to produce plenty of milk.

- Nurse with the nipple and the areola (brown area surrounding the nipple) in the baby's mouth, not just the nipple.

- Breastfeed on demand. Since breast milk is more easily digested than formula, breastfed babies eat more frequently than bottle-fed babies. Babies nurse less frequently as they get older and start solid foods. Watch your baby, not the clock, for signs of hunger, such as being more alert or active, mouthing (putting hands or fists to mouth and making sucking motion with mouth), or rooting (turning head in search of nipple). Crying is a late sign of hunger.

Chapter 26

Keeping Your Breasts Healthy

Breast cancer is the most common form of cancer in women in the U.S. today. Every woman is at risk, but many women don't know this fact: although there is no certain way to prevent the disease, there are ways that each woman can protect her health. This chapter encourages you to learn about breast cancer, and to help all women in your life do the same.

Early Detection of Breast Cancer

- Get a yearly mammogram (breast x-ray), starting at age 40 (or as directed by your doctor).

- Have your breasts examined by a doctor or nurse each year, starting at age 20.

- Learn the normal feel of your breasts, and check them yourself each month.

When detected early—often before it can be felt—breast cancer can be treated successfully. About 96 percent of women treated for breast cancer that is found early are alive five years later. Most women can be treated without losing their breast.

Reprinted with permission from *How to Take Charge of Your Breast Health*, a brochure published by the National Alliance of Breast Cancer Organizations (NABCO). © 2002 NABCO. All rights reserved. For additional information, call 888-80-NABCO, or visit www.nabco.org.

There are other steps to take for good breast health. Researchers are still exploring the benefits of leading an active lifestyle and maintaining a lifelong healthy weight. We now know that being overweight after menopause appears to increase breast cancer risk and that women who maintain a healthy weight or lose excess weight have a lower risk of breast cancer than overweight women.

Weight gain at certain places in your body (in your midsection) can affect your breast health. Many studies confirm that maintaining a lifelong healthy weight is good for your overall health and for your heart and bones.

Other Breast Cancer Prevention Strategies

- Maintain a diet low in fat that includes fruits, vegetables, and whole grains. Eating low-fat, high-fiber foods also has other proven health benefits, including reducing the risk of heart disease, colon cancer, and stroke.

- Exercise regularly. Exercise helps prevent osteoporosis and heart disease, and several studies have shown that regular exercise may reduce your breast cancer risk. Walk, bike, or do other activities that raise your heart rate, at least three times a week

- Avoid alcohol. Regular use of even small amounts of liquor, beer, or wine can increase breast cancer risk.

- Learn the pros and cons of postmenopausal hormone therapy and oral contraceptives (birth control pills). In a number of studies, medications that add estrogen to your body also increased breast cancer risk when taken for several years. Women who have a strong family history of breast cancer are often advised to avoid hormones. Each woman should discuss a range of approaches with her doctor, and make an informed decision based on her own personal history, symptoms, and needs.

- Know your family health history. Having close relatives—both female and male—with breast, ovarian, or other cancers may influence your own breast cancer risk. Learn as much as you can about your family's health and review this history with your doctor.

- Don't smoke. Smoking causes several types of cancer, heart disease, and other illnesses. It affects the health of others and can limit a woman's options for treatment and breast reconstruction.

Taking these steps will benefit your overall health and help you look and feel your best.

Chapter 27

Understanding Breast Changes

Introduction

Breast cancer is hard to ignore. It is the most common form of cancer among American women, and almost everyone knows at least one person who has been treated for it.

Understandably, women are concerned about getting breast cancer, and this concern prompts them to watch for breast changes. Breast changes are common. Even though most are not cancer, they can be worrisome.

About Breast Lumps and Other Changes

Over her lifetime, a woman can encounter a broad variety of breast conditions. These include normal changes that occur during the menstrual cycle as well as several types of benign lumps. What they have in common is that they are not cancer. Even for breast lumps that require a biopsy, some 80 percent prove to be benign.

Each breast has 15 to 20 sections, called lobes, each with many smaller lobules. The lobules end in dozens of tiny bulbs that can produce milk. Lobes, lobules, and bulbs are all linked by thin tubes called ducts. These ducts lead to the nipple, which is centered in a dark area of skin called the areola. The spaces between the lobules and ducts

Excerpted from "Understanding Breast Changes: A Health Guide for Women," National Cancer Institute, September 1998. Available online at http://www.cancer.gov. Reviewed and revised by David A. Cooke, M.D. on June 30, 2003.

are filled with fat. There are no muscles in the breast, but muscles lie under each breast and cover the ribs.

These normal features can sometimes make the breasts feel lumpy, especially in women who are thin or who have small breasts. In addition, from the time a girl begins to menstruate, her breasts undergo regular changes each month. Many doctors believe that nearly all breasts develop some lasting changes, beginning when the woman is about 30 years old. Eventually, about half of all women will experience symptoms such as lumps, pain, or nipple discharge. Generally these disappear with menopause.

Some studies show that the chances of developing benign breast changes are higher for a woman who has never had children, has irregular menstrual cycles, or has a family history of breast cancer. Benign breast conditions are less common among women who take birth control pills or who are overweight. Because they generally involve the glandular tissues of the breast, benign breast conditions are more of a problem for women of child-bearing age, who have more glandular breasts.

Types of Benign Breast Changes

Common benign breast changes fall into several broad categories. These include generalized breast changes, solitary lumps, nipple discharge, and infection and/or inflammation.

Generalized Breast Changes

Generalized breast lumpiness is known by several names, including fibrocystic disease changes and benign breast disease. Such lumpiness, which is sometimes described as ropy or granular, can often be felt in the area around the nipple and areola and in the upper-outer part of the breast. Such lumpiness may become more obvious as a woman approaches middle age and the milk-producing glandular tissue of her breasts increasingly gives way to soft, fatty tissue. Unless she is taking replacement hormones, this type of lumpiness generally disappears for good after menopause.

The menstrual cycle also brings cyclic breast changes. Many women experience swelling, tenderness, and pain before and sometimes during their periods. At the same time, one or more lumps or a feeling of increased lumpiness may develop because of extra fluid collecting in the breast tissue. These lumps normally go away by the end of the period.

During pregnancy, the milk-producing glands become swollen and the breasts may feel lumpier than usual. Although very uncommon, breast cancer has been diagnosed during pregnancy. If you have any questions about how your breasts feel or look, talk to your doctor.

Solitary Lumps

Benign breast conditions also include several types of distinct, solitary lumps. Such lumps, which can appear at any time, may be large or small, soft or rubbery, fluid-filled or solid.

Cysts are fluid-filled sacs. They occur most often in women ages 35 to 50, and they often enlarge and become tender and painful just before the menstrual period. They are usually found in both breasts. Some cysts are so small they cannot be felt; rarely, cysts may be several inches across. Cysts are usually treated by observation or by fine needle aspiration. They show up clearly on ultrasound.

Fibroadenomas are solid and round benign tumors that are made up of both structural (fibro) and glandular (adenoma) tissues. Usually, these lumps are painless and found by the woman herself. They feel rubbery and can easily be moved around. Fibroadenomas are the most common type of tumors in women in their late teens and early twenties, and they occur twice as often in African-American women as in other American women.

Fibroadenomas have a typically benign appearance on mammography (smooth, round masses with a clearly defined edge), and they can sometimes be diagnosed with fine needle aspiration. Although fibroadenomas do not become malignant, they can enlarge with pregnancy and breast-feeding. Most surgeons believe that it is a good idea to remove fibroadenomas to make sure they are benign.

Fat necrosis is the name given to painless, round, and firm lumps formed by damaged and disintegrating fatty tissues. This condition typically occurs in obese women with very large breasts. It often develops in response to a bruise or blow to the breast, even though the woman may not remember the specific injury. Sometimes the skin around the lumps looks red or bruised. Fat necrosis can easily be mistaken for cancer, so such lumps are removed in a surgical biopsy.

Sclerosing adenosis is a benign condition involving the excessive growth of tissues in the breast's lobules. It frequently causes breast pain. Usually the changes are microscopic, but adenosis can produce lumps, and it can show up on a mammogram, often as calcifications. Short of biopsy, adenosis can be difficult to distinguish from cancer. The usual approach is surgical biopsy, which furnishes both diagnosis and treatment.

Nipple Discharge

Nipple discharge accompanies some benign breast conditions. Since the breast is a gland, secretions from the nipple of a mature woman are not unusual, nor even necessarily a sign of disease. For example, small amounts of discharge commonly occur in women taking birth control pills or certain other medications, including sedatives and tranquilizers. If the discharge is being caused by a disease, the disease is more likely to be benign than cancerous.

Nipple discharges come in a variety of colors and textures. A milky discharge can be traced to many causes, including thyroid malfunction and oral contraceptives or other drugs. Women with generalized breast lumpiness may have a sticky discharge that is brown or green.

The doctor will take a sample of the discharge and send it to a laboratory to be analyzed. Benign sticky discharges are treated chiefly by keeping the nipple clean. A discharge caused by infection may require antibiotics.

One of the most common sources of a bloody or sticky discharge is an intraductal papilloma, a small, wartlike growth that projects into breast ducts near the nipple. Any slight bump or bruise in the area of the nipple can cause the papilloma to bleed. Single (solitary) intraductal papillomas usually affect women nearing menopause. If the discharge becomes bothersome, the diseased duct can be removed surgically without damaging the appearance of the breast.

Multiple intraductal papillomas, in contrast, are more common in younger women. They often occur in both breasts and are more likely to be associated with a lump than with nipple discharge. Multiple intraductal papillomas, or any papillomas associated with a lump, need to be removed.

Infection and/or Inflammation

Infection and/or inflammation, including mastitis and mammary duct ectasia, are characteristic of some benign breast conditions.

Mastitis (sometimes called postpartum mastitis) is an infection most often seen in women who are breastfeeding. A duct may become blocked, allowing milk to pool, causing inflammation, and setting the stage for infection by bacteria.

The breast appears red and feels warm, tender, and lumpy. In its earlier stages, mastitis can be cured by antibiotics. If a pus-containing abscess forms, it will need to be drained or surgically removed.

Mammary duct ectasia is a disease of women nearing menopause. Ducts beneath the nipple become inflamed and can become clogged. Mammary duct ectasia can become painful, and it can produce a thick and sticky discharge that is grey to green in color. Treatment consists of warm compresses, antibiotics, and, if necessary, surgery to remove the duct.

A word of caution: If you find a lump or other change in your breast, don't use this chapter to try to diagnose it yourself. There is no substitute for a doctor's evaluation.

Benign Breast Conditions and the Risk for Breast Cancer

Most benign breast changes do not increase a woman's risk for getting cancer. Recent studies show that only certain very specific types of microscopic changes put a woman at higher risk. These changes feature excessive cell growth, or hyperplasia.

About 70 percent of the women who have a biopsy showing a benign condition have no evidence of hyperplasia. These women are at no increased risk for breast cancer.

About 25 percent of benign breast biopsies show signs of hyperplasia, including conditions such as intraductal papilloma and scalloping adenosis. Hyperplasia slightly increases the risk of developing breast cancer. The remaining 5 percent of benign breast biopsies reveal both excessive cell growth—hyperplasia—and cells that are abnormal—atypical. A diagnosis of atypical hyperplasia, as it is called, moderately increases breast cancer risk.

If You Find a Lump

If you discover a lump in one breast, check the other breast. If both breasts feel the same, the lumpiness is probably normal. You should, however, mention it to your doctor at your next visit.

But if the lump is something new or unusual and does not go away after your next menstrual period, it is time to call your doctor. The same is true if you discover a discharge from the nipple or skin changes such as dimpling or puckering. If you do not have a doctor, your local medical society may be able to help you find one in your area.

You should not let fear delay you. It is natural to be concerned if you find a lump in your breast. But remember that four-fifths of all breast lumps are not cancer. The sooner any problem is diagnosed, the sooner you can have it treated.

Chapter 28

Breast Problems and Disorders

Chapter Contents

Section 28.1

Common Benign Lumps

Reprinted from "Benign Breast Changes," a *Facts for Life* fact sheet, with the permission of the Susan G. Komen Breast Cancer Foundation. © 2002. For more information about breast health or breast cancer, call the Susan G. Komen Breast Cancer Foundation's Toll-Free Helpline at 1.800 I'M AWARE® (1.800.462.9273) or visit the website at http://www.komen.org.

Fibrocystic Breast Changes

Have you ever felt a bumpy texture or lumpiness in your breasts? This lumpiness and tenderness or pain at certain times of the month is called fibrocystic breast changes. These changes are a normal part of the menstrual cycle. You are most likely to notice them in the premenstrual phase of your cycle, or if you are past menopause, when taking hormones. Fibrocystic changes do not increase your chance of getting breast cancer. In contrast, a breast change that should be checked is one that does not change with your cycle. Any persistent lump or thickening should be checked by your trained medical professional.

Benign Breast Problems

Many breast problems—such as a prominent breast lump, breast pain, or infection—are usually benign (not cancerous). All the same, if you have any of the breast changes listed below, be sure to have your breasts checked by a trained medical professional.

Have You Found a New Breast Lump?

Do not panic, but have it checked by a trained medical professional right away. Even if you have had cysts or fibroadenomas in the past, do not assume that a new lump will be the same. The lump may not turn out to be cancerous, but it is best to make sure.

Warning Signs to Heed

If you notice any of these things in your breast, see a trained medical professional:

- lump, hard knot, or thickening
- unusual swelling, warmth, redness, or darkening
- change in the size or shape

Table 28.1. Breast Problems

Types of Breast Changes	Found Most Often in	Relationship to Cancer
Cyst (a fluid-filled sac that feels like a soft lump or a tender spot)	women ages 30 to 50; postmenopausal women taking hormones	typically is not cancerous; does not increase your chance of getting breast cancer in the future; a rare type of cancer that occurs in about 1 percent of cysts
Fibroadenoma (a smooth, rubbery, or hard lump that moves easily within the breast tissue)	teenagers and young women; African American women; sometimes found in postmenopausal women taking hormones	typically is not cancerous; if the lump contains certain types of cells, you may have a three times greater chance of developing breast cancer; a rare type of cancer that occurs in about 1 percent of fibroadenomas
Cancer (a hard lump that may or may not be tender)	women who are over age 40 and women with a strong family history	
Cyclical (breast tenderness that varies over the breast cycle)	menstruating women; postmenopausal women taking hormones	not associated with breast cancer
Non-cyclical (constant pain in one spot that does not vary over the menstrual cycle)	women of all ages and ethnicities	often from a new or enlarging cyst; about 10 percent of women with non-cyclical pain have cancer
Non-breast-origin (pain in the chest or ribs under the chest)	women of all ages and ethnicities	not related to breast cancer, but may be another medical problem that should be checked

- dimpling or puckering of the skin
- an itchy, scaly sore or rash on the nipple
- pulling in of the nipple or other parts
- nipple discharge that starts suddenly
- pain in one spot that does not vary with your monthly cycle

Certain breast problems, such as infections, nipple discharge, or itchy nipples usually are not cancerous but can look just like symptoms of some rare types of breast cancer.

No matter what the diagnosis, if you feel sure that something is wrong, ask for a biopsy or get a second opinion. After all, no one knows your body better than you.

Resources

Book

Dr. Susan Love's Breast Book, 3rd ed. By Susan A. Love with Karen Lindsey. 2000 (Addison-Wesley).
See Chapters 6 through 9.

Internet

American Cancer Society
Website: http://www.cancer.org
See topic: Benign Breast Conditions

Note: This list of resources is made available solely as a suggested resource. Please note that it is not a complete listing of materials or information available on breast health and breast cancer. This information is not meant to be used for self-diagnosis or to replace the services of a medical professional. Further, The Susan G. Komen Breast Cancer Foundation does not endorse, recommend or make any warranties or representations regarding the accuracy, completeness, timeliness, quality or non-infringement of any of the materials, products, or information provided by the organizations referred to in this list.

Section 28.2

Mastalgia (Breast Pain)

"Breast Pain: What does it mean?" by M. Ellen Mahoney, M.D., Community Breast Health Project Newsletter, October 1999. Reprinted with permission of the Community Breast Health Project, www.cbhp.org.

Pain is the most common breast problem seen by primary care doctors.

Breast tenderness and swelling is so prevalent a premenstrual symptom that many women and practitioners alike consider it to be normal. However, many women experience intervals during their lives when the pain is more constant and becomes severe enough to cause concern.

As with almost any medical problem, the workup for a patient complaining of breast pain begins with a good history and physical. Is the pain clearly cyclical and limited to the week prior to menstruation? Is it noncyclical? If cyclical, has it changed in character, becoming more severe or involving most of the month? Are there new medications, new activities, or a change in diet that can account for the change? When the complaint is pain, the physician will make an effort to determine the location of the pain in the breast tissue itself or in the chest wall.

Cyclical Breast Pain

In the past, cyclical breast pain and swelling has been referred to as fibrocystic disease. Since all women experience cyclical tenderness and swelling at some time in their lives, we now try to avoid the use of the term disease to describe these normal changes. Premenstrual syndrome is certainly tied to the complex cycle of various hormones that are regulated by feedback loops and interactions between them. The exact nature of the hormonal imbalance remains a point of controversy. Not all patients need therapy; often all the patient needs is education about the nature of the phenomenon and its variability.

If part of the discomfort is due to the pull of breasts heavy with an unaccustomed amount of fluid, a proper supportive bra may help.

Women who wear underwires may find they are more comfortable in a sports bra, and others may find switching to underwires actually provides better support for them. Some doctors have prescribed diuretics to be taken in the last week of the cycle, but whenever the efficacy has been studied objectively there is no proven reduction in breast swelling and pain associated with temporarily reducing total body water. Some women feel relief from non-steroidal anti-inflammatory drugs like ibuprofen. Claims have been made for vitamin E and the B vitamins, which may help a small percentage of those affected. Other women have found a degree of relief in taking evening primrose oil, which has a high essential fatty acid composition. It seems to have few side effects, but should not be taken by women who are or may become pregnant.

Complete abstention from caffeine and related chemicals has been advised in the past, but there is little objective evidence that it helps many women. About 15% of women appear to be sensitive to coffee, tea, cola and chocolate, and their breasts feel better if they do not indulge, especially in the second half of the cycle. If patients want to test to see if they are one of the 15%, they should stay away from all of the foods mentioned for 3 months. If they do not improve symptomatically, they should return to their normal intake. There is much misunderstanding about these matters, and consequently many sleepy women with sore breasts fighting the urge to drink coffee or to have a hot fudge sundae, thinking that they are reducing their risk of breast cancer! By the way, read the labels and posters. Many popular coffee outlets sell decaffeinated coffees that actually contain a substantial amount of caffeine.

Most physicians prefer to begin treatment with the remedies listed above because they do not interfere with normal physiology, nor induce any changes in the hormonal production feedback loops. However, sometimes more aggressive therapy may be necessary. Oral contraceptives can sometimes cause severe breast pain, but some women will also find that using birth control pills to regularize their cycle can actually lead to a reduction of pain after about 4 months of use. In more severe cases stronger drugs are needed, including danazol, bromocriptine, and even tamoxifen. A program of education, patience, and conservative measures brings relief to the vast majority of women.

Noncyclical Breast Pain

Pain that does not fluctuate with menstruation is called noncyclical breast pain. Here the history and physical are even more important.

If the pain comes from a site clearly inside the breast on physical examination, the possibilities include hematoma, fat necrosis, ruptured cyst, infection, or tumor.

A hematoma is a deep bruise, and the patient usually knows the cause, especially once she is asked. There can be an associated lump caused by a collection of clotted blood.

Fat necrosis is also usually caused by trauma. However, unlike with hematoma, the trauma causing fat necrosis can be minor, and since there is no bruise, the origins of the trauma may not be remembered. In fat necrosis, a portion of fat loses its blood supply and the body's resulting attempt to clean up the dead cells is accompanied by inflammation, which can cause a sudden painful lump.

Though not dangerous, fat necrosis can be very worrisome because it can be impossible to distinguish from cancer on physical exam and on mammography. It will eventually resolve over several weeks, whereas cancer will not, but in almost all cases a biopsy is done before that time because of the heightened concern. It is *not* true that the presence of pain eliminates the worry about cancer.

A ruptured cyst can cause the same type of painful lump by the same mechanism as fat necrosis. The lump can also be indistinguishable from cancer and a biopsy is usually necessary, though some physicians will advise a wait of 4 weeks to see if it resolves.

Another cause of breast pain is infection, which is common while breastfeeding, but uncommon at other times of life. One course of antibiotics (7 to 10 days) is reasonable, but if the symptoms do not resolve completely a biopsy must be done to rule out inflammatory cancer.

If noncyclical breast pain is not localized to the breast, other causes must be sought. Some patients may have pain referred to the breast from an inflamed gall bladder, a ruptured disc in the neck, an unexpected pregnancy, and a recent weight-training program. Sometimes the cause of the pain can be traced to the sudden unaccustomed use of heavier backpacks. Costochondritis, a common cause of breast pain, can be traced to the joint between the ribs and the sternum in the center of the chest wall. A recent viral upper respiratory infection may be the cause of costochondritis. Pneumonia or other disease of the lung can produce symptoms in the breast. Angina pectoris can seem to originate in the breast rather than the heart and is associated with pain on exertion or with cold weather. Esophageal pain or spasm can also be referred to the breast. This type of pain is alleviated by antacid treatment.

Young women who have cyclical breast pain should be followed clinically until symptoms abate, or while successive measures are tried. They do not need breast imaging. If there is a particular painful spot, an ultrasound can sometimes be performed to try to locate the rare single simple cyst, which can then be drained for relief. The older patient should also be evaluated for breast imaging, depending on her coincidental need for screening and the index of suspicion regarding her current situation. Remember that with all presenting breast problems, the screening guideline criteria do not apply, since they were developed for women who have no breast symptoms. Once there is an established problem, the task is no longer one of screening, but of diagnosis, and strict age guidelines no longer apply.

Chapter 29

Breast Surgeries and Procedures

Chapter Contents

Section 29.1

Information about Biopsies

Excerpted from "Understanding Breast Changes: A Health Guide for Women," National Cancer Institute, published September 1998. Available online at http://www.cancer.gov; accessed August 2003. Reviewed and revised by David A. Cooke, M.D. on June 30, 2003.

The only certain way to learn whether a breast lump or mammographic abnormality is cancerous is by having a biopsy, a procedure in which tissue is removed by a surgeon or other specialist and examined under a microscope by a pathologist. A pathologist is a doctor who specializes in identifying tissue changes that are characteristic of disease, including cancer.

Tissue samples for biopsy can be obtained by either surgery or needle. The doctor's choice of biopsy technique depends on such things as the nature and location of the lump, as well as the woman's general health.

Surgical biopsies can be either excision or incision. An excision biopsy removes the entire lump or suspicious area. Excision biopsy is currently the standard procedure for lumps that are smaller than an inch or so in diameter. In effect, it is similar to a lumpectomy, surgery to remove the lump and a margin of surrounding tissue. Lumpectomy is usually used in combination with radiation therapy as the basic treatment for early breast cancer.

An excision biopsy is typically performed in the outpatient department of a hospital. A local anesthetic is injected into the woman's breast. Sometimes she is given a tranquilizer before the procedure. The surgeon makes an incision along the contour of the breast and removes the lump along with a small margin of normal tissue. Because no skin is removed, the biopsy scar is usually small.

The procedure typically takes less than an hour. After spending an hour or two in the recovery room, the woman goes home the same day.

An incision biopsy removes only a portion of the tumor (by slicing into it) for the pathologist to examine. Incision biopsies are generally reserved for tumors that are larger. They too are usually performed under local anesthesia, with the woman going home the same day.

Whether or not a surgical biopsy will change the shape of your breast depends partly on the size of the lump and where it is located in the breast, as well as how much of a margin of healthy tissue the surgeon decides to remove. You should talk with your doctor beforehand, so you understand just how extensive the surgery will be and what the cosmetic result will be.

Needle biopsies can be performed with either a very fine needle or a cutting needle large enough to remove a small nugget of tissue.

Fine needle aspiration uses a very thin needle and syringe to remove either fluid from a cyst or clusters of cells from a solid mass. Accurate fine needle aspiration biopsy of a solid mass takes great skill, gained through experience with numerous cases.

Core needle biopsy uses a somewhat larger needle with a special cutting edge. The needle is inserted, under local anesthesia, through a small incision in the skin, and a small core of tissue is removed. This technique may not work well for lumps that are very hard or very small. Core needle biopsy may cause some bruising, but rarely leaves an external scar, and the procedure is over in a matter of minutes.

At some institutions with extensive experience, aspiration biopsy is considered as reliable as surgical biopsy; it is trusted to confirm the malignancy of a clinically suspicious mass or to confirm a diagnosis that a lump is not cancerous. Should the needle biopsy results be uncertain, the diagnosis is pursued with a surgical biopsy. Some doctors prefer to verify all aspiration biopsy results with a surgical biopsy before proceeding with treatment.

Localization biopsy (also known as needle localization) is a procedure that uses mammography to locate and a needle to biopsy breast abnormalities that can be seen on a mammogram but cannot be felt (nonpalpable abnormalities). Localization can be used with surgical biopsy, fine needle aspiration, or core needle biopsy.

For a surgical biopsy, the radiologist locates the abnormality on a mammogram (or a sonogram) just prior to surgery. Using the mammogram as a guide, the radiologist inserts a fine needle or wire so the tip rests in the suspicious area—typically, an area of microcalcifications. The needle is anchored with a gauze bandage, and a second mammogram is taken to confirm that the needle is on target. The woman, along with her mammograms, goes to the operating room, where the surgeon locates and cuts out the needle-targeted area. The more precisely the needle is placed, the less tissue needs to be removed.

Sometimes the surgeon will be able to feel the lump during surgery. In other cases, especially where the mammogram showed only microcalcifications, the abnormality can be neither seen nor felt. To make sure the surgical specimen in fact contains the abnormality, it is x-rayed on the spot. If this specimen x-ray fails to show the mass or the calcifications, the surgeon is able to remove additional tissue.

Stereotactic localization biopsy is a newer approach that relies on a three-dimensional x-ray to guide the needle biopsy of a nonpalpable mass. With one type of equipment, the patient lies face down on an examining table with a hole in it that allows the breast to hang through; the x-ray machine and the maneuverable needle "gun" are set up underneath. Alternatively, specialized stereo tactic equipment can be attached to a standard mammography machine.

The breast is x-rayed from two different angles, and a computer plots the exact position of the suspicious area. (Because only a small area of the breast is exposed to the radiation, the doses are similar to those from standard mammography.) Once the target is clearly identified, the radiologist positions the gun and advances the biopsy needle into the lesion.

Section 29.2

Lumpectomy

Reprinted with permission of the nonprofit organization breastcancer.org, dedicated to providing the most reliable, complete, and up-to-date information about breast cancer. Published October 2001. Available online at http://www.breastcancer.org; accessed July 2003.

Any form of surgery that removes only part of the breast is considered breast-conserving or breast preservation surgery. You may hear your surgeon use any one of several names: biopsy, lumpectomy, partial mastectomy, re-excision, quadrantectomy, wedge resection. Technically, a lumpectomy is a partial mastectomy, because part of the breast is removed. But how much of the breast is removed can vary greatly.

Quadrantectomy, for example, means that a quarter of your breast will be removed. Be sure your surgeon discusses his or her plan of action with you, so that you have a clear understanding of how much of your breast may be gone after surgery.

Lumpectomy

Lumpectomy is the most common form of breast cancer surgery today. The surgeon removes only the part of your breast containing the tumor (the lump) and some of the normal tissue that surrounds it. All the tissue removed from your breast is examined carefully to see if cancer cells are present in the margins—the normal tissue surrounding the tumor.

If cancer cells are found in the margins, extending out to the edge of the breast tissue that was removed, your surgeon will do additional surgery (called re-excision) to remove the remaining cancer. Most women receive five to seven weeks of radiation therapy after lumpectomy, in order to eliminate any cancer cells that may be present in the remaining breast tissue.

The combination of lumpectomy and radiation is commonly called breast-conserving therapy.

Is Lumpectomy Good Breast Cancer Treatment?

A general principle of cancer treatment is that almost always, the whole breast must be treated for breast cancer. This can be accomplished by:

- mastectomy (removal of the whole breast) or
- lumpectomy and radiation therapy to the rest of the breast

A great deal of research has been done in recent years to determine if lumpectomy is as good an option as mastectomy for treating breast cancer.

The evidence shows that lumpectomy followed by radiation is likely to be equally as effective as mastectomy for women with:

- only one site of cancer in their breast, and
- a tumor under four centimeters, removed with clear margins (no cancer cells in the tissue surrounding the tumor)

Doctors in some parts of the United States may be more old-fashioned and less likely to offer lumpectomy with radiation as an option for their patients, particularly their older patients. Such doctors may urge mastectomy, even for women who should be offered the choice. Don't let hidden biases or unchanging attitudes keep you from getting the best care. Find a surgeon who keeps current, and whose techniques aren't limited to what used to be the standard of care twenty or thirty years ago.

Is Lumpectomy and Radiation Right for You?

While lumpectomy and radiation is an excellent option for many women with breast cancer, it's not the best treatment for everyone. You may have to rule out lumpectomy if:

- You have already had radiation to the same breast for an earlier breast cancer.

- You have extensive cancer in the breast or have two or more separate areas of cancer in the same breast.

- You have a small breast and a large tumor, so that removing the tumor would be extremely disfiguring.

- Multiple attempts to remove the tumor have not been able to completely remove the cancer and obtain clear margins.

- You have a connective tissue disease, such as lupus or vasculitis, that would make you sensitive to the side effects of radiation.

- You are pregnant and so should not have radiation therapy.

- You are not willing to commit to the daily schedule of radiation therapy, or distance makes it impossible.

- You believe you would have greater peace of mind with a mastectomy.

Re-excision

Re-excision lumpectomy—also called simply re-excision—involves going back into the area where you have had either a lumpectomy or excisional biopsy (the two terms refer to the same procedure) and taking out the tissue that used to surround your tumor. Your surgeon will do a re-excision if the margins of resection show cancer cells close to the edge of the tissue removed during the first surgery. It is important to remove a margin or zone of cancer-free tissue completely surrounding the original tumor, to try to be sure that all the cancer is gone. You may hear your surgeon refer to this as clearing the margins.

Section 29.3

Breast Reduction

If You're Considering Breast Reduction

Women with very large, pendulous breasts may experience a variety of medical problems caused by the excessive weight—from back and neck pain and skin irritation to skeletal deformities and breathing problems. Bra straps may leave indentations in their shoulders. And unusually large breasts can make a woman—or a teenage girl— feel extremely self-conscious.

Breast reduction, technically known as reduction mammaplasty, is designed for such women. The procedure removes fat, glandular tissue, and skin from the breasts, making them smaller, lighter, and firmer. It can also reduce the size of the areola, the darker skin surrounding the nipple. The goal is to give the woman smaller, better-shaped breasts in proportion with the rest of her body.

If you're considering breast reduction, this will give you a basic understanding of the procedure—when it can help, how it's performed, and what results you can expect. It can't answer all of your questions, since a lot depends on your individual circumstances. Please be sure to ask your doctor if there is anything about the procedure you don't understand.

The Best Candidates for Breast Reduction

Breast reduction is usually performed for physical relief rather than simply cosmetic improvement. Most women who have the surgery are troubled by very large, sagging breasts that restrict their activities and cause them physical discomfort.

In most cases, breast reduction isn't performed until a woman's breasts are fully developed; however, it can be done earlier if large breasts are causing serious physical discomfort. The best candidates are those who are mature enough to fully understand the procedure and have realistic expectations about the results. Breast reduction is not recommended for women who intend to breastfeed.

All Surgery Carries Some Uncertainty and Risk

Breast reduction is not a simple operation, but it's normally safe when performed by a qualified plastic surgeon. Nevertheless, as with any surgery, there is always a possibility of complications, including bleeding, infection, or reaction to the anesthesia. Some patients develop small sores around their nipples after surgery; these can be treated with antibiotic creams. You can reduce your risks by closely following your physician's advice both before and after surgery.

The procedure does leave noticeable, permanent scars, although they'll be covered by your bra or bathing suit. (Poor healing and wider scars are more common in smokers.) The procedure can also leave you with slightly mismatched breasts or unevenly positioned nipples. Future breastfeeding may not be possible, since the surgery removes many of the milk ducts leading to the nipples.

Some patients may experience a permanent loss of feeling in their nipples or breasts. Rarely, the nipple and areola may lose their blood supply and the tissue will die. (The nipple and areola can usually be rebuilt, however, using skin grafts from elsewhere on the body.)

Planning Your Surgery

In your initial consultation, it's important to discuss your expectations frankly with your surgeon, and to listen to his or her opinion. Every patient—and every physician, as well—has a different view of what is a desirable size and shape for breasts.

The surgeon will examine and measure your breasts, and will probably photograph them for reference during surgery and afterward. (The photographs may also be used in the processing of your insurance coverage.) He or she will discuss the variables that may affect the procedure-such as your age, the size and shape of your breasts, and the condition of your skin. You should also discuss where the nipple and areola will be positioned; they'll be moved higher during the procedure, and should be approximately even with the crease beneath your breasts.

Your surgeon should describe the procedure in detail, explaining its risks and limitations and making sure you understand the scarring that will result. The surgeon should also explain the anesthesia he or she will use, the facility where the surgery will be performed, and the costs. (Some insurance companies will pay for breast reduction if it's medically necessary; however, they may require that a certain amount of breast tissue be removed. Check your policy, and have your surgeon write a "predetermination letter" if required.)

Preparing for Your Surgery

Your surgeon may require you to have a mammogram (breast x-ray) before surgery. You'll also get specific instructions on how to prepare for surgery, including guidelines on eating and drinking, smoking, and taking or avoiding certain vitamins and medications.

Some surgeons suggest that their patients diet before the operation. Breast reduction doesn't usually require a blood transfusion. However, if a large amount of breast tissue will be removed, your physician may advise you to have a unit of blood drawn ahead of time. That way, if a transfusion should be needed, your own blood can be used.

While you're making preparations, be sure to arrange for someone to drive you home after your surgery and to help you out for a few days if needed.

Where Your Surgery Will Be Performed

Breast reduction surgery may be performed in a hospital, an out-patient surgery center, or an office-based surgical suite. If you are admitted to the hospital, your stay will be a short one. The surgery itself usually takes two to four hours, but may take longer in some cases.

Type of Anesthesia

Breast reduction is nearly always performed under general anesthesia. You'll be asleep through the entire operation.

The Surgery

Techniques for breast reduction vary, but the most common procedure involves an anchor-shaped incision that circles the areola, extends downward, and follows the natural curve of the crease beneath the breast. The surgeon removes excess glandular tissue, fat, and skin, and moves the nipple and areola into their new position. He or she then brings the skin from both sides of the breast down and around the areola, shaping the new contour of the breast. Liposuction may be used to remove excess fat from the armpit area.

In most cases, the nipples remain attached to their blood vessels and nerves. However, if the breasts are very large or pendulous, the nipples and areolas may have to be completely removed and grafted into a higher position. (This will result in a loss of sensation in the nipple and areolar tissue.)

Stitches are usually located around the areola, in a vertical line extending downward, and along the lower crease of the breast. In some cases, techniques can be used that eliminate the vertical part of the scar. And occasionally, when only fat needs to be removed, liposuction alone can be used to reduce breast size, leaving minimal scars.

After Your Surgery

After surgery, you'll be wrapped in an elastic bandage or a surgical bra over gauze dressings. A small tube may be placed in each breast to drain off blood and fluids for the first day or two.

You may feel some pain for the first couple of days—especially when you move around or cough—and some discomfort for a week or more. Your surgeon will prescribe medication to lessen the pain.

The bandages will be removed a day or two after surgery, though you'll continue wearing the surgical bra around the clock for several weeks, until the swelling and bruising subside. Your stitches will be removed in one to three weeks.

If your breast skin is very dry following surgery, you can apply a moisturizer several times a day, but be sure to keep the suture area dry.

Your first menstruation following surgery may cause your breasts to swell and hurt. You may also experience random, shooting pains for a few months. You can expect some loss of feeling in your nipples and breast skin, caused by the swelling after surgery. This usually fades over the next six weeks or so. In some patients, however, it may last a year or more, and occasionally it may be permanent.

Getting Back to Normal

Although you may be up and about in a day or two, your breasts may still ache occasionally for a couple of weeks. You should avoid lifting or pushing anything heavy for three or four weeks.

Your surgeon will give you detailed instructions for resuming your normal activities. Most women can return to work (if it's not too strenuous) and social activities in about two weeks. But you'll have much less stamina for several weeks, and should limit your exercises to stretching, bending, and swimming until your energy level returns. You'll also need a good athletic bra for support.

You may be instructed to avoid sex for a week or more, since sexual arousal can cause your incisions to swell, and to avoid anything but gentle contact with your breasts for about six weeks.

A small amount of fluid draining from your surgical wound, or some crusting, is normal. If you have any unusual symptoms, such as bleeding or severe pain, don't hesitate to call your doctor.

Your New Look

Although much of the swelling and bruising will disappear in the first few weeks, it may be six months to a year before your breasts settle into their new shape. Even then, their shape may fluctuate in response to your hormonal shifts, weight changes, and pregnancy.

Your surgeon will make every effort to make your scars as inconspicuous as possible. Still, it's important to remember that breast reduction scars are extensive and permanent. They often remain lumpy and red for months, then gradually become less obvious, sometimes eventually fading to thin white lines. Fortunately, the scars can usually be placed so that you can wear even low-cut tops.

Of all plastic surgery procedures, breast reduction results in the quickest body-image changes. You'll be rid of the physical discomfort of large breasts, your body will look better proportioned, and clothes will fit you better.

However, as much as you may have desired these changes, you'll need time to adjust to your new image—as will your family and friends. Be patient with yourself, and with them. Keep in mind why you had this surgery, and chances are that, like most women, you'll be pleased with the results.

Section 29.4

Mastectomy

Reprinted with permission of the nonprofit organization breastcancer.org, dedicated to providing the most reliable, complete, and up-to-date information about breast cancer. Published October 2001. Available online at http://www.breastcancer.org; accessed July 2003.

For a long time, a procedure called a radical mastectomy was the only treatment available to women with breast cancer. No matter what stage of breast cancer you had, mastectomy was your only option. Catching a cancer early didn't give you the benefit of having a less radical, more cosmetically acceptable treatment option. Things have changed a great deal since then. Mastectomy no longer has to be as extensive, scarring, or disfiguring. It can actually be different operations for different people, in different situations.

In a simple or total mastectomy, the surgeon removes the entire breast but does not take out any axillary lymph nodes (nodes in the underarm area, also called the axilla). No muscles are removed from beneath your breast. Occasionally, lymph nodes may be removed because they are actually located within the breast tissue taken during surgery. A total mastectomy is appropriate for women with ductal carcinoma in situ or DCIS, and for women seeking prophylactic mastectomies—that is, breast removal in order to prevent any possibility of breast cancer occurring.

A modified radical mastectomy removes the entire breast and includes a procedure called axillary dissection, in which levels I and II (of three levels) of the axillary lymph nodes in the underarm area) are also removed. Most women who have mastectomies today have modified radical mastectomies.

Radical mastectomy includes removal of the entire breast, all underarm lymph nodes, and chest wall muscles under the breast. Although it was common in the past, radical mastectomy is now rarely performed because modified radical mastectomy has proven to be just as effective and less disfiguring. Today radical mastectomy is recommended only when cancer has spread to the chest muscles under the breast.

Is Mastectomy Right for You?

Mastectomy may be right for you if:

- Cancer is found in more than one part of your breast.

- Your breast is small or is shaped so that a lumpectomy would leave you with very little breast tissue or a very deformed breast.

- Radiation therapy after surgery is not appropriate for you.

- You believe you would have greater peace of mind with a mastectomy.

When Is Radiation Added to Mastectomy?

Radiation may be recommended after mastectomy if:

- The tumor is larger than five centimeters.

- The removed tissue has a positive margin of resection.

- Four or more lymph nodes were involved.

- The cancer is multi-centered—it occurred in a number of locations within the breast.

Section 29.5

Preventive Mastectomy

National Cancer Institute, Cancer Information Service, June 1, 2001.
Available online at http://cis.nci.nih.gov; accessed August 2003.

Preventive mastectomy (also called prophylactic mastectomy) is the surgical removal of one or both breasts in an effort to prevent or reduce the risk of breast cancer. Total mastectomy, an operation to remove the entire breast and nipple, is the procedure of choice. Subcutaneous mastectomy, an operation to remove the breast tissue but spare the nipple, is recommended less often because of the possibility of leaving cancerous breast tissue behind. It is important that a woman who is considering preventive mastectomy talk with a doctor about her risk of developing breast cancer (with or without a mastectomy), the surgical procedure, and potential complications. She should also discuss her feelings about mastectomy, alternatives to surgery, and follow-up care. A woman may also wish to get a second medical opinion to help with the decision.

Reasons for Preventive Mastectomy

Preventive mastectomy may be considered for several reasons. Women who have already had one breast removed due to cancer may consider this procedure in an effort to avoid developing a new cancer in the other breast. Preventive mastectomy may also be an option for women with a strong family history of breast cancer, especially if several close relatives developed the disease before age 50. Women in families with hereditary breast cancer who test positive for a known cancer-causing gene alteration may also consider this surgery. In addition, preventive mastectomy is sometimes considered for women who have had lobular carcinoma in situ, a condition that increases their risk of developing breast cancer in the same and/or in the opposite breast. Rarely, preventive mastectomy may be considered for women with diffuse and indeterminate breast microcalcifications (tiny deposits of calcium in the breast) or for women whose breast tissue is very dense. (This is particularly important in women who have already had a mastectomy in the other breast.) Dense breast tissue is linked to an elevated risk of breast cancer and also makes diagnosing breast abnormalities difficult. Multiple biopsies, which may be necessary for diagnosing abnormalities in dense breasts, cause scarring and further complicate examination of the breast tissue.

Although having a preventive mastectomy can reduce the risk, no one can be certain that this procedure will protect a woman from breast cancer. Because it is impossible for a surgeon to remove all breast tissue, breast cancer can still develop in the small amount of remaining tissue. All women are different, so the procedure should be considered in the context of each woman's unique risk factors and her level of concern.

Breast Reconstruction

Many women who choose to have preventive mastectomy decide to have breast reconstruction (plastic surgery to restore the shape of the breast). Before performing this type of procedure, the plastic surgeon carefully examines the breasts and discusses the appropriate types of reconstruction.

Doctors do not always agree on the most effective way to manage the care of women who have a strong family history of breast cancer and/or have other risk factors for the disease. Some doctors may recommend preventive mastectomy, while others may prescribe tamoxifen, a medication that has been shown to decrease the chances of getting breast cancer in women at high risk for the disease. Some doctors may advise very close monitoring (periodic mammograms, regular checkups that include a clinical breast examination performed by a health care professional, and monthly breast self-examination) to increase the chance of detecting breast cancer at an early stage. Although the effects are not proven, doctors may also encourage women at high risk to limit their consumption of alcohol, eat a low-fat diet, engage in regular exercise, and avoid hormone replacement therapy.

Section 29.6

Breast Augmentation

Excerpted from "Breast Implants: An Update" from the U.S. Food and Drug Administration, Center for Devices and Radiological Health, August 2000. Available online at http://www.fda.gov; accessed July 2003.

There are three types of breast implants, all of which are intended for breast augmentation, breast reconstruction, and/or revision (replacement) of a breast implant. The saline-filled implant has an external silicone shell and is filled with sterile saline (salt water). The silicone gel-filled implant also has an external silicone shell but is filled with silicone gel. An alternative breast implant may have a different shell material and/or a different filler.

While many women believe breast implants cause debilitating systemic illnesses, such as autoimmune disease, this is not proven at this time. However, most women with breast implants will experience some local complications such as rupture, pain, capsular contracture (a tightening of the scar tissue or capsule the body forms around the breast implant), disfigurement, and serious infection. These may lead to nonsurgical medical treatments and repeat surgeries.

Breast Implant Risks

There are risks or complications associated with any surgical procedure, such as the effects of anesthesia, infection, swelling, redness, bleeding, and there are complications specific to breast implants. These complications are described below.

- **Capsular Contracture:** Capsular contracture is when the scar tissue or capsule that normally forms around the implant tightens and squeezes the implant. It may be more common following infection, hematoma (collection of blood), and seroma (collection of watery portion of blood).

- **Deflation/Rupture/Leakage:** Breast implants are not lifetime devices and cannot be expected to last forever. Some implants deflate or rupture in the first few months after being implanted and some deflate after several years; others are intact 10 or more years after the surgery.

- **Additional Surgeries:** You should understand there is a high chance that you will need to have additional surgery at some point to replace or remove your implant(s) due to problems such as deflation, capsular contracture, infection, shifting, and calcium deposits. Many women decide to have the implants replaced, but some women do not. Those who do not have their implants replaced may have cosmetically undesirable dimpling and/or puckering of the breast following removal of the implant.

- **Pain:** Women may feel pain of varying severity (degrees) and duration (length of time) following breast implant surgery. In addition, improper size, placement, surgical technique, or capsular contracture may result in pain associated with nerve entrapment or interference with muscle motion. You should tell your doctor if you have pain.

- **Dissatisfaction with Cosmetic Results:** Dissatisfying results such as wrinkling, asymmetry, implant displacement (shifting), incorrect size, unanticipated shape, implant palpability, scar deformity, hypertrophic (irregular, raised scar) scarring, and/or sloshing may occur. Careful surgical planning and technique can minimize but not always prevent such results. Additionally, for saline-filled implants that have a valve, you also might be able to feel the valve of the implant with your hand. Repeated surgeries to improve the appearance of the breasts and/or to remove ruptured or deflated prostheses may result in an unsatisfactory cosmetic outcome.

- **Infection:** Infection can occur with any surgery. Most infections resulting from surgery appear within a few days to weeks after the operation. However, infection is possible at any time after surgery. Infections with an implant present are harder to treat than infections in normal body tissues. If an infection does not respond to antibiotics, the implant may have to be removed, and another implant may be placed after the infection has cleared up. In rare instances, Toxic Shock Syndrome has been noted in women after breast implant surgery, and it is a life-threatening condition. Symptoms include sudden fever, vomiting, diarrhea, fainting, dizziness, and/or sunburn-like rash. A doctor should be seen immediately for diagnosis and treatment.

- **Hematoma/Seroma:** Hematoma is a collection of blood inside a body cavity, and seroma is a collection of the watery portion of the blood around the implant or around the incision. Postoperative hematoma and seroma may contribute to infection and/ or capsular contracture. Swelling, pain, and bruising may result. If a hematoma occurs, it will usually be soon after surgery; however, this can also occur at any time after injury to the breast. While the body absorbs small hematomas and seromas, large ones will require the placement of surgical drains for proper healing. A small scar can result from surgical draining. Implant deflation/rupture can occur from surgical draining if damage to the implant occurs during the draining procedure.

- **Changes in Nipple and Breast Sensation:** Feeling in the nipple and breast can increase or decrease after implant surgery. The range of changes varies from intense sensitivity to no feeling in the nipple or breast following surgery. Changes in feeling can be temporary or permanent and may affect sexual response or the ability to nurse a baby.

- **Calcium Deposits in the Tissue Around the Implant:** Deposits of calcium can be seen on mammograms and can be mistaken for possible cancer, resulting in additional surgery to biopsy and/or remove the implant to distinguish these deposits from cancer. Calcium deposits may be felt as nodules (hard knots) under the skin around the implant.

- **Delayed Wound Healing:** In some cases, the incision site fails to heal normally or takes longer to heal.

- **Extrusion:** An unstable or compromised tissue covering and/or interruption of wound healing may result in extrusion of the implant, which is when the breast implant comes through the skin. The additional surgery needed to correct this complication can result in unacceptable scarring or loss of breast tissue.

- **Necrosis:** Necrosis is the formation of dead tissue around the implant. This may prevent wound healing and require surgical correction and/or implant removal. Permanent scar and/or deformity may occur following necrosis. Factors associated with increased necrosis include infection, use of steroids in the surgical pocket, smoking, chemotherapy/radiation, and excessive heat or cold therapy.

- **Breast Tissue Atrophy/Chest Wall Deformity:** The pressure of the breast implant may cause the breast tissue to thin and shrink. This can occur while implants are still in place or following implant removal without replacement.

- **Interference with Mammography:** Interference with mammography due to breast implants may delay or hinder the early detection of breast cancer either by hiding suspicious lesions (wounds or injuries or tumors) or by making it more difficult to include them in the image. Implants increase the difficulty of both taking and reading mammograms.

- **Galactorrhea:** Sometimes after breast implant surgery, you may begin producing breast milk. In some cases, the milk production stops spontaneously or when medication is given to suppress milk production. In other cases, removal of the implant(s) may be needed.

Other Illnesses

Some women with breast implants have reported health problems that they believe are related to their implants, but most studies of these illnesses have failed to show an association with breast implants. There also have been concerns about possible, but unproven, effects on health.

Most of the health concerns about breast implants are related to silicone gel. Even if a silicone gel-filled breast implant does not rupture, small amounts of the silicone fluid or oil may bleed out of the implant and migrate into the surrounding tissue. There has been concern that this escaped silicone fluid or oil might cause harmful effects, including connective tissue disease and related disorders and/or cancer.

Section 29.7

Breast Reconstruction after Breast Removal

Reprinted with permission from the American Society of Plastic Surgery®.
© 2003. For additional information, visit www.plasticsurgery.org, or to find
a plastic surgeon in your area, call the ASPS Plastic Surgeon Referral
Service at 1-888-4-PLASTIC (1-888-475-2784).

If You're Considering Breast Reconstruction

Reconstruction of a breast that has been removed due to cancer
or other disease is one of the most rewarding surgical procedures
available today. New medical techniques and devices have made it
possible for surgeons to create a breast that can come close in form
and appearance to matching a natural breast. Frequently, reconstruction is possible immediately following breast removal (mastectomy), so the patient wakes up with a breast mound already in place,
having been spared the experience of seeing herself with no breast
at all.

But bear in mind, post-mastectomy breast reconstruction is not a
simple procedure. There are often many options to consider as you and
your doctor explore what's best for you.

This information will give you a basic understanding of the procedure—when it's appropriate, how it's done, and what results you can
expect. It can't answer all of your questions, since a lot depends on
your individual circumstances. Please be sure to ask your surgeon if
there is anything you don't understand about the procedure.

The Best Candidates for Breast Reconstruction

Most mastectomy patients are medically appropriate for reconstruction, many at the same time that the breast is removed. The best
candidates, however, are women whose cancer, as far as can be determined, seems to have been eliminated by mastectomy.

Still, there are legitimate reasons to wait. Many women aren't
comfortable weighing all the options while they're struggling to
cope with a diagnosis of cancer. Others simply don't want to have any

more surgery than is absolutely necessary. Some patients may be advised by their surgeons to wait, particularly if the breast is being rebuilt in a more complicated procedure using flaps of skin and underlying tissue. Women with other health conditions, such as obesity, high blood pressure, or smoking, may also be advised to wait.

In any case, being informed of your reconstruction options before surgery can help you prepare for a mastectomy with a more positive outlook for the future.

All Surgery Carries Some Uncertainty and Risk

Virtually any woman who must lose her breast to cancer can have it rebuilt through reconstructive surgery. But there are risks associated with any surgery and specific complications associated with this procedure.

In general, the usual problems of surgery, such as bleeding, fluid collection, excessive scar tissue, or difficulties with anesthesia, can occur although they're relatively uncommon. And, as with any surgery, smokers should be advised that nicotine can delay healing, resulting in conspicuous scars and prolonged recovery. Occasionally, these complications are severe enough to require a second operation.

If an implant is used, there is a remote possibility that an infection will develop, usually within the first two weeks following surgery. In some of these cases, the implant may need to be removed for several months until the infection clears. A new implant can later be inserted.

The most common problem, capsular contracture, occurs if the scar or capsule around the implant begins to tighten. This squeezing of the soft implant can cause the breast to feel hard. Capsular contracture can be treated in several ways, and sometimes requires either removal or scoring of the scar tissue, or perhaps removal or replacement of the implant.

Reconstruction has no known effect on the recurrence of disease in the breast, nor does it generally interfere with chemotherapy or radiation treatment, should cancer recur. Your surgeon may recommend continuation of periodic mammograms on both the reconstructed and the remaining normal breast. If your reconstruction involves an implant, be sure to go to a radiology center where technicians are experienced in the special techniques required to get a reliable x-ray of a breast reconstructed with an implant.

Women who postpone reconstruction may go through a period of emotional readjustment. Just as it took time to get used to the loss of

273

a breast, a woman may feel anxious and confused as she begins to think of the reconstructed breast as her own.

Planning Your Surgery

You can begin talking about reconstruction as soon as you're diagnosed with cancer. Ideally, you'll want your breast surgeon and your plastic surgeon to work together to develop a strategy that will put you in the best possible condition for reconstruction.

After evaluating your health, your surgeon will explain which reconstructive options are most appropriate for your age, health, anatomy, tissues, and goals. Be sure to discuss your expectations frankly with your surgeon. He or she should be equally frank with you, describing your options and the risks and limitations of each. Post-mastectomy reconstruction can improve your appearance and renew your self-confidence—but keep in mind that the desired result is improvement, not perfection.

Your surgeon should also explain the anesthesia he or she will use, the facility where the surgery will be performed, and the costs. In most cases, health insurance policies will cover most or all of the cost of post-mastectomy reconstruction. Check your policy to make sure you're covered and to see if there are any limitations on what types of reconstruction are covered.

Preparing for Your Surgery

Your oncologist and your plastic surgeon will give you specific instructions on how to prepare for surgery, including guidelines on eating and drinking, smoking, and taking or avoiding certain vitamins and medications.

While making preparations, be sure to arrange for someone to drive you home after your surgery and to help you out for a few days, if needed.

Where Your Surgery Will Be Performed

Breast reconstruction usually involves more than one operation. The first stage, whether done at the same time as the mastectomy or later on, is usually performed in a hospital.

Follow-up procedures may also be done in the hospital. Or, depending on the extent of surgery required, your surgeon may prefer an outpatient facility.

Types of Anesthesia

The first stage of reconstruction, creation of the breast mound, is almost always performed using general anesthesia, so you'll sleep through the entire operation.

Follow-up procedures may require only a local anesthesia, combined with a sedative to make you drowsy. You'll be awake but relaxed, and may feel some discomfort.

Types of Implants

If your surgeon recommends the use of an implant, you'll want to discuss what type of implant should be used. A breast implant is a silicone shell filled with either silicone gel or a salt-water solution known as saline.

Because of concerns that there is insufficient information demonstrating the safety of silicone gel-filled breast implants, the Food & Drug Administration (FDA) has determined that new gel-filled implants should be available only to women participating in approved studies. This currently includes women who already have tissue expanders, who choose immediate reconstruction after mastectomy, or who already have a gel-filled implant and need it replaced for medical reasons. Eventually, all patients with appropriate medical indications may have similar access to silicone gel-filled implants.

The alternative saline-filled implant, a silicone shell filled with salt water, continues to be available on an unrestricted basis, pending further FDA review.

As more information becomes available, these FDA guidelines may change. Be sure to discuss current options with your surgeon. (Above guidelines are current as of July 1992.)

The Surgery

While there are many options available in post-mastectomy reconstruction, you and your surgeon should discuss the one that's best for you.

Skin expansion. The most common technique combines skin expansion and subsequent insertion of an implant.

Following mastectomy, your surgeon will insert a balloon expander beneath your skin and chest muscle. Through a tiny valve mechanism buried beneath the skin, he or she will periodically inject a salt-water solution to gradually fill the expander over several weeks or months. After the skin over the breast area has stretched enough, the expander may be removed in a second operation and a more permanent implant will be inserted. Some expanders are designed to be left in place as the final implant. The nipple and the dark skin surrounding it, called the areola, are reconstructed in a subsequent procedure.

Some patients do not require preliminary tissue expansion before receiving an implant. For these women, the surgeon will proceed with inserting an implant as the first step.

Flap reconstruction. An alternative approach to implant reconstruction involves creation of a skin flap using tissue taken from other parts of the body, such as the back, abdomen, or buttocks.

In one type of flap surgery, the tissue remains attached to its original site, retaining its blood supply. The flap, consisting of the skin, fat, and muscle with its blood supply, are tunneled beneath the skin to the chest, creating a pocket for an implant or, in some cases, creating the breast mound itself, without need for an implant.

Another flap technique uses tissue that is surgically removed from the abdomen, thighs, or buttocks and then transplanted to the chest by reconnecting the blood vessels to new ones in that region. This procedure requires the skills of a plastic surgeon who is experienced in microvascular surgery as well.

Regardless of whether the tissue is tunneled beneath the skin on a pedicle or transplanted to the chest as a microvascular flap, this type of surgery is more complex than skin expansion. Scars will be left at both the tissue donor site and at the reconstructed breast, and recovery will take longer than with an implant. On the other hand, when the breast is reconstructed entirely with your own tissue, the results are generally more natural and there are no concerns about a silicone implant. In some cases, you may have the added benefit of an improved abdominal contour.

Follow-up procedures. Most breast reconstruction involves a series of procedures that occur over time. Usually, the initial reconstructive operation is the most complex. Follow-up surgery may be required to replace a tissue expander with an implant or to reconstruct the nipple and the areola. Many surgeons recommend an additional operation to enlarge, reduce, or lift the natural breast to match the reconstructed breast. But keep in mind, this procedure may leave scars on an otherwise normal breast and may not be covered by insurance.

After Your Surgery

You are likely to feel tired and sore for a week or two after reconstruction. Most of your discomfort can be controlled by medication prescribed by your doctor.

Depending on the extent of your surgery, you'll probably be released from the hospital in two to five days. Many reconstruction options require a surgical drain to remove excess fluids from surgical sites immediately following the operation, but these are removed within the first week or two after surgery. Most stitches are removed in a week to 10 days.

Getting Back to Normal

It may take you up to six weeks to recover from a combined mastectomy and reconstruction or from a flap reconstruction alone. If implants are used without flaps and reconstruction is done apart from the mastectomy, your recovery time may be less.

Reconstruction cannot restore normal sensation to your breast, but in time, some feeling may return. Most scars will fade substantially over time, though it may take as long as one to two years, but they'll never disappear entirely. The better the quality of your overall reconstruction, the less distracting you'll find those scars.

Follow your surgeon's advice on when to begin stretching exercises and normal activities. As a general rule, you'll want to refrain from any overhead lifting, strenuous sports, and sexual activity for three to six weeks following reconstruction.

Your New Look

Chances are your reconstructed breast may feel firmer and look rounder or flatter than your natural breast. It may not have the same contour as your breast before mastectomy, nor will it exactly match your opposite breast. But these differences will be apparent only to you. For most mastectomy patients, breast reconstruction dramatically improves their appearance and quality of life following surgery.

Part Four

Sexuality and
Reproductive Issues

Chapter 30

A Woman's Guide to Sexuality

We are all sexual.
Our sexuality includes:

- our bodies and how our bodies work
- our genders—male or female
- our sexual orientations—straight, lesbian, or bisexual
- our values about life, love, and the people our lives touch.

Our sexuality influences how we feel about all of those things and how we experience love, compassion, joy, sorrow, and pleasure.

Some of the most difficult choices you will make as a woman will be about sex. They will affect your decisions about school, career, lifestyle, relationship, and family. No one else can make them for you. Whatever sexual choices you make, choose the ones that help you feel proud in your mind, body, and spirit.

Sex, Love, and Relationships—in the Real World

We live in a very sexual world. Sex seems to be everywhere. It is used to sell videos, magazines, records, and movies. We watch actors play women and men who are swept away by passion. There are seldom any real consequences. Great fantasies! But anyone who expects real life to be that way is in for a big surprise. The only kind of sex that has no serious consequences is masturbation.

There's a difference between sexual desire and love. Sexual desire is a powerful physical excitement. Love is a powerful caring for someone else. It can also be physically exciting. Love can exist without sexual desire, and sexual desire can exist without love. Many people are happiest when both love and sexual desire are shared by both partners.

Having sex with another person is very personal and very intimate. You can't have sex without getting involved in someone else's life—even if it's a one-night stand. No matter how brief, sexual relationships are partnerships. Sex partners who understand this are honest and caring with one another. They have regard for one another's feelings and are willing to talk openly about their own. They also share responsibility for birth control and protect one another from sexually transmitted infections like HIV, gonorrhea, syphilis, herpes, genital warts, and chlamydia.

Not all women are interested in sexual relationships with men. They may be interested in relationships with other women. No one knows for sure what makes women lesbian, bisexual, or heterosexual. We do know that people don't decide their sexual orientations. Our sexual identities develop as naturally as the rest of what makes us who we are.

Lesbians and bisexuals do not have to deal with pregnancy as a consequence of having sex with other women. Any woman of reproductive age who has sex with men, even occasionally, needs to use contraception if they don't want to become pregnant.

The benefits and risks of sexual relationships are much the same for women, regardless of sexual orientation—with one exception. Lesbians and bisexual women are often subjected to harassment and discrimination based on their sexual orientation.

If you want to talk with someone about your sexuality, whether you're lesbian, bisexual, or heterosexual, try a trusted friend, teacher, counselor, or someone at Planned Parenthood.

Enjoying Your Sexuality

Enjoying your sexuality is more than just having sex. Women enjoy their bodies, their femininity, and their fantasies. They take pride in their sensuality and their capacity for multiple orgasm—whether or not they have sex partners. They value their potential to give life and cherish their desires for physical connection and emotional intimacy.

It is healthy for women to be comfortable with their bodies and know what gives them pleasure. Outside images can frustrate what being a woman means to you. For example, the standard American fashion mannequin is five feet, eight inches tall and wears a size six dress. The average American woman is five feet, four inches tall and wears a size 12. Women who struggle to look like mannequins may injure their health. Differences in body type, height, and weight are normal—and healthy.

Every woman has different feelings about sexual pleasure. For example, some women do not like to have their breasts touched by their sex partners. Others find it very exciting. Exploring your own body to discover what you like and what you don't like can help you understand your sexuality.

Women are entitled to sexual pleasure. Our society can make women feel bad about their sexual desires. But guilt and shame about sexual feelings are unhealthy. It is healthier for you to enjoy your sexuality without shame. Many women learn about their sexual pleasure by masturbating. Understanding what gives you sexual pleasure may make having sex with a partner easier and more rewarding. Many women masturbate throughout their lives—whether or not they are in relationships.

Every woman has her own sexual values. Don't let others impose their values on you. Only you will know what sex means for you. Is it about finding a life partner? Is it about satisfying a physical need? Is it about developing a relationship? Is it waiting until marriage? It is all of these? The meaning of sex may change over your lifetime.

Sexual intercourse can really complicate things. It is important to be ready before getting involved. It can be very unsatisfying to have sex only because you think you must.

Sexual Relationships

Self-respect is the key to a healthy and rewarding sex life. We cannot expect others to respect us if we do not respect ourselves. Being your own woman means doing what you know deep down is right for you. Sometimes your friends give you lots of support. But sometimes they can try to pressure you into doing things you're not ready to do. It's important to be honest with yourself about what makes you comfortable and what doesn't—what you want and what you don't want.

Women who respect themselves are less likely to get involved in sexual activities that wound their pride, are unpleasant, or hurt them. Some women try to put up with discomfort or pain, hoping they'll get used to it. They may not know what to expect from sex play. If sex hurts, use more lubrication, try a different position or some other form of sex play, or ask your partner to be more gentle.

Some people put up with abuse to protect their relationships. This is very unhealthy and dangerous. That is why physical and sexual abuse are illegal in any relationship. Alcohol or other drugs can lower your inhibitions and increase your risk for abuse.

Avoid regrets—trust your feelings about becoming sexually involved. Our society does not help a woman understand her real feelings about sex. Thinking about your answers to each of these questions may help you understand some of yours:

- What are my sexual desires?

- What are my sexual limits—am I clear with myself about what I will do and won't do?

- Do I want to have sex?

- What do I want to get out of it?

- Will I get what I want?

- What does my partner want? Why?

- Could I get hurt?

- Will this relationship be honest, equal, respectful, and responsible?

- Am I prepared for any physical or emotional outcome?

Don't let your partner rush you. If things are moving too fast, slow them down. If you feel pressured or overwhelmed, take a break. Worthwhile partners will care about your feelings. They will support your need to take your time. They will be proud to protect you from sexually transmitted infections and unintended pregnancy. It is wrong for a partner to pressure you, ask you to take risks, or ignore your feelings. It is not a good sign if your partner keeps secrets.

Communication is very important. People often think very differently about sex and what it means. For example, many people expect that having sexual intercourse will increase their intimacy. In fact, having sex does not guarantee intimacy. It can even be a barrier to intimacy. Or sometimes, one partner is having sex just to have sex while the other is hoping for a lifetime relationship.

Sex cannot take the place of conversation. Partners who talk with one another about their real feelings don't hurt each other as much as those who keep their feelings to themselves. Talking about what they expect from sex helps couples decide whether or not they should have sex together.

Get good advice about how to handle sex and relationships from people you can trust. Try to benefit from the experience of older friends and family members.

Getting the Facts

Women are becoming more open about issues of sexuality with friends, parents, and with their partners. They have the good sense to find out as much as they can about sex and sexuality, not only for their own sake, but also so they can inform friends who need information. They can get the facts from their public library, health care provider, or reproductive and family health center.

Women often take part in discussion groups about reproduction, birth control, femininity, health care, pregnancy, sexually transmitted infections, and relationships. Some are for women only. There's no pressure, and everything that's discussed is confidential. Women can relax and talk with people who have similar concerns.

To find such discussion groups, check with your public library, your temple, church, or mosque, community center, a YWCA, or your local Planned Parenthood health center.

Being sexually active can be exciting and rewarding. It can also be very risky. There are a lot of things to consider. If you know you're not ready to have sex, waiting until you are ready may be one of the best decisions you will ever make.

Chapter 31

Sexually Transmitted Diseases

What are sexually transmitted diseases (STDs)? Why do women need to be concerned about them?

STDs, once called venereal diseases, are among the most common diseases in the United States. STDs are diseases that you get by having sexual contact (vaginal, oral, or anal) with someone who already has an STD. Caused by a number of bacteria and viruses, more than 20 STDs affect both women and men. While some STDs can be cured, other STDs are lifelong (can't be cured). STDs can affect a person's physical health, emotional health, and quality of life. While rare, STDs can cause life-threatening conditions, particularly when they are not treated. Experts believe that having an STD can increase a person's chances for getting infected with HIV, the virus that causes AIDS.

It is very common for women to have no symptoms with STDs, mostly in the early stages of illness. This can result in not getting treatment until the illness is severe, when symptoms do become present. Not getting treated early can cause serious problems like infertility (not being able to get pregnant). Some STDs can also be passed, during pregnancy or birth, to a baby. These are some reasons why it is so important for women to learn about STDs—the ways they are spread, their symptoms, how they can be treated, and how they

Excerpted from the U.S. Department of Health and Human Services, National Women's Health Information Center (NWHIC), October 2002. Available online at http://www.4woman.gov; accessed July 2003.

can be prevented. This chapter gives an overview of the most common STDs that affect women.

What are the most important things for a woman to know about STDs?

- STDs affect everyone. STDs affect women and men of all ages, racial/ethnic backgrounds, and income levels. Teenagers and young adults get STDs more often than any other age group. This is because they tend to have sex more often and have more sex partners.

- The number of people getting STDs is going up. The number of people getting STDs has gone up over the last 20 years, and the numbers continue to rise. This is due, in part, to young people becoming sexually active at earlier ages and marrying later. And today, sexually active people tend to have more than one sex partner during their lives. This can end up increasing a person's chances of being exposed to an STD.

- You can have an STD, have no symptoms, and still pass it to another person. Much of the time STDs cause no symptoms, especially in women. When and if symptoms develop, they may be confused with symptoms of other diseases that aren't STDs. Even if you have no symptoms of an STD, you can still pass the infection on to another person. This is why it is so important to get tested. Talk with your health care provider about getting tested for STDs, particularly if you have more than one sex partner. Remember, you don't have to have symptoms to get tested.

- STDs can cause lifelong and severe health problems. Health problems tend to be more severe and more frequent for women than men. This may be because women most often have no symptoms and seek care only when serious problems develop. STDs can affect women in different ways. Some STDs are linked to cancer of the cervix. One STD, human papillomavirus (HPV), causes genital warts and cervical and other genital cancers.

- A mother can pass an STD to her baby before, during, or right after birth. Some of these infections can be easily cured. But others can harm a newborn, causing lifelong damage or even death. STDs are most successfully treated if caught early. There are tests to tell if you have an STD and many treatments for STDs. When you have an STD, getting treated right away is best. It is important to know that even with treatment that cures an STD, you can still get the STD again.

How can I keep from getting STDs?

- The best way to prevent any STD is to practice abstinence (don't have sex). Delaying having sex for the first time is another way to reduce your chances of getting an STD. Studies show that the younger people are when having sex for the first time, the more likely it is that they will get an STD. The risk of getting an STD also becomes greater over time, as the number of a person's sex partners increases.

- Have a sexual relationship with one partner who doesn't have any STDs, where you are faithful to each other (meaning that you only have sex with each other and no one else).

- Practice safer sex. This means protecting yourself with a condom **every** time you have vaginal, anal, or oral sex. For vaginal sex, use a latex male condom or a female polyurethane condom. For anal sex, use a latex male condom. If needed, use only water-based lubricants with male and female condoms. For oral sex, use a dental dam—a device used by dentists, made out of a rubbery material, that you place over the opening to the vagina before having oral sex. If you don't have a dental dam, you can cut an unlubricated male condom open and place it over the opening to the vagina. Even though it may be embarrassing, if you don't know how to use a male or female condom, talk to your health care provider. The biggest reason condoms don't work is because they are not used correctly.

- Be aware that condoms don't provide complete protection against STDs. But, they do decrease your chances of getting an STD. Know also that other methods of birth control, like birth control pills, shots, implants, or diaphragms don't protect you from STDs. If you use one of these methods, be sure to also use a condom every time you have sex.

- Limit your number of sexual partners. Your risk of getting an STD increases with the number of partners you have.

- Don't share needles or drug injection equipment. This includes illegal drugs like heroin and cocaine and legal drugs like steroids and vitamins. If you get a tattoo or body piercing, make sure the needles are sterile (clean).

- Learn how to talk with your partner about STDs and using condoms. It's up to you to make sure you are protected. You can also talk with your health care provider about this.

- When you are sexually active, especially if you have more than one partner, get regular exams for STDs from a health care provider. Many tests for STDs can be done during an exam. And, the earlier an STD is found, the easier it is to treat.

- Learn the common symptoms of STDs. Seek medical help right away if you think you may have an STD.

- Don't douche. Douching removes some of the normal bacteria in the vagina that protects you from infection. This can increase your risk for getting some STDs.

Table 31.1. Common Sexually Transmitted Diseases (continued on next page)

STD	Symptoms
Bacterial Vaginosis (BV)	Vaginal discharge that can be white, gray, or thin and have an odor. Burning or pain when urinating. Itching around the outside of the vagina. Can have no symptoms.
Chlamydia	Most people have no symptoms. Vaginal discharge. Burning when urinating.
Genital Herpes	Small red bumps, blisters, or open sores on the penis, vagina, or areas close by. Vaginal discharge. Fever, headache, and muscle aches. Pain when urinating. Itching, burning, or swollen glands in genital area. Pain in legs, buttocks, or genital area. Can have no symptoms.
Gonorrhea	Women often have no symptoms. Pain or burning when urinating. Yellowish and sometimes bloody vaginal discharge. Bleeding between menstrual periods. Heavy bleeding with periods. Pain when having sex. Lower abdominal pain.
Hepatitis	Mild fever. Headache and muscle aches. Tiredness. Loss of appetite. Nausea, vomiting, and diarrhea. Dark-colored urine and pale bowel movements. Stomach pain. Skin and whites of eyes turning yellow (jaundice). Can have no symptoms.

What should I do if I have an STD?

Sometimes a person may be too scared or embarrassed to ask for information or help. But, keep in mind most STDs are easy to treat. Early treatment of STDs is important. The quicker you seek treatment, the less likely the STD will cause you severe harm. And the sooner you tell your sex partners about having an STD, the less likely they are to spread the disease to others (because they can get treated). For pregnant women, early treatment also reduces the chances of passing the STD to a baby.

Doctors, local health departments, and STD and family planning clinics have information about STDs. The American Social Health Association (ASHA) has free information and keeps lists of clinics and doctors who provide treatment for STDs. Call ASHA at (800) 227-8922.

Table 31.1. Common Sexually Transmitted Diseases (continued from previous page)

STD	Symptoms
HIV Infection and AIDS	Can have no symptoms for 10 years or more. Lack of energy or fatigue. Weight loss. Frequent low-grade fevers and night sweats. Frequent yeast infections (in the mouth). Skin rashes or flaky skin that is hard to get rid of. Women can have vaginal yeast infections and other STDs; pelvic inflammatory disease (PID); and menstrual cycle changes.
Human Papillomavirus (HPV)	Genital warts that sometimes can be hard to see. Can have no symptoms.
Syphilis	Painless sores (chancres) and skin rash. Mild fever. Feeling very tired. Headache and sore throat. Hair loss. Swollen lymph glands throughout the body. Can have no symptoms.
Trichomoniasis	Yellow, green, or gray vaginal discharge with a strong odor. Discomfort during sex and when urinating. Irritation and itching of the genital area. Lower abdominal pain (rare).
Vaginal Yeast Infections	Itching, burning, and irritation of the vagina. Pain when urinating or with intercourse. Cottage-cheesy looking vaginal discharge.

You can get information from the phone line without leaving your name.

If you have an STD or think you may have an STD:

- Get it treated right away. Studies suggest that having an STD increases your risk for getting infected with HIV, the virus that causes AIDS.

- Follow your health care provider's orders and finish all the medicine that you are given. Even if the symptoms go away, you still need to finish all of the medicine.

- Avoid having any sexual activity while you are being treated for an STD.

- Be sure to tell your sexual partners, so they can be treated too.

- Get a follow-up test to make sure that the infection has been cured (for those STDs that can be cured; some are lifelong infections).

- If you are pregnant, be sure to tell your doctor. Some medicines aren't safe to take when pregnant, and you may need a different drug to treat the STD.

- If you are breastfeeding, talk with your doctor about the risk of passing the STD to your baby while breastfeeding.

Chapter 32

Sexual Dysfunction

Chapter Contents

Section 32.1

Sexual Problems

American College of Obstetricians and Gynecologists.
Sexuality and Sexual Problems. (Patient Education Pamphlet No.
AP072). Washington, DC. © ACOG 2000.

Women—whether married or single, young or old—differ greatly in their sexual interest and response. A woman's sexual function is not limited to sexual intercourse. Her sexuality also includes the way she thinks and feels about herself as a woman.

Some women have trouble with sex at some time in their lives. They often find it hard to talk about their sexual concerns—even with their partner, a trusted friend, or their doctor.

Sexuality

Sexual identity is shaped and reshaped throughout life. A number of key factors affect your sexual development. These include early role models, religious teachings, and early sexual experiences—both good and bad.

Sexual Problems

A woman's progress through the sexual response cycle varies greatly from one time to another. No one pattern is more "normal" than another. If any of the stages of the cycle does not occur, though, it may cause a sexual problem.

The sexual response cycle: A woman's body follows a regular pattern when she has sex. There are four stages:

- desire
- arousal
- orgasm
- resolution

Sexual response depends on a complex interplay—physical and emotional—between two people.

294

Sexual problems can be linked to a physical condition, such as pregnancy or an illness. They also can relate to daily stress, poor communication between partners, unrealistic ideas about sexual performance, or problems with trust and commitment.

Lack of desire. Lack of interest in sex—or lack of desire—is the most common sexual problem in women. With a low level of sexual desire, a woman may have a hard time getting aroused.

Many women find that the stresses of daily living—such as concerns about work, family, and money—can create a lack of desire.

Lack of orgasm. Most women are able to have an orgasm during sexual activity. Some may reach orgasm by masturbation or by having their partner arouse them with their hands or with oral sex.

Problems with reaching orgasm can stem from negative feelings about sex learned in childhood. Women who have suffered a trauma related to sex, such as sexual abuse, may not be able to reach orgasm.

If a woman has no orgasm during sex, it does not mean it was a failure. Sharing love, closeness, warmth, and tenderness are often enough.

Painful sex. Dyspareunia is a term for pain during or after sex. This may include pain during entry into the vagina, pain during deep thrusting, or pain after sex. The pain can be on the surface or deep, along the middle of the pelvis, or on one or both sides.

The most common cause is that the vagina is not well lubricated. Vaginismus also can cause pain during sex. This is a spasm of the pubic muscles and lower vagina. It makes entering the vagina painful.

Conditions That Can Affect Your Sexual Function

Some conditions can have a big impact on sexuality. They may be short-term, such as the flu or pregnancy, or may persist over time and require the couple to adjust.

Pregnancy. In most cases, sexual activity doesn't have to change during pregnancy. Sex does not harm the fetus unless certain conditions are present.

Menopause. As women approach menopause, they may lose desire slowly, have a hard time getting aroused, and feel pain during sex. The lack of estrogen that occurs after menopause makes the vagina dry.

Cancer. Women with cancer often worry about how the disease will affect their sex life. Surgery, radiation, and chemotherapy can be painful and sap the woman's energy. She may struggle with fears of death, disfigurement, or the partner's rejection.

Chronic illness. Diseases that persist for a lifetime, such as diabetes, arthritis, or heart disease, can have a major impact on a woman's self-image and her ability to feel sexual. Some medications can affect her desire or make it hard to reach orgasm.

Male Factor. If a male partner is having sexual problems, pleasure for both partners may be affected. Many men have trouble with impotence—not being able to achieve or keep an erection—at some time in their lives.

Impotence is usually caused by physical or medical factors.

If You Think You Have a Problem

Nearly every couple has a problem with sex at some time in their lives. Some problems go away on their own or can be worked out with patience and a caring and informed partner. Others may take more effort and a change of approach.

If you think you may have a health condition that is stopping you from enjoying sex, see your doctor. Any pain in the pelvic, genital or vaginal area is a sign that there may be a problem.

Your doctor may be able to help you. Your doctor also can refer you to other experts. Sex counseling for individuals or couples is often short term and works well.

Finally

Being able to express yourself sexually lasts a lifetime. It should be nurtured—it's a key part of feeling fulfilled. For all women, talking about sexual needs and concerns is a process that should never end. Sexual problems are common. If you are having a problem with sex, know there are many people with the skills and understanding to help.

Section 32.2

Dyspareunia (Painful Intercourse)

What Is Dyspareunia?

Dyspareunia is the medical term for pain during intercourse. You may hear your doctor use this word or see it in other written material.

Pain during intercourse can be caused by a wide variety of reasons. Examples include an allergic reaction to a personal hygiene product or hormonal changes related to aging. Sometimes, emotional issues may also play a role.

The Causes of Pain during Intercourse

- Tipped or retroverted uterus—Some women with a tipped uterus experience pain during intercourse. This happens when the penis hits the cervix or uterus during sex. This condition is known as collision dyspareunia.

- Endometriosis—The tissue lining the uterus—the endometrium—may grow outside the uterus causing deep pain during sex.

- Infection—Bacterial or yeast infections are among the most common causes of pain during intercourse.

- Lack of estrogen—During menopause, the vaginal walls thin and the amount of vaginal lubrication decreases.

- Vulvodynia—In this condition, the vulva is hypersensitive and extremely tender on touch.

- Drug side effects—Common drugs including those for allergy, high blood pressure, or depression may affect the amount of vaginal lubrication, as well as the level of sexual arousal and desire.

- Physical problems—Scar tissue from abdominal surgery or from delivering a baby can distort the anatomy and cause significant pain during intercourse. A cyst on an ovary can also cause pain.

- Pelvic floor myalgia—Pelvic floor muscle spasms are involuntary muscle spasms and can result in difficult and uncomfortable sex.

- Emotional issues—Sometimes, past issues such as sexual abuse or communication problems in a relationship can translate into sexual difficulties.

Pain during sex may be caused by other reasons as well. Only consultation with a physician or another health care professional will help you find out why you hurt and help you find a solution.

Section 32.3

Getting Help for Female Sexual Problems

"Female Sexual Problems" reprinted with permission of the American Association for Marriage and Family Therapy, 2002. By Dixie A. Guidner, M.R.E. © 2002.

In Western society we are bombarded with messages about sexuality from the popular media, and yet it can be embarrassing to talk about our personal sexuality, especially any sexual concerns we may have. Sexual problems can have a ripple effect on many other areas of our lives including intimate relationships with a partner, the family, and work, and our general well being. At the same time all of our life interactions and activities can affect our sexuality The media tends to present sex as easy, good, and spontaneous, and it implies that we should always be in the mood for it. If only sex were that simple.

If you and your partner are experiencing problems with sex, you are not alone. Recent studies reveal that nearly 40 percent of women of all ages report having sexual problems. It just isn't the kind of thing people want to admit. But you deserve to have a pleasurable sex life and there are professionals who can help.

What are female sexual problems?

There are a variety of sexual problems that women experience, either alone or with a partner. The term "sex" is not limited just to intercourse, and can also refer to a variety of intimate sexual activities such as fondling, self-stimulation (masturbation), and oral sex. Sexual problems are generally defined as any problem that occurs in the course of sexual activity, including:

- Not being in the mood
- Trouble becoming aroused, which usually involves being too dry
- Difficulty having orgasms
- Pain during sex or pain related to sexual activity

Most women experience these from time to time. It is when they are persistent that they become problematic for the woman and her partner. You should seek help more promptly if you are experiencing physical pain.

What causes female sexual problems?

Sexual problems can be influenced by a wide variety of factors. There are two main components-biological and psychological-and usually they interact. Biological problems usually involve such things as hormonal imbalances, infections (like yeast infections), or diseases (like diabetes or multiple sclerosis) that have potential side effects like pain during sex or excessive dryness. There are certain times in a woman's life when she is more prone to sexual problems because of hormonal changes. For example, some women experience a range of sexual responses right after childbirth and during menopause. Also, some commonly prescribed medications, like certain antidepressants, can lead to sexual side effects.

There is also the psychological aspect. This can include such things as the many conflicting cultural messages one learns about sexuality. Gender messages are especially influential, impacting how a woman views her sexual self, including body image, roles, power, and her view of her partner.

From birth throughout her life every woman is developing a unique sexual story influenced by culture, gender, family of origin, and personal experiences. The story takes on the beliefs and meanings that she attributes to her sexuality.

Couples must negotiate their personal sexual stories as they develop their own style of sexual communication and activity. This should be an ongoing process, since everyday life problems may get in the way of intimacy and sexuality. Job worries, pressures of juggling work and family, substance abuse, depression, and financial worries can all influence how you feel sexually. In our fast paced world, having a lot on your mind, as most people do, can get in the way even when you want to focus on being intimate.

Over time psychological troubles can create biological problems and vice versa. It all starts to blur together so you can't even really pinpoint where the issues started. You just know you want help.

How do you know when to seek help?

It really depends on the woman and her partner. Sometimes a problem seems to go away pretty quickly on its own. But, if this is something that is really worrying or frustrating you or your partner and does not seem to go away no matter what you try, or if you are experiencing considerable pain or discomfort, it may be time to consider professional help.

How do you get help?

Help is available through both individual or couples therapy. Many people will use a combination of the two. When a couple begins therapy, the therapist may refer one or both partners to a physician to rule out any medical conditions that could be contributing to the problem. The therapist or physician should fully inform you of the reasons for the medical procedure. A physician can also help with issues surrounding medication, like experimenting with the dosage of your medication to reduce sexual side effects. There are some hormonal treatments for women that are helpful during and after menopause. For now, there are no drugs available to help improve women's sexual functioning like there are for men, though some may be available in the next few years.

Therapy can help women, either alone or with a partner, who are experiencing sexual problems. Most therapists are used to talking to couples about their sexual lives and will not be embarrassed if you bring it up. The therapist is there to help the woman and her partner gain understanding of some of the relationship dynamics and background issues that may be influencing the problem. The therapist can also provide you with information about human sexuality and sexual functioning, and answer your questions.

Chapter 33

Birth Control (Contraception)

Chapter Contents

Section 33.1

Birth Control Methods

Text reprinted from the National Women's Health Information Center, U.S. Department of Health and Human Services, Office on Women's Health (http://www.4women.gov/faq/birthcont.htm), November 2002, and "FDA Approves Seasonale Oral Contraceptive," *FDA Talk Paper*, U.S. Food and Drug Administration, September 5, 2003. Table reprinted from the U.S. Food and Drug Administration, www.fda.gov, August 2002.

What Is the Best Method of Birth Control (or Contraception)?

All women and men should have control over if and when they become parents. Making decisions about birth control, or contraception, is not easy—there are many things to think about. Learning about birth control methods you or your partner can use to prevent pregnancy and talking with your health care provider are two good ways to get started.

There is no best method of birth control. Each method has its own pros and cons. Some methods work better than others do at preventing pregnancy.

Researchers are always working to develop or improve birth control methods. The birth control method you choose should take into account:

- your overall health;
- how often you have sex;
- the number of sexual partners you have;
- if you want to have children;
- how well each method works (or is effective) in preventing pregnancy;
- any potential side effects; and
- your comfort level with using the method.

Bear in mind that NO method of birth control prevents pregnancy all of the time. Birth control methods can fail. But you can greatly increase a method's success rate by using it correctly all of the time. The only way to be sure you never get pregnant is to not have sex (abstinence).

FDA Approved New Oral Contraceptive in September 2003

The FDA has approved Seasonale, a new choice in oral contraceptives for women for prevention of pregnancy. Seasonale is a 91-day oral contraceptive regimen. Tablets containing the active hormones are taken for 12 weeks (84 days), followed by one week (7 days) of placebo (inactive) tablets. Conventional oral contraceptive use is based on a 28-day regimen (21 days of active tablets followed by 7 days of placebo tablets). Seasonale contains a progestin (levonorgestrel) and an estrogen (ethinyl estradiol), which are active ingredients in already approved oral contraceptives.

Under Seasonale's dosing regimen the number of expected menstrual periods that a woman usually experiences are reduced from once a month to about once every three months. As with the conventional 28-day regimen, women will have their period while taking the placebo tablets.

Although Seasonale users have fewer scheduled menstrual cycles, the data from clinical trials show that many women, especially in the first few cycles of use, had more unplanned bleeding and spotting between the expected menstrual periods than women taking a conventional 28-day cycle oral contraceptive.

Like other available oral contraceptives, Seasonale is effective for prevention of pregnancy when used as directed. The risks of using Seasonale are similar to the risks of other conventional oral contraceptives and include an increased risk of blood clots, heart attack, and stroke. The labeling also carries the warning that cigarette smoking increases the risk of serious cardiovascular side effects from use of combination estrogen and progestin containing contraceptives. Birth control pills do not protect against HIV infection (AIDS) or other sexually transmitted diseases.

Since Seasonale users can expect to have fewer periods, the label also advises women to consider the possibility that they may be pregnant if they miss any scheduled periods. Women should discuss contraceptive use and the precautions and warnings for use of the drug with their doctors.

Seasonale is manufactured by Barr Laboratories of Pomona, New York.

Table 33.1. Birth Control Guide. (continued on next page)

Failure Rate: Number of pregnancies expected per 100 women per year.
Some Risks: Serious medical risks from contraceptives are rare.

Male Condom Latex/Polyurethane

FDA Approval Date: Latex: Use started before premarket approval was required; Polyurethane: cleared in 1989; available starting 1995

Description: A sheath placed over the erect penis blocking the passage of sperm.

Failure Rate: 11

Some Risks: Irritation and allergic reactions (less likely with polyurethane)

Protection from Sexually Transmitted Diseases (STDs): Except for abstinence, latex condoms are the best protection against STDs, including herpes and AIDS.

Convenience: Applied immediately before intercourse; used only once and discarded. Polyurethane condoms are available for those with latex sensitivity.

Availability: Nonprescription

Female Condom

FDA Approval Date: 1993

Description: A lubricated polyurethane sheath shaped similarly to the male condom. The closed end has a flexible ring that is inserted into the vagina.

Failure Rate: 21

Some Risks: Irritation and allergic reactions

Protection from Sexually Transmitted Diseases (STDs): May give some STD protection; not as effective as latex condom.

Convenience: Applied immediately before intercourse; used only once and discarded.

Availability: Nonprescription

Diaphragm with Spermicide

FDA Approval Date: Use started before premarket approval was required.

Description: A dome-shaped rubber disk with a flexible rim that covers the cervix so that sperm cannot reach the uterus. A spermicide is applied to the diaphragm before insertion.

Failure Rate: 17

Some Risks: Irritation and allergic reactions, urinary tract infection; risk of toxic shock syndrome, a rare but serious infection, when kept in place longer than recommended.

Protection from Sexually Transmitted Diseases (STDs): None

Convenience: Inserted before intercourse and left in place at least six hours after; can be left in place for 24 hours, with additional spermicide for repeated intercourse.

Availability: Prescription

Table 33.1. (continued) Birth Control Guide. (continued on next page)

Failure Rate: Number of pregnancies expected per 100 women per year.
Some Risks: Serious medical risks from contraceptives are rare.

Cervical Cap with Spermicide

FDA Approval Date: 1988

Description: A soft rubber cup with a round rim, which fits snugly around the cervix.

Failure Rate: 17

Some Risks: Irritation and allergic reactions, abnormal Pap test; risk of toxic shock syndrome, a rare but serious infection, when kept in place longer than recommended.

Protection from Sexually Transmitted Diseases (STDs): None

Convenience: May be difficult to insert; can remain in place for 48 hours without reapplying spermicide for repeated intercourse.

Availability: Prescription

Sponge with Spermicide

FDA Approval Date: 1983 (not currently marketed in the United States)

Description: A disk-shaped polyurethane device containing the spermicide nonoxynol-9.

Failure Rate: 14-28

Some Risks: Irritation and allergic reactions, difficulty in removal; risk of toxic shock syndrome, a rare but serious infection, when kept in place longer than recommended.

Protection from Sexually Transmitted Diseases (STDs): None

Convenience: Inserted before intercourse and protects for repeated acts of intercourse for 24 hours without additional spermicide; must be left in place for at least six hours after intercourse; must be removed without 30 hours of insertion. Is discarded after use.

Availability: Nonprescription; not currently marketed in the United States

Spermicide Alone

FDA Approval Date: Use started before premarket approval was required. Starting November 2002, only one active ingredient will be allowed.

Description: A foam, cream, jelly, film, suppository, or tablet that contains nonoxynol-9, a sperm-killing chemical.

Failure Rate: 20-50 (studies have shown varying failure rates)

Some Risks: Irritation and allergic reactions, urinary tract infections

Protection from Sexually Transmitted Diseases (STDs): None

Convenience: Instructions vary; check labeling. Inserted between 5 and 90 minutes before intercourse and usually left in place at least six to eight hours after.

Availability: Nonprescription

Table 33.1. (continued) Birth Control Guide. (continued on next page)

Failure Rate: Number of pregnancies expected per 100 women per year.
Some Risks: Serious medical risks from contraceptives are rare.

Oral Contraceptives—Combined Pill

FDA Approval Date: First in 1960; most recent in 2000

Description: A pill that suppresses ovulation by the combined actions of the hormones estrogen and progestin.

Failure Rate: 1

Some Risks: Dizziness; nausea; changes in menstruation, mood, and weight; rarely cardiovascular disease, including high blood pressure, blood clots, heart attack, and strokes

Protection from Sexually Transmitted Diseases (STDs): None, except some protection against pelvic inflammatory disease

Convenience: Must be taken on daily schedule, regardless of frequency of intercourse.

Availability: Prescription

Oral Contraceptives—Progestin-Only Minipill

FDA Approval Date: 1973

Description: A pill containing only the hormone progestin that reduces and thickens cervical mucus to prevent sperm from reaching the egg.

Failure Rate: 2

Some Risks: Irregular bleeding, weight gain, breast tenderness, less protection against ectopic pregnancy

Protection from Sexually Transmitted Diseases (STDs): None

Convenience: Must be taken on daily schedule, regardless of frequency of intercourse.

Availability: Prescription

Patch (Ortho Evra)

FDA Approval Date: 2001

Description: Skin patch worn on the lower abdomen, buttocks, or upper body that releases the hormones progestin and estrogen into the bloodstream.

Failure Rate: 1 (appears to be less effective in women weighing more than 198 pounds)

Some Risks: Similar to oral contraceptives—combined pill

Protection from Sexually Transmitted Diseases (STDs): None

Convenience: New patch is applied once a week for 3 weeks. Patch is not worn during the fourth week, and woman has a menstrual period.

Availability: Prescription

Table 33.1. (continued) Birth Control Guide. (continued on next page)

Failure Rate: Number of pregnancies expected per 100 women per year.

Some Risks: Serious medical risks from contraceptives are rare.

Vaginal Contraceptive Ring (NuvaRing)

FDA Approval Date: 2001

Description: A flexible ring about 2 inches in diameter that is inserted into the vagina and releases the hormones progestin and estrogen

Failure Rate: 1

Some Risks: Vaginal discharge, vaginitis, irritation. Similar to oral contraceptives—combined pill

Protection from Sexually Transmitted Diseases (STDs): None

Convenience: Inserted by the woman; remains in the vagina for 3 weeks, then is removed for 1 week. If ring is expelled and remains out for more than 3 hours, another birth control method must be used until ring has been used continuously for 7 days.

Availability: Prescription

Post-Coital Contraceptives (Preven and Plan B)

FDA Approval Date: 1998-1999

Description: Pills containing either progestin alone or progestin plus estrogen

Failure Rate: Almost 80 percent reduction in risk of pregnancy for a single act of un-protected sex

Some Risks: Nausea, vomiting, abdominal pain, fatigue, headache

Protection from Sexually Transmitted Diseases (STDs): None

Convenience: Must be taken within 72 hours of having unprotected intercourse.

Availability: Prescription

Injection (Depo-Provera)

FDA Approval Date: 1992

Description: An injectable progestin that inhibits ovulation, prevents sperm from reaching the egg, and prevents the fertilized egg from implanting in the uterus.

Failure Rate: Less than 1

Some Risks: Irregular bleeding, weight gain, breast tenderness, headaches

Protection from Sexually Transmitted Diseases (STDs): None

Convenience: One injection every three months.

Availability: Prescription

Table 33.1. (continued) Birth Control Guide. (continued on next page)

Failure Rate: Number of pregnancies expected per 100 women per year.

Some Risks: Serious medical risks from contraceptives are rare.

Injection (Lunelle)

FDA Approval Date: 2000

Description: An injectable form of progestin and estrogen

Failure Rate: less than 1

Some Risks: Changes in menstrual cycle, weight gain. Similar to oral contraceptives—combined

Protection from Sexually Transmitted Diseases (STDs): None

Convenience: Injection given once a month

Availability: Prescription

Implant (Norplant)

FDA Approval Date: 1990

Description: Six matchstick-sized rubber rods that are surgically implanted under the skin of the upper arm, where they steadily release the contraceptive steroid levonorgestrel

Failure Rate: Less than 1

Some Risks: Irregular bleeding, weight gain, breast tenderness, headaches, difficulty in removal

Protection from Sexually Transmitted Diseases (STDs): None

Convenience: Implanted by health-care provider in minor outpatient surgical procedure; effective for up to five years.

Availability: Prescription. In July 2002, Norplant's manufacturer announced that it will no longer distribute the Norplant system. Women using the system should contact their doctors about what their contraceptive options will be after the five-year expiration date of their Norplant systems.

IUD (Intrauterine Device)

FDA Approval Date: 1976

Description: A T-shaped device inserted into the uterus by a health professional.

Failure Rate: Less than 1

Some Risks: Cramps, heavy bleeding, pelvic inflammatory disease, infertility, perforation of uterus

Protection from Sexually Transmitted Diseases (STDs): None

Convenience: After insertion by physician, can remain in place for up to one or 10 years, depending on type.

Availability: Prescription

Table 33.1. (continued) Birth Control Guide.

Failure Rate: Number of pregnancies expected per 100 women per year.

Some Risks: Serious medical risks from contraceptives are rare.

Periodic Abstinence

FDA Approval Date: N/A

Description: To deliberately refrain from having sexual intercourse during times when pregnancy is more likely.

Failure Rate: 20

Some Risks: None

Protection from Sexually Transmitted Diseases (STDs): None

Convenience: Requires frequent monitoring of body functions (for example, body temperature for one method.)

Availability: Instructions from health care provider

Surgical Sterilization—Female

FDA Approval Date: N/A

Description: The woman's fallopian tubes are blocked so the egg and sperm can't meet in the fallopian tube, preventing conception.

Failure Rate: Less than 1

Some Risks: Pain, bleeding, infection, other postsurgical complications

Protection from Sexually Transmitted Diseases (STDs): None

Convenience: One-time surgical procedure

Availability: Surgery

Surgical Sterilization—Male

FDA Approval Date: N/A

Description: Sealing, tying, or cutting a man's vas deferens so that the sperm can't travel from the testicles to the penis.

Failure Rate: Less than 1

Some Risks: Pain, bleeding, infection, other minor postsurgical complications

Protection from Sexually Transmitted Diseases (STDs): None

Convenience: One-time surgical procedure

Availability: Surgery

Note: Failure rates in this chart are based on information from clinical trials submitted to the Food and Drug Administration during product reviews. This number represents the percentage of women who become pregnant during the first year of use of a birth control method. For methods that the FDA does not review, such as periodic abstinence, numbers are estimated from published literature. For comparison, about 85 out of 100 sexually active women who wish to become pregnant would be expected to become pregnant in a year. The most effective way to avoid both pregnancy and sexually transmitted disease is to practice total abstinence (refrain from sexual contact).

This chart is a summary; it is not intended to be used alone. All product labeling should be followed carefully, and a health-care professional should be consulted for some methods.

Source: Food and Drug Administration.

Section 33.2

Emergency Contraception

Excerpted from the U.S. Department of Health and Human Services, National Women's Health Information Center (NWHIC), November 2002. Available online at http://www.4woman.gov; accessed July 2003.

Emergency contraception, or emergency birth control, is used to keep a woman from getting pregnant when she has had unprotected vaginal intercourse. Unprotected can mean that no method of birth control was used. It can also mean that a birth control method was used but did not work—like a condom breaking. Other things can happen as well that put a woman at risk for getting pregnant. A woman may have forgotten to take her birth control pills. She may have been abused or forced to have sex when she did not want to. Emergency contraception should never be used as a regular method of birth control. There are effective methods of birth control that women can use on a regular basis to prevent pregnancy.

Emergency contraception keeps a woman from getting pregnant by stopping:

- ovulation, or stopping the ovaries from releasing eggs that can be fertilized;

- fertilization, or stopping the egg from being fertilized by the sperm;

- implantation, or stopping a fertilized egg from attaching itself to the wall of the uterus.

If you are already pregnant, emergency contraception will **not** work. If you have an ectopic pregnancy, where the pregnancy develops outside of the uterus, it will also not work. This can be a serious condition that can be fatal. Signs of ectopic pregnancy include extreme pain on one or both sides of the lower abdomen, spotting blood, and feeling dizzy or faint. If you think you have an ectopic pregnancy, go to an emergency room right away.

Chapter 34

Abortion

Chapter Contents

Section 34.1

Medical Abortion

What is medical abortion?

Medical abortion is a way to end pregnancy without surgery. Recent studies show that medical abortion works up to 63 days after the last period begins.

How does medical abortion work?

There are three steps. At the first step, your clinician will give you an injection of methotrexate or a dose of mifepristone in tablet form. At the second step, you will take another medication called misoprostol in tablet form. At the third step, you will return to your clinician for a follow-up visit.

Step One

- Methotrexate—stops the pregnancy in the uterus. It can also stop those that develop in the fallopian tube, which are called ectopic pregnancies.

- Mifepristone—blocks the hormone progesterone. Without progesterone, the lining of the uterus breaks down, ending the pregnancy.

Methotrexate and mifepristone affect the body differently. A clinician can help you decide which is best for you.

Step Two

- Misoprostol—causes the uterus to contract and empty.

Step Three

- Follow up. Your clinician needs to make sure the abortion is complete. You will need an ultrasound or blood test.

How long does it take?

- With methotrexate—About 50 percent of women have the abortion the same day they take misoprostol. It happens within a week for another 35 to 40 percent. The whole process can take up to 14 days.

- With mifepristone—About 10 percent of women will have the abortion before they take misoprostol. Most others will have it within four hours of taking misoprostol. For others, bleeding begins in 24 hours. The whole process can take about a week.

It's important to remember that choosing medical abortion means that you will need to visit your clinician's office more than one time.

How effective is it?

Medical abortion with methotrexate is about 90 percent effective. With mifepristone, it is from 92 to 95 percent effective. Methotrexate and misoprostol can cause serious birth defects. If the medical abortion does not work, a surgical abortion must be done.

What do I need to do to have a medical abortion?

During the first visit, you will need to have counseling; sign a consent form; give a medical history; have laboratory tests; and have a physical exam—including an ultrasound

You will take the first medicine at the clinic. You and your clinician will plan the next step according to what is best for you. You may take the second medication at home. Or you may need to return to the clinic.

After you take misoprostol you will start to bleed heavily within hours or days. This is the abortion.

How does it feel?

For most women, medical abortion is like an early miscarriage. You might feel strong cramps; feel nauseous or vomit; have diarrhea; or feel temporary abdominal pain.

Acetaminophen—such as Tylenol or Excedrin—can reduce most of these symptoms. Painkillers such as ibuprofen—for example, Motrin or Advil—can also reduce symptoms. You may see large blood clots or tissue at the time of the abortion. You may have some bleeding for up to four weeks after.

313

Call a clinician if you:

- soak more than two maxi pads an hour, more than two hours in a row

- bleed heavily for more than 12 hours in a row

- pass clots larger than lemons for two hours or more

- run a temperature over 101.4 degrees Fahrenheit for more than four hours

- feel strong nausea or throw up for more than four hours

- are in pain, even with painkillers

- have an allergic reaction to the medicine

You may need a clinic visit. Rarely, women need surgical abortion or hospitalization.

Why do some women prefer medical abortion?

- No anesthesia or surgery.
- Can be done early.
- They can begin treatment as soon as they know they are pregnant.
- Less cramping than with surgery.
- More control.
- They may feel it is less invasive.
- More natural.
- They may feel it is more like miscarriage.
- More privacy.
- They may have the abortion at home.

Ninety-six percent of women in clinical trials would recommend medical abortion to a friend.

Who can choose medical abortion?

You may choose medical abortion if you are up to 63 days pregnant. But you must agree to have a surgical abortion if the medical treatment fails. You also need access to a telephone, transportation, and backup medical care.

Medical abortion is not recommended if:

- you are more than 63 days pregnant
- take anti-clotting medication or have blood clotting disorders
- have severe heart, liver, or kidney problems
- have seizures more than once a week
- take any medicine that should not be combined with methotrexate, mifepristone, or misoprostol
- cannot return for follow-up visits
- are unwilling or unable to have a surgical abortion if the medical abortion is incomplete
- have an allergy to the medications

Will I need to prepare for the follow-up visit?

Yes. After you take the medicine and before your follow-up exam:

- Do not take a vitamin with folic acid. It can interfere with methotrexate.
- Do not take aspirin.
- Do not drink alcoholic drinks.
- Do not take anti-coagulant (anti-clotting) drugs.

What if I'm still pregnant after taking the medicine?

Your clinician will help you decide. You may: wait two to six weeks and check again; take more misoprostol; or need a surgical abortion.

When will I get my period?

Abortion begins a new menstrual cycle. You should have a regular period in four to eight weeks.

When can I have sex again?

Don't have vaginal intercourse or insert anything into the vagina for one week after the abortion. You can get pregnant very soon after the abortion. Discuss birth control options with your clinician.

Where can I get a medical abortion?

Contact Planned Parenthood at 1-800-230-PLAN, other women's health care centers, or your private clinician. Planned Parenthood centers that do not provide medical abortion can refer you to someone who does.

How much does it cost?

Medical abortion involves two or three office visits, testing, and exams. Cost varies—from $350 to $575. Costs may be more or less depending on locale and what ever additional tests, visits, or exams are needed.

Section 34.2

Surgical Abortion

What is surgical abortion?

Surgical abortion is a way to end pregnancy.

How does it work?

The three most common methods are manual vacuum aspiration, dilation and suction curettage, and dilation and evacuation. The method used depends on how long you have been pregnant—the number of days since the first day of your last period.

Manual vacuum aspiration—or MVA, empties the uterus with gentle suction of a manual syringe. It is often used for very early surgical abortion. It can be done as soon as you know you are pregnant and up to 10 weeks after your last period.

Dilation and suction curettage—also known as D&C, or vacuum aspiration, gently empties the uterus with machine-operated suction.

A curette (narrow metal loop) may be used to clean the walls of the uterus. This method is used for early surgical abortion. It is performed from six to 14 weeks after your last period.

Dilation and evacuation—also known as D&E, is a two-part procedure. The cervix is slowly opened. The procedure is completed with medical instruments, suction, and curettage. After 24 weeks of pregnancy, abortions are usually performed only for serious health reasons.

How long does it take?

MVA and D&C take about 10 minutes. A D&E takes between 10 and 20 minutes. Allow more time for the whole process, which also includes counseling, a physical exam, forms to read and sign, and a recovery period.

How effective is it?

Surgical abortion is nearly 100 percent effective. It fails to end a pregnancy one out of 500 times. This can happen due to unusual conditions: there can be more than one chamber in the uterus or the pregnancy may not be in the uterus.

What do I need to do to get a surgical abortion?

You will need to: have counseling; sign a consent form give a medical history; have laboratory tests; and have a physical exam—which may include an ultrasound

You may need special counseling or arrangements if you: are extremely uncomfortable about having the procedure; are extremely overweight; have certain kinds of sexually transmitted infections; have an infection in your uterus; have seizures more than once a week; are running a fever; have certain serious health problems; or have problems with anesthesia.

How does it feel?

Most women feel pain similar to menstrual cramps. For others, abortion is more uncomfortable.

Local painkillers are usually used. Some clinics use a kind that allows you to be awake but deeply relaxed. Others offer general anesthesia so you can sleep through the procedure. This, however, increases the medical risks and how long you must remain at the clinic.

Abortion with local anesthetic after 24 weeks of pregnancy is about as painful as labor during birth.

How is MVA performed?

- Your vagina is washed with an antiseptic.

- The clinician may inject a painkiller into or near your cervix.

- The opening of the cervix may be stretched with dilators. Or you may be given a medication, or you may have a special dilator inserted the night before to open your cervix.

- A tube is inserted through the cervix into the uterus. A hand-held pump gently empties the uterus.

How is a D&C performed?

- Your vagina is washed with an antiseptic.

- The clinician may recommend sedation and may inject a painkiller into or near your cervix.

- The opening of the cervix is stretched with dilators. Or you may be given a medication or you may have a special dilator inserted the night before to open your cervix.

- A tube is inserted into the uterus. This tube is attached to a suction machine.

- The suction machine is turned on. The uterus is emptied by gentle suction.

- A curette may be used.

How is a D&E performed?

- Your vagina is washed with an antiseptic.

- You may be given medication or have a special dilator inserted the night before to open your cervix. You may also be given antibiotics to prevent infection.

- You may be sedated and may be given intravenous painkillers.

- A local anesthetic is injected into or near the cervix.

- The dilator is removed.

- The fetus and other products of conception are removed from the uterus with medical instruments, suction, and curette.

What are the health risks of abortion?

In the first 20 weeks, abortion is much safer than giving birth. Complications from early abortion include:

- Allergic reactions to the drugs. Tell your clinician what medications or recreational drugs you take. It will be strictly confidential.

- Incomplete abortion. This occurs in less than one out of 100 D&C abortions. It occurs in one out of 200 D&Es.

- Blood clots in the uterus.

- Infection. Usually antibiotics clear up the infection. In rare cases, a repeat procedure, hospitalization, or surgery is needed.

- Very heavy bleeding. You may need medication, a D&C, or, rarely, surgery. Very rarely, blood transfusions are required.

- A cut or torn cervix. This occurs in fewer than one out of 100 early abortions.

- Organ injury. In about one of 1,000 early abortions, an instrument goes through the wall of the uterus. In even fewer cases, this leads to infection, heavy bleeding, or both. In D&E this happens three of 1,000 times. Surgery, or very rarely, hysterectomy, may be needed.

- Death occurs in one of 100,000 abortions. Childbirth carries seven times more risk.

What happens after the abortion?

- After very early and early abortions, you will rest in a recovery room for about an hour.

- If you have an Rh-negative blood type, you will receive an injection to protect future pregnancies.

- You will receive written after-care instructions and a 24-hour emergency phone number.

- Call your clinician if you have heavy bleeding, pain, or fever.

- You can discuss birth control with your counselor.

- You will make a follow-up appointment in two to four weeks.

How will I feel later?

You may have cramps. You may want to relax for the rest of the day. You may shower as soon as you wish. Do not take baths, douche, or use vaginal medications. You can usually return to work or other normal activities the next day. Recovery after later abortions may take longer.

Will I bleed for a long time?

You may bleed off and on for a couple of weeks. Some women have cramps and pass a few large blood clots for up to 10 days. Use sanitary pads—not tampons.

When will I get my period?

Abortion begins a new menstrual cycle. You should have a regular period in four to eight weeks.

When can I have sex again?

Don't have vaginal intercourse or insert anything into the vagina for one week after the abortion. You can get pregnant very soon after the abortion. Discuss birth control options with your clinician.

Where can I get a surgical abortion?

Contact Planned Parenthood at 1-800-230-PLAN, other women's health centers, or your private clinician. Or call the National Abortion Federation at 1-800-772-9100.

How much does abortion cost?

Fees depend on how long you've been pregnant and where you go. At health centers, the cost ranges from about $225 to $575 for abortion in the first trimester. Hospitals generally cost more.

Chapter 35

Infertility

Chapter Contents

Section 35.1

Frequently Asked Questions about Infertility

Reprinted with permission of the American Society for Reproductive Medicine, http://www.asrm.org. © 2000.

Quick Facts about Infertility

- Infertility is *not* an inconvenience; it is a disease of the reproductive system that impairs the body's ability to perform the basic function of reproduction.

- Infertility affects about 6.1 million people in the U.S.—about 10% of the reproductive age population.

- Infertility affects men and women equally. Most infertility cases—85% to 90%—are treated with conventional medical therapies such as medication or surgery.

- While vital for some patients, in vitro fertilization and similar treatments account for less than 5% of infertility services, and only three hundredths of one percent (.003%) of U.S. health care costs.

What is infertility?

Infertility is a disease of the reproductive system that impairs one of the body's most basic functions: the conception of children. Conception is a complicated process that depends upon many factors: on the production of healthy sperm by the man and healthy eggs by the woman; unblocked fallopian tubes that allow the sperm to reach the egg; the sperm's ability to fertilize the egg when they meet; the ability of the fertilized egg (embryo) to become implanted in the woman's uterus; and sufficient embryo quality.

Finally, for the pregnancy to continue to full term, the embryo must be healthy and the woman's hormonal environment adequate for its development. When just one of these factors is impaired, infertility can result.

What causes infertility?

No one can be blamed for infertility any more than anyone is to blame for diabetes or leukemia. In rough terms, about one third of infertility cases can be attributed to male factors, and about one third to factors that affect women. For the remaining one third of infertile couples, infertility is caused by a combination of problems in both partners or, in about 20% of cases, is unexplained.

The most common male infertility factors include azoospermia (no sperm cells are produced) and oligospermia (few sperm cells are produced). Sometimes, sperm cells are malformed or they die before they can reach the egg. In rare cases, infertility in men is caused by a genetic disease such as cystic fibrosis or a chromosomal abnormality.

The most common female infertility factor is an ovulation disorder. Other causes of female infertility include blocked fallopian tubes, which can occur when a woman has had pelvic inflammatory disease or endometriosis (a sometimes painful condition causing adhesions and cysts). Congenital anomalies (birth defects) involving the structure of the uterus and uterine fibroids are associated with repeated miscarriages.

How is infertility diagnosed?

Couples are generally advised to seek medical help if they are unable to achieve pregnancy after a year of unprotected intercourse. The doctor will conduct a physical examination of both partners to determine their general state of health and to evaluate physical disorders that may be causing infertility. Usually both partners are interviewed about their sexual habits in order to determine whether intercourse is taking place properly for conception.

If no cause can be determined at this point, more specific tests may be recommended. For women, these include an analysis of body temperature and ovulation, x-ray of the fallopian tubes and uterus, and laparoscopy. For men, initial tests focus on semen analysis.

How is infertility treated?

Most infertility cases—85 to 90 percent—are treated with conventional therapies, such as drug treatment or surgical repair of reproductive organs.

What is in vitro fertilization?

In infertile couples where women have blocked or absent fallopian tubes, or where men have low sperm counts, in vitro fertilization (IVF) offers a chance at parenthood to couples who until recently would have had no hope of having a "biologically related" child.

In IVF, eggs are surgically removed from the ovary and mixed with sperm outside the body in a Petri dish ("in vitro" is Latin for "in glass"). After about 40 hours, the eggs are examined to see if they have become fertilized by the sperm and are dividing into cells. These fertilized eggs (embryos) are then placed in the women's uterus, thus bypassing the fallopian tubes.

IVF has received a great deal of media attention since it was first introduced in 1978, but it actually accounts for less than five percent of all infertility treatment in the United States.

Is in vitro fertilization expensive?

The average cost of an IVF cycle in the United States is $12,400. Like other extremely delicate medical procedures, IVF involves highly trained professionals with sophisticated laboratories and equipment, and the cycle may need to be repeated to be successful. While IVF and other assisted reproductive technologies are not inexpensive, they account for only three hundredths of one percent (0.03%) of U.S. health care costs.

Does in vitro fertilization work?

Yes. IVF was introduced in the U.S. in 1981 and from 1985 through 1998 ASRM [American Society for Reproductive Medicine] and its affiliate, the Society for Assisted Reproductive Technology (SART), have counted more than 91,000 births of babies conceived through IVF. Through the end of 2000, more than 212,000 babies have been born in the U.S. as a result of reported ART [assisted reproductive technology] procedures. IVF currently accounts for about 98% of procedures with GIFT [gamete intrafallopian transfer], ZIFT [zygote intrafallopian transfer] and combination procedures making up the remainder. The average live delivery rate for IVF in 1998 was 29.1 per cent per retrieval—a little better than the 20% chance in any given month that a reproductively healthy couple has of achieving a pregnancy and carrying it to term.

Do insurance plans cover infertility treatment?

The degree of services covered depends on where you live and the type of insurance plan you have. Fourteen states currently have laws that require insurers to either cover or offer to cover some form of infertility diagnosis and treatment. Those states are Arkansas, California, Connecticut, Hawaii, Illinois, Maryland, Massachusetts, Montana,

New Jersey, New York, Ohio, Rhode Island, Texas and West Virginia. HOWEVER, the laws vary greatly in their scope of what is and is not required to be covered. For more information about the specific laws for each of those states, please call your state's Insurance Commissioner's office or to learn about pending insurance legislation in your state, please contact your State Representatives.

Whether or not you live in a state with an infertility insurance law, you may want to consult with your employer's director of human resources to determine the exact coverage your plan provides. If that isn't an option, an excellent resource for determining coverage is, "Infertility Insurance Advisor—An Insurance Counseling Program for Infertile Couples." This booklet is available for a small fee from RESOLVE, an infertility patient advocacy and information organization.

The desire to have children and be parents is one of the most fundamental aspects of being human. People should not be denied insurance coverage for medically appropriate treatment to fulfill this goal.

Section 35.2

Disorders Associated with Infertility

Excerpted from "Disorders Associated with Infertility," 2003, National Institute of Child Health and Human Development available online at http://www.nichd.nih.gov; accessed August 2003.

Many disorders that affect a woman's ability to get pregnant. Some of these conditions include:

- Polycystic Ovary Syndrome (PCOS)
- Endometriosis
- Premature Ovarian Failure (POF)
- Uterine Fibroids

Polycystic Ovary Syndrome (PCOS)

PCOS is the most common cause of female infertility. A woman's ovaries have follicles, which are tiny, fluid-filled sacs that hold the eggs. When an egg is mature, the follicle breaks open to release the egg so it can travel to the uterus for fertilization. In women with PCOS, immature follicles bunch together to form large cysts or lumps. The eggs mature within the bunched follicles, but the follicles don't break open to release them. As a result, women with PCOS often don't have menstrual periods, or they only have periods now and then.

Because the eggs are not released, most women with PCOS have trouble getting pregnant. Researchers estimate that 5 percent to 10 percent of women in the United States have PCOS.

Women with PCOS may also have other health problems, such as abnormally high levels of insulin, obesity, high blood pressure, and heart disease. A small number of these women will also gain weight and notice an increase in their hair growth.

Endometriosis

Endometriosis occurs when tissue like that which lines the inside of the uterus grows outside the uterus. The two most common symptoms, pain and infertility, can deeply affect a woman's quality of life. In many cases, women who receive treatment for their endometriosis pain are able to get pregnant. But this is not the case for all women. Researchers estimate that nearly 5.5 million women in North America have endometriosis.

Endometriosis is not a cancerous condition. Also, current research does not prove an association between endometriosis and uterine, cervical, endometrial, or ovarian cancers.

Premature Ovarian Failure (POF)

Health care providers use the term POF to describe a stop in normal functioning of the ovaries in a woman under the age of 40. (Women's ovary function naturally begins to decline at age 40). In POF, the ovaries stop making eggs and stop making certain hormones. An estimated 250,000 women under age 40 have POF in the United States.

The most common first symptom of POF is having irregular periods. Health care providers sometimes overlook irregular or skipped periods as being related to stress. But a woman's monthly cycle is actually an important sign of her health, in the same way that blood pressure or temperature are signs of health. If you have irregular periods or skip periods, you should tell your health care provider, so that he or she can begin to find the cause of these problems.

Women with POF often have difficulty becoming pregnant because their ovaries aren't working correctly. There is currently no proven medical treatment that improves a woman's ability to have a baby naturally if she has POF. But, between 5 percent and 10 percent of women with POF do become pregnant, even though they have not had any fertility treatment. Sometimes pregnancy can occur decades after the initial diagnosis. Researchers cannot explain why some women with POF get pregnant, while others do not.

Women with POF are at greater risk for certain other health conditions, including Addison disease, a condition in which the body does not respond well to physical stresses. This condition can be dangerous for women who don't know they have it.

Uterine Fibroids

Uterine fibroids are the most common, non-cancerous tumors in women of childbearing age. These tumors are made of muscle cells and other tissues that grow within the wall of the uterus.

Fibroids can grow in different locations, including:

- Just underneath the lining of the uterus, called submucosal

- In between the muscles of the uterus, called intramural

- On the outside of the uterus, called subserosal

Uterine fibroids are the cause of more than 200,000 hysterectomies each year.

The most common symptoms of fibroids are heavy bleeding or painful periods, bleeding between periods, a full feeling in the lower abdomen (sometimes called pelvic pressure), and urinating often. In some cases, fibroids may make it difficult for a woman to get pregnant naturally, although researchers don't know exactly why.

Uterine fibroids are not cancerous, nor are they associated with cancer. In very rare instances, less than 0.1 percent of cases, fibroids do develop into cancer.

Section 35.3

Healthy Couples Usually
Conceive Naturally within Two Years

"Don't Turn to Assisted Reproduction Too Quickly Warns US Expert,"
July 3, 2002, National Institute of Environmental and Health Sciences.

For would-be parents worried because they had difficulty conceiving, a new study presented at Europe's leading reproductive medicine conference shows that most healthy couples concerned because the woman was not pregnant after a year of trying will conceive during the second year.

A U.S. team from the National Institute of Environmental Health Sciences in North Carolina who analyzed data on 782 couples from seven European cities, concluded that even when the woman was aged between 35 and 39, fewer than 1 in 10 failed to conceive after 2 years unless the male partner was over 40.

Lead investigator Dr. David Dunson suggested that couples should be patient and doctors should not intervene too fast with assisted reproductive techniques unless there are known reasons for a couple not conceiving naturally within a year.

He told the annual conference of the European Society of Human Reproduction and Embryology that recent research undertaken by his team showed that fertility in women started to decline as early as the late 20s and for men from their late 30s . But, this was due primarily to declines in the per menstrual cycle conception rate and not to an increase in the proportion of couples unable to achieve an unassisted pregnancy.

Now his team has extended their research using data from the European Fecundability Study to see what the implications are for fertility rates overall.

"On average the time to pregnancy increases with the age of the woman. The percentage failing to conceive within a year ranged from 8% for 19- to 26-year-olds to 13 to 14% for 27 to 34-year-olds to 18% for 35- to 39-year-olds."

"But, regardless of age, most of the women who failed to conceive within the first 12 cycles conceived in the next 12. Only 3% of 19 to

26-year-olds, 6% of 27 to 34-year-olds and 9% of 35 to 39-year-olds failed to conceive in the second year, provided the male partner was aged under 40. Starting in the late 30s though, male age was also important: it meant that the percentage of failures after one year for women aged 35 to 39 rose from 18% to 28% if the male partner was over 40. After the second year the figure was 9% with male partners under 40 and 16% with male partners over 40."

Dr. Dunson said there were clear increases with age in the number of menstrual cycles needed to achieve pregnancy and in the probability of being classified as clinically infertile—a definition applied after a year of trying to conceive.

But, their research had clearly shown that among outwardly healthy couples with no known conditions associated with infertility, most who failed to conceive naturally within the first year will conceive naturally in the second year—regardless of age.

"So, in the absence of clinical indicators of infertility in addition to a long time to pregnancy, it may be appropriate to delay assisted reproduction until the couple has failed to conceive naturally in 18 to 24 months. There is a large amount of normal variability in fertility and many couples having below average, but normal fertility may fail to conceive within a year. This is particularly true for older couples, many of whom fail to conceive within the first year but are successful in the second."

He said it was important for doctors to avoid recommending assisted reproduction too soon due to well-documented side effects. "Fertility treatment, such as IVF and ICSI [intracytoplasmic sperm injection], can result in an increased risk of multiple pregnancies, pregnancy complications, low birth weight, major birth defects and long-term disability among surviving infants. In addition, the chance of success with ART decreases with age, while the side effects increase in prevalence."

Section 35.4

Diabetes Drug May Prevent Miscarriage in Women with Polycystic Ovary Syndrome

"Oral Diabetes Drug Shows Promise in Preventing Miscarriage in Common Infertility Disorder," February 27, 2002, National Institutes of Health, National Institute of Child Health and Human Development.

The anti-diabetes drug metformin appears to reduce the likelihood of early miscarriage in women with a common form of female infertility, according to a study funded by the National Institute of Child Health and Human Development (NICHD). The study appears in the February [2002] issue of the *Journal of Clinical Endocrinology and Metabolism*.

The drug, metformin, increases the body's sensitivity to insulin and is used to treat non-insulin-dependent diabetes. Metformin also has proven successful in treating some of the symptoms of Polycystic Ovary Syndrome (PCOS), the most common form of female infertility in which women fail to ovulate.

"This is a very promising lead," said Duane Alexander, M.D., Director of the NICHD. "The next step is to confirm these results in a larger, randomized trial."

PCOS affects from 5 to 10 percent of American women of reproductive age (as many as 5 million in all), explained the study's senior author, John E. Nestler, M.D., chairman of endocrinology at the Medical College of Virginia at Virginia Commonwealth University in Richmond. Dr. Nestler's group is part of NICHD's Specialized Cooperative Centers Program in Reproduction Research.

The ovaries of women with PCOS appear to be filled with numerous small cysts, Dr. Nestler added. The cyst-like appearance results from an accumulation of immature ovarian follicles, the bubble-like structures which, upon maturation, rupture and release of the egg. The features of PCOS may include failure to ovulate or menstruate, abnormally high levels of insulin, obesity, high blood pressure, hardening of the arteries, and high triglyceride levels. PCOS patients also have high levels of the male hormone testosterone, which may cause them to grow excess facial or body hair. Also, PCOS patients have a higher than normal risk of developing non-insulin-dependent, type 2 diabetes.

In the article, the study authors noted that women with PCOS often have a history of recurrent miscarriage. In earlier studies, Dr. Nestler's group had shown that metformin reduces the high testosterone levels of PCOS patients and also increases the chances that they can become pregnant. Similarly, other research by the group showed that, in women with PCOS, metformin increases blood flow to the uterus and brings about changes in the lining of the uterus that make it more capable of supporting a fetus.

In the current study, Dr. Nestler and his coworkers evaluated a group of women under the care of Venezuelan endocrinologist Daniela J. Jakubowicz. Dr. Nestler's group had earlier learned that it was Dr. Jakubowicz's practice to prescribe metformin during the pregnancies of patients under treatment for PCOS. After analyzing records of patients treated by Dr. Jakubowicz, Dr. Nestler and his coworkers found that of the 68 pregnancies that were treated with metformin, 6 pregnancies (8.8 percent) ended in miscarriage. By comparison, of the 31 pregnancies in the group that did not receive metformin, 13 pregnancies (41.9 percent) ended in miscarriage.

Only one child born in the metformin group had a birth defect. This child, a boy, had chondrodysplasia, a genetic disorder in which the limbs fail to keep pace with the growth of the body. More studies would need to be conducted to confirm the current study's results and assess the drug's safety for use during pregnancy.

The study results do not mean that physicians should begin treating PCOS patients with metformin during their pregnancies, said the project officer for NICHD's Specialized Cooperative Centers in Reproduction Research, Dr. Louis DePaolo. Although metformin has not been shown to cause any problems during pregnancy in animal studies, its use throughout pregnancy has not been rigorously studied in human beings.

Chapter 36

Pregnancy and Delivery

Chapter Contents

Section 36.1

Are You Ready for Pregnancy?

Excerpted from "Before You're Pregnant: 10 Steps to Getting Healthy
Before Pregnancy," "Before You're Pregnant: Are You Ready Emotionally?" and "Before You're Pregnant: Ka-ching! Financial Planning for
Baby," which are reprinted with permission from the March of Dimes.
© 2000 March of Dimes. All rights reserved. For additional information, contact the March of Dimes at their website at www.marchof
dimes.com.

Are You Ready Physically?

The physical health of the mom and dad before pregnancy affect
the health of their future baby. There are specific things you can do
to help your baby even before you're pregnant.

Take folic acid. Take a multivitamin with 400 micrograms of folic
acid every day before pregnancy and during early pregnancy when
the baby's brain and spinal cord are developing. Look on the label of
the vitamin bottle to see if it contains the necessary amount of folic
acid.

Eat a healthy diet that includes foods that contain folate, the natural form of the vitamin. Such foods include fortified breakfast cereals, beans, leafy green vegetables, and orange juice.

Get a pre-pregnancy checkup. Your health care provider can
help you stay as healthy as possible. She or he can explain how pregnancy might affect you, review any medications you are taking, and
make sure you are up to date on immunizations.

Your doctor or nurse may ask to test you for HIV and other sexually transmitted infections (STIs), as well as immunity to certain childhood diseases, like chicken pox and rubella. It's a good idea to have
these tests done before pregnancy.

Eat right, maintain a healthy weight, and get fit. You'll feel
better and start your pregnancy off right if you eat a variety of nutri-
tious foods every day. Avoid foods high in fat and sugar. Also, cut back

on caffeine. Drinking more than two cups of coffee, tea, or caffeinated soda a day may make it harder for you to get pregnant.

If you're overweight, lose weight before you start trying to get pregnant. If you're underweight, it may be easier to get pregnant if you reach a healthier weight. Once you start trying to get pregnant, don't try to lose weight; you could harm your baby.

Exercise is a good way to help maintain or lose weight, build fitness, and reduce stress. If you aren't already exercising, now is a good time to start. Talk to your health care provider about activities that are both safe and beneficial.

Stop smoking and avoid secondhand smoke. Smoking may make it harder for you to get pregnant. Smoking during pregnancy can put your baby at risk for certain serious health problems. Research has shown that smoking slows the growth of the baby.

The best time to stop smoking is before you get pregnant. If you need help, ask your health care provider for advice. Smoke from other people's cigarettes can also be harmful. Avoid secondhand smoke before you're pregnant and when you're pregnant.

Stop drinking alcohol. Drinking any kind of alcohol (liquor, wine, beer, wine coolers, etc.) puts your baby at risk for miscarriage and serious physical and mental problems. If you need help to stop drinking, ask your health care provider.

Don't use illegal drugs. Taking street drugs can put your baby at risk for miscarriage, preterm delivery, and serious physical and mental problems. Stop using any illegal drugs before you try to get pregnant and stay clean throughout your pregnancy. If you need help to stop, ask your health care provider. But don't stop taking any prescription medications without first talking with you provider.

Avoid infections. Some infections can harm a developing baby. Wash your hands frequently. Stay away from potentially unsafe food. Cook all meat and eggs thoroughly. Wash all fruits and vegetables well. Avoid unpasteurized milk products.

Avoid handling cat litter or soil; they can contain a parasite that causes an infection called toxoplasmosis. This infection can harm your baby.

Stay away from children with colds or common childhood illnesses. Discard contaminated tissues and wash your hands afterwards. Don't share drinking glasses.

335

Avoid sexually transmitted infections. Have sex with only one person who doesn't have other sex partners and/or use a condom when having sex. If your partner has sores in his or her genital area, don't have sex at this time. Ask your health care provider for advice.

Avoid hazardous substances and chemicals. Some cleaning products, pesticides, solvents, and lead in drinking water from old pipes can be dangerous to your baby. Avoid chemicals and paint. Reduce your risk by wearing rubber gloves and working in a well-ventilated area. Ask your health care provider for advice about hazardous substances and chemicals.

Learn about genetics. Your health care provider will take your health history and ask about the health of members of your family. Based on this information, your doctor or nurse may recommend that you see a genetic counselor to learn about your risk of having a baby with a birth defect.

Avoid stress. Stress isn't good for you or your baby—before, during, or after pregnancy. Too much stress may increase the risk of preterm labor, low birthweight, and possibly miscarriage.

Don't forget to help Dad get healthy, too! To improve your chances of getting pregnant, it's important for your partner to take care of himself, exercise, eat right, and stop smoking, drinking, or taking illegal drugs.

Are You Ready Emotionally?

What You Need to Know

Being a parent is a full-time job. There is no right or wrong time to have a baby—it's up to you and your partner. Before you get pregnant, think about the emotional and lifestyle issues you will face as a parent. It's important for you and your partner to agree on most of the major issues, or begin discussing your differences, before you conceive.

What You Can Do

Ask yourself these ten questions:

- Why do you want to have a baby? Have you made up your own mind? Is your partner, a parent, or someone else pressuring you?

336

- How will a child affect your relationship with your partner? Are you both ready to become parents?

- If you're not in a relationship, are you prepared to raise a child alone? Who will help you?

- How will a baby affect your future educational or career plans?

- Do you and your partner have religious or ethnic differences? Have you discussed how you will handle these differences and how they might affect your child?

- What will you do for child care?

- Are you prepared to parent a child who is sick or has special needs?

- Are you ready to give up sleeping in on weekend mornings? Are you ready to find child care every time you want to go out without your baby?

- Do you enjoy spending time with children? Can you see yourself as a parent?

- What did you like about your childhood? What didn't you like? What do you want for your child?

Are You Ready Financially?

What You Need to Know

Many new parents are surprised by how expensive a baby can be. But if you plan ahead, these new costs will be easier to manage.

What You Can Do

- Take a look at your budget. How will having a baby affect your income and expenses?

- Check the leave policy where you work. How much maternity or paternity leave do you get?

- Check your health insurance. Does it cover medical care for you during pregnancy and for your newborn baby?

- Make saving a habit.

- Review or purchase long-term disability and life insurance coverage.

- Check out special benefits that you may qualify for such as Medicaid and the WIC program.

Section 36.2

Prenatal Care

"Prenatal Care," is reprinted with permission from the March of Dimes. © 2000 March of Dimes. All rights reserved. For additional information, contact the March of Dimes at their website at www.marchofdimes. com.

Prenatal care is the care you get while you are pregnant. This care can be provided by a doctor, midwife, or other health care professional.

The goal of prenatal care is to monitor the progress of a pregnancy and to identify potential problems before they become serious for either mom or baby.

As soon as you think you are pregnant, call your health care provider to find out when you should come in for your first prenatal care appointment.

During your pregnancy, make sure you attend all of your prenatal care appointments, even if you're feeling fine.

Sometimes getting to an appointment may be difficult or it may seem like a waste of time. For the sake of your baby, though, make getting prenatal care a priority.

Why Prenatal Care?

All women need prenatal care. Young or old, first baby or fifth, all mothers-to-be benefit from regular care during their pregnancy. Babies born to mothers who receive late or no prenatal care are nearly twice as likely to be born low birthweight as babies born to mothers who receive early prenatal care.

Ask your friends who've been pregnant before about prenatal care. At least one of them will probably tell you about a problem they had that was caught at a prenatal care appointment. If they didn't have any problems, they will probably tell you about the peace of mind that prenatal care brought to them. It is reassuring to find out that you and your baby are doing just fine.

A *typical prenatal care schedule.*

A typical prenatal care schedule for a low-risk woman with a normally progressing pregnancy is:

- **Weeks 4 to 28:** 1 visit per month (every 4 weeks)
- **Weeks 28 to 36:** 2 visits per month (every 2 weeks)
- **Weeks 36 to birth:** 1 visit per week

A woman with a chronic medical condition or a high-risk pregnancy may have to see her health care provider more often. Make sure you go to all your prenatal care appointments, even if you're feeling fine.

What happens at a prenatal care visit?

During your first prenatal care visit, your provider will ask you a lot of questions and do some tests. Most of your other visits will be much shorter.

At the first visit your health care provider will:

- Ask you about your health, your partner's health, and the health of your close family members. Don't worry if you don't know all the answers.
- Do a physical exam and a pelvic (internal) exam.
- Weigh you.
- Check your blood pressure.
- Ask for a urine sample.
- Do some blood tests to check for anemia and see if you have had certain infections. You will be asked if you want a test for HIV, the virus that causes AIDS.
- Do a Pap smear to check for cervical cancer and other tests for vaginal infections
- Figure out your due date: an estimate of the day your baby will be born. Most babies are born within two weeks (before or after) their due date.

During later prenatal visits your provider will:

- Weigh you.

- Check your blood pressure.

- Ask for a urine sample to check for protein and sugar.

- Measure your belly to see how the baby is growing (middle and late pregnancy).

- Check your hands, feet, and face for swelling.

- Listen for the baby's heartbeat (after the 12th week of pregnancy).

- Feel your abdomen to gauge the baby's position (later in pregnancy).

- Do any tests that are needed, such as blood tests or ultrasound.

- Ask you if you have any questions or concerns. It's a good idea to write down your questions and bring a list with you so you don't forget.

Remember, the things you tell your health care provider are confidential. That means that he or she can't tell anyone else what you say without your permission. So don't be afraid to talk about issues that might be uncomfortable or embarrassing. It's OK to tell your provider if you smoke, drink alcohol, or take any drugs, or if your partner hurts or scares you. Your provider needs to know all about you and your lifestyle so that he or she can give you and your baby the best care.

No one knows exactly why women who get early and regular prenatal care have healthier pregnancies and healthier babies. But we do know it works. So go. Do it for yourself and your baby.

Section 36.3

Healthy Pregnancy, Healthy Baby

U.S. Food and Drug Administration, *FDA Consumer*, March-April 1999.
By Rebecca D. Williams.

Worries and pregnancy seem to go hand in hand. Fortunately, however, most women of childbearing age are healthy and most pregnancies are considered low-risk.

For most women, the surest way to have a healthy baby is to live a healthy lifestyle. The March of Dimes suggests the following precautions:

- Get early prenatal care, even before you're pregnant.
- Eat a well-balanced diet, including a vitamin supplement that contains folic acid.
- Exercise regularly with your doctor's permission.
- Avoid alcohol, cigarettes, and illicit drugs, and limit caffeine.
- Avoid x-rays, hot tubs, and saunas.
- Avoid infections.

Avoid Infections

Many infections during pregnancy can be dangerous to an unborn child. Urinary tract infections and any sexually transmitted diseases need to be treated immediately.

Cat litter and raw meat may contain the parasite *Toxoplasma gondii*, which can cause toxoplasmosis infection. It's rare for a pregnant woman to get the infection, but if she does, her baby could be at risk for serious illness or death. Get someone else to change the kitty litter if possible, or wear a face mask and rubber gloves for protection.

Problems also may arise when a pregnant woman eats undercooked or raw foods, or cooked foods that have been cross-contaminated with bacteria from raw food nearby. Food poisoning can cause meningitis, pneumonia, or even death to an unborn child, plus the vomiting and diarrhea involved leave the mother exhausted and dehydrated.

The Naughty Stuff

Nearly everyone knows pregnant women shouldn't take illicit drugs, but it's the legal ones—alcohol and tobacco—that are more commonly the source of pregnancy problems.

Smokers put their babies at a significantly higher risk of preterm birth, low birth weight, and stillbirth compared with nonsmokers. After birth, the babies of mothers who smoked during pregnancy are more likely to have poor lung development, asthma and respiratory infections, and to die of sudden infant death syndrome (SIDS).

If a woman quits smoking early in pregnancy, however, she can still improve her chances of having a healthy baby. Expectant fathers or other members of the family should quit, too, because studies suggest breathing secondhand smoke may be dangerous as well.

Alcohol, too, can damage a developing fetus. Alcohol travels rapidly to the bloodstream, so when an expectant mother drinks, her baby drinks also. Alcohol is known to cause mental retardation and facial abnormalities in babies, a condition called fetal alcohol syndrome. The Institute of Medicine estimates some 12,000 children with fetal alcohol syndrome are born in the United States each year. No one knows what amount of alcohol is safe during pregnancy; therefore, the U.S. Surgeon General recommends pregnant women avoid alcohol altogether.

A few other activities are known to be dangerous during pregnancy. X-rays can expose the fetus to radiation and potentially cause birth defects. Hot tubs and saunas can raise the core temperature of a pregnant woman's body and could potentially harm the fetus. Warm baths, however, are fine if the water is kept at body temperature.

Exercise

There's increasing medical evidence to show that exercise, even a vigorous workout, is healthy during pregnancy. A pregnant woman should check with her doctor before exercising, however. If she gets the OK to work out, she should do so at least three times a week for 20 minutes each time, recommends the American College of Obstetrics and Gynecology. Walking, swimming, riding a stationary bicycle, and joining a prenatal aerobics class are all excellent exercise choices for a pregnant woman. Exercises that require jerky, bouncy movements and being outside in hot weather are not good choices. Don't try deep knee bends, sit-ups (or any exercise that requires you to lie on your back after the first trimester), and toe touches. Other sports to avoid include downhill skiing, rock climbing, and horseback riding.

Wear a supportive bra and properly fitting athletic shoes while exercising. Stop if you feel dizzy, faint, overheated, or in pain. Drink plenty of water. Staying in shape will help you keep up your stamina during your own impending marathon—labor! And, afterward, the more muscle mass you have, the quicker you'll regain your pre-pregnancy shape and be able to pack away those maternity pants.

Rebecca D. Williams is a writer in Oak Ridge, Tennessee.

Section 36.4

Pregnancy and Nutrition

Excerpted from the publication by the U.S. Department of Health and Human Services, National Women's Health Information Center (NWHIC), 2000. Available online at http://www.4woman.gov; accessed May 2003.

How should my diet change now that I am pregnant?

Even before pregnancy begins, nutrition is a primary factor in the health of mother and baby. If you are eating a well-balanced diet before you become pregnant, you will only need to make a few changes to meet the nutritional needs of pregnancy.

According to the American College of Obstetricians and Gynecologists (ACOG), pregnant women should increase their usual servings of a variety of foods from the four basic food groups to include the following:

- Four or more servings of fruits and vegetables for vitamins and minerals

- Four or more servings of whole-grain or enriched bread and cereal for energy

- Four or more servings of milk and milk products for calcium

- Three or more servings of meat, poultry, fish, eggs, nuts, dried beans and peas for protein

Eating a well-balanced diet while you are pregnant will help to keep you and your baby healthy. Most physicians agree that the Recommended Daily Allowances (RDAs), except those for iron, can be obtained through a proper diet.

Should I take a multi-vitamin during my pregnancy?

The nutritional requirements for pregnant women vary based on individual needs. Discuss whether you need to take a multi-vitamin with your doctor.

What about folic acid?

Pregnancy doubles a woman's need for folate (folic acid or folacin). Folic acid has been shown to be important in preventing neural tube defects, such as spina bifida and anencephaly and is essential to the formation of red blood cells. Severe folate deficiency can result in a condition called megaloblastic anemia, which occurs most often in the last trimester of pregnancy. In this condition, the mother's heart, liver, and spleen may become enlarged, which can threaten the life of the fetus. Folic acid can be found in many foods, including kidney beans, leafy green vegetables, peas, and liver. Women in their childbearing years should consume plenty of these foods. In fact, folate is so important to the health of women and their babies that the Food and Drug Administration (FDA) recently required the addition of folic acid to prepackaged bread and cereals.

Section 36.5

Pregnancy and the Drug Dilemma

Excerpted from "Pregnancy and the Drug Dilemma,"
by Michelle Meadows, U.S. Food and Drug Administration
(http://www.fda.gov), *FDA Consumer*, May-June 2001.

Experts say that while they have certainly learned some useful information for successful drug treatment in pregnancy, their knowledge is limited for the most part. That goes for information in the literature and on the labels doctors use to make clinical decisions, says Beth Conover, a genetic counselor who coordinates the Teratogen Information Service at the University of Nebraska Medical Center. Teratogen is a term that refers to any substance with the potential to cause birth defects.

Conover says advising patients and doctors about medication use in pregnancy is like working in shades of gray. "Parents want someone to assure them their babies will be OK, and of course that's what we want to do," she says. "But it's very hard to prove absolute safety. We would need extensive, long-term studies to do that, and we don't have them in many cases."

The reality, of course, is that pregnant women get sick, whether it's with pneumonia or cancer. Or, they come to pregnancy with chronic conditions that require treatment. So despite some areas of uncertainty, health professionals must look to the resources they do have to make clinical decisions.

Dianne Kennedy, a regulatory health project manager with the Food and Drug Administration's Center for Drug Evaluation and Research (CDER), says withholding all medication during pregnancy is not the answer. Too many conditions pose more of a health risk if left untreated, she adds. In fact, medication use in pregnancy is common, and the number of prescriptions tends to rise with the mother's age.

In addition to general questions about safety, almost no information is available to help doctors know what the best dose of a particular medicine is for pregnant women. Changes in the body's physiology during pregnancy have the potential to require that doses be increased or decreased.

How do health care professionals make decisions about drug treatment? "Generally, we use medicine when we have to and try to do the best we can," says Conover "That means looking carefully at the data we do have."

Animal studies look for possible adverse reproductive effects in humans by giving animals higher doses of a drug. Experts also consider how a drug works and its likely effects, reported experiences with similar drugs, and adverse event reports.

Additionally, pregnancy registries have grown over the years. These registries follow women taking a certain drug until their pregnancy ends, allowing researchers to use the results to assess risks to mothers and their babies.

The stage of pregnancy also influences clinical decisions. For example, after 24 weeks of pregnancy, the antibiotic tetracycline can cause permanent staining of a baby's teeth. And ACE (angiotensin converting enzyme) inhibitors, a group of drugs that treat high blood pressure, can damage a baby's kidneys in the second and third trimesters of pregnancy.

Depending on the risks, doctors may adapt treatment by switching a pregnant woman to a similar drug that is safer or prescribing medicine only during a certain portion of the pregnancy. "For example, if a depressed woman is taking lithium, she may be able to briefly discontinue the medication during the period of the baby's heart formation," Conover says. "Lithium use in pregnancy carries a small risk of fetal heart defects."

Section 36.6

Ectopic Pregnancy

This information was provided by KidsHealth, one of the largest resources online for medically reviewed health information written for parents, kids, and teens. For more articles like this one, visit www.KidsHealth.org, or www.TeensHealth.org. © 2001 The Nemours Center for Children's Health Media, a division of The Nemours Foundation.

Ectopic pregnancy is the leading cause of first-trimester maternal death in the United States. According to the U.S. Centers for Disease Control and Prevention (CDC), the rate of ectopic pregnancy in the United States—2% of all pregnancies—increased fivefold since 1970.

But despite these frightening statistics, deaths from ectopic pregnancy are rare, at fewer than one in 2,500 cases—thanks in part to early detection efforts. The earlier an abnormal pregnancy is diagnosed, the better the mother's chances of survival.

What Is an Ectopic Pregnancy?

Ectopic means "out of place." In an ectopic pregnancy, a fertilized egg has implanted outside the uterus. The egg settles in the fallopian tubes more than 95% of the time. This is why ectopic pregnancies are commonly called "tubal pregnancies." The egg can also implant in the ovary, abdomen, or the cervix, so you may see these referred to as cervical or abdominal pregnancies. None of these areas has as much space or nurturing tissue as a uterus for a pregnancy to develop. As the fetus grows, it will eventually burst the organ that contains it. This can cause severe bleeding and endanger the mother's life. A classical ectopic pregnancy never develops into a live birth.

Signs and Symptoms

Ectopic pregnancy can be difficult to diagnose because symptoms often mirror those of a normal early pregnancy. These can include missed periods, breast tenderness, nausea, vomiting, or frequent urination.

347

Pain is usually the first red flag. You might feel pain in your pelvis, abdomen, or, in extreme cases, even your shoulder or neck (if blood from a ruptured ectopic pregnancy builds up and irritates certain nerves). Most women describe the pain as sharp and stabbing. It may concentrate on one side of the pelvis, and it may come and go or vary in intensity.

Any of the following additional symptoms can suggest an ectopic pregnancy:

- vaginal spotting or bleeding
- dizziness or fainting (caused by blood loss)
- low blood pressure (caused by blood loss)
- lower back pain

What Causes an Ectopic Pregnancy?

An ectopic pregnancy results from a fertilized egg's inability to work its way quickly enough down the fallopian tube into the uterus. An infection or inflammation of the tube may have partially or entirely blocked it.

Pelvic inflammatory disease (PID) is the most common of these infections. Endometriosis (when cells from the lining of the uterus detach and grow elsewhere in the body) or scar tissue from previous abdominal or fallopian surgeries can also cause blockages. More rarely, birth defects or abnormal growths can alter the shape of the tube and impede the egg's progress.

How Is It Diagnosed?

If you arrive in the emergency room complaining of abdominal pain, you'll likely be given a urine pregnancy test. Although these tests aren't sophisticated, they are fast—and speed can be crucial in treating ectopic pregnancy.

If you already know you're pregnant, or if the urine test comes back positive, you'll probably be given a quantitative hCG test. This blood test measures levels of the hormone human chorionic gonadotropin (hCG), which is produced by the placenta. hCG appears in the blood and urine as early as 10 days after conception, and its levels double every 2 days for the first 10 weeks of pregnancy. If hCG levels are lower than expected for your stage of pregnancy, doctors are one step closer to diagnosing ectopic pregnancy.

The doctor will also give you a pelvic exam to locate the areas causing pain, to check for an enlarged, pregnant uterus, or to find any masses in your abdomen. You'll probably also get an ultrasound examination, which shows whether the uterus contains a developing fetus or if masses are present elsewhere in the abdominal area. The ultrasound, however, may not be able to detect every ectopic pregnancy.

A less commonly performed test, a culdocentesis, may be used to look for internal bleeding. In this test, a needle is inserted into the space at the very top of the vagina, behind the uterus and in front of the rectum. Any blood or fluid found there likely comes from a ruptured ectopic pregnancy.

Even with the best equipment, it is hard to see a pregnancy less than 6 weeks along. If your doctor can't diagnose ectopic pregnancy but can't rule it out, he or she may ask you to return every 2 days to measure your hCG levels. If these levels don't rise as quickly as they should, the doctor will continue to monitor you carefully until 6 weeks, when an ultrasound can be used.

Options for Treatment

Treatment of an ectopic pregnancy varies, depending on its size and location and whether you want the ability to conceive again.

An early ectopic pregnancy can sometimes be treated with an injection of methotrexate, which dissolves the fertilized egg and allows your body to reabsorb it. This nonsurgical approach minimizes scarring of your pelvic organs.

If the pregnancy is further along, you will likely need surgery to remove the abnormal pregnancy. In the past this was a major operation, requiring general anesthesia and a large incision across the pelvic area. This may still be necessary in cases of emergency or extensive internal injury.

However, the pregnancy may sometimes be removed using laparoscopy, a less invasive surgical procedure. The surgeon makes a small incision in the lower abdomen, and then inserts a laparoscope. This long, hollow tube with a lighted end allows the doctor to view internal organs and insert other instruments as needed. Sometimes a second small abdominal incision is made for the instruments. The ectopic pregnancy is then surgically removed and any damaged organs are repaired or removed. General or regional anesthesia may be used.

Whatever your treatment, the doctor will want to see you regularly afterward to make sure your hCG levels return to zero. This may take up to 12 weeks. An elevated hCG could mean that some ectopic tissue was missed. This tissue may have to be removed using methotrexate or additional surgery.

Future Pregnancies

Approximately 30% of women who have had ectopic pregnancies will have difficulty becoming pregnant again. Your prognosis depends mainly on the extent of the damage and the surgery that was done.

If the fallopian tube has been spared, chances of a future successful pregnancy are 60%. Even if one fallopian tube has been removed, chances of having a successful pregnancy with the other tube can be greater than 40%.

The likelihood of a repeat ectopic pregnancy increases with each subsequent ectopic pregnancy. Once you have had one ectopic pregnancy, you face an approximate 15% chance of having another.

Am I at Risk for an Ectopic Pregnancy?

The risk of ectopic pregnancy is highest for women who are between 35 and 44 years old and have had:

- PID
- previous ectopic pregnancy
- surgery on a fallopian tube
- infertility problems or medication to stimulate ovulation

Some birth control methods can also increase your risk of ectopic pregnancy. If you get pregnant while using progesterone-only oral contraceptives, progesterone intrauterine devices (IUDs), or the morning after pill, you are more likely to have an ectopic pregnancy.

When to Call Your Doctor

If you believe you're at risk for an ectopic pregnancy, meet with your doctor to discuss your options before you become pregnant. There is nothing anyone can do to prevent ectopic pregnancy, but you can make sure it's detected early. You and your doctor may want to plan on checking your hormone levels starting at 10 days or scheduling an ultrasound at 6 weeks to ensure that your pregnancy is developing normally.

Call your doctor immediately if you are pregnant and experiencing any of the signs or symptoms of ectopic pregnancy. When it comes to detecting an ectopic pregnancy, "better safe than sorry" is more than just a cliché.

Note: All information on KidsHealth is for educational purposes only. For specific medical advice, diagnoses, and treatment, consult your doctor.

Section 36.7

Pregnancy Loss: Miscarriage and Molar Pregnancy

American College of Obstetricians and Gynecologists. *Early Pregnancy Loss: Miscarriage and Molar Pregnancy.* (Patient Education Pamphlet No. AP090). Washington, DC. © ACOG 2002.

A normal pregnancy is about 40 weeks. The loss of a pregnancy before 20 weeks is called early pregnancy loss. Often, the loss is a miscarriage (sometimes called spontaneous abortion by doctors). A rare form of pregnancy loss is molar pregnancy.

Miscarriage

Miscarriages occur in about 15 percent to 20 percent of pregnancies. Most occur in the first 13 weeks of pregnancy.

Miscarriage can be caused by any one of a number of things before, during, or after this process.

The cause of miscarriage often is not known. Most factors that cause a miscarriage are genetic.

Genetic Factors

More than half of miscarriages in the first 13 weeks of pregnancy are caused by problems with the chromosomes of the fetus.

Factors of the Woman's Health

Infections may affect the uterus and fetus and, as a result, end the pregnancy. Problems with the woman's hormones also can cause very early miscarriage. If the woman has a chronic disease, such as diabetes that is not controlled, she may have a higher risk for miscarriage.

Lifestyle Factors

Pregnant women who smoke are more likely to have vaginal bleeding during pregnancy. Their risk of miscarriage is higher than that of women who don't smoke. Heavy alcohol use and illegal drug use also increase the risk of miscarriage. This is especially true in early pregnancy.

What Doesn't Cause Miscarriage

Most aspects of daily life do not increase the risk of miscarriage. For instance, there is no proof that working, exercising, having sex, or having used birth control pills before getting pregnant increases a woman's risk.

Symptoms of Miscarriage

Bleeding is the most common sign of miscarriage. This is why bleeding during early pregnancy is called threatened miscarriage.

Sometimes mild cramping of the lower stomach or a low backache may occur along with bleeding.

If you have heavy bleeding and think you have passed fetal tissue, place it in a clean container and take it to the doctor for inspection.

After a Miscarriage

Often when miscarriage occurs early in pregnancy, tissue is left in the uterus. If there is concern about heavy bleeding or infection, this tissue will be removed. The tissue that remains may be removed by dilation and curettage (D&C).

If your blood is Rh negative, you should ask your doctor whether you need a blood product called Rh immune globulin. This prevents you from developing antibodies that could affect a future Rh-positive baby.

Molar Pregnancy

Molar pregnancy, also called gestational trophoblastic disease (GTD), is rare. It results in the growth of abnormal tissue. In the

United States, molar pregnancy occurs in 1 of every 1,000 to 1,200 pregnancies.

Types of Molar Pregnancy

There are two types of molar pregnancy—complete and partial.

Symptoms and Diagnosis

Most molar pregnancies cause symptoms that signal a problem. The most common symptom is vaginal bleeding during the first trimester.

Other signs of molar pregnancy, such as a uterus that is too large for the stage of the pregnancy or cysts (fluid-filled sacs or pouches) on the ovaries, can be found by your doctor.

Treatment

To treat a molar pregnancy, the cervix is dilated, either under general or local anesthesia, and the tissue is removed by D&C. About 90 percent of women whose molar pregnancies are removed require no further treatment.

After the pregnancy has been removed, abnormal cells may remain. This is called persistent GTD. It occurs in as many as 10 percent of women after a molar pregnancy. Sometimes chemotherapy may be needed to remove the abnormal cells that remain.

Coping with the Loss

For many women, emotional healing takes a good deal longer than physical healing. The feelings of loss can be intense.

Grief can involve a wide range of feelings. Your feelings of grief may differ from those of your partner. You are the one who has felt the physical changes of pregnancy. Your partner also may grieve, but he may not express his feelings in the same way you do.

If either of you is having trouble handling the feelings that go along with this loss, talk to your doctor.

Finally

Don't blame yourself for the pregnancy loss. In most cases it is not likely that it could have been prevented. Losing a pregnancy often doesn't mean that a woman can't have more children or that there is something wrong with her health. Most women who miscarry can have a healthy pregnancy later.

Section 36.8

Labor and Delivery

"What Happens during Labor?" © 2003, Childbirth Solutions, Inc. Written by Pam Cass, Former Vice President of Childbirth Solutions, Inc. and Doula, DONA Certified Childbirth Solutions.com. Reprinted with permission.

Every woman giving birth is embarking on a wondrous journey. Fortunately, it's a journey that countless women before them have taken so the territory is not entirely uncharted. In preparation for labor, thousands of women participate in childbirth education classes every year in the United States. Many more pore over books and ask their care provider what they can expect. Almost every woman at some point approaches another woman who has completed the journey to get some insight. They are all looking for the same information and asking the same questions: What is labor like? How long will it last? What will it feel like? How can I cope?

While it is true that every woman experiences this journey in an individual way the basic sequence of events is the same for all. This overview should give you an idea of the physical steps all must go through in order to complete the process of labor and birth. It will also show you what to expect emotionally and give you tips on how to cope each step of the way.

This chapter is designed to give you an overview of a "normal" labor and birth. Therefore, it is a completely intervention-free birth.

Prodromal Labor

Often in the past prodromal labor has been given the misnomer false labor, yet every woman experiencing it has said in frustration "There's nothing false about what I'm feeling!" The misunderstanding has arisen because prodromal labor can feel very much like active labor, yet is not consistently progressive; it does not lead without a break to the birth of the baby. It does, though, serve an important function in the birth process. Prodromal labor does the preliminary work of preparing the uterus, baby, and cervix for birth. All of this work has to be done before the baby can be born. Some women's bodies do it all without her being aware of it. However, some women's bodies draw a great deal of attention to the work being done.

"This is driving me crazy," one pregnant mother sighed. "I've been having contractions off and on now for three days. Just when I think it's time to call my midwife, they completely stop again!"

Length

- Prodromal labor contractions may begin hours or even days before active labor.

Contractions

- The contractions may feel like Braxton Hicks contractions or they may be quite a bit stronger.

- They are irregular in length, frequency, and intensity. The key word here is irregular. In general though, they are not longer than a minute and not more frequent than 7 to 10 minutes apart. They shouldn't be so intense that they take your breath away.

- They may or may not be affected by your activity. The wisest course is to vary your activity level, alternating periods of mild activity with rest.

Physical Effects

- The cervix is moving from a posterior (back) position to an anterior (forward) position.

- The cervix is softening.

- The cervix is beginning its effacement or thinning. It may thin anywhere from 0% to 50% during this stage.

- You may lose your mucous plug from the cervix.

- Your cervix may begin to dilate, opening anywhere from 1 to 4 centimeters.

Emotional Effects

- You may be quite excited when you first feel these contractions, especially if they are stronger than any you've had until now.

- As time goes on and the contractions continue without any apparent progress you may feel let down and eventually become quite tired and discouraged.

Active Labor (First Stage): Latent Phase

The latent phase is the beginning of active labor and will carry you about halfway through the birth of your baby. This phase of the active stage of labor begins when your contractions become progressively longer, stronger, and closer together and ends when your cervix is about 4 or 5 centimeters dilated.

Length

- The latent phase of active labor can last anywhere from a few hours to 10 hours or more.

Contractions

- They will grow longer, stronger, and closer together.

- The timing of these contractions can vary widely from woman to woman. Some start with contractions 30 minutes apart, others start right out at 7 or even as few as 5 minutes apart.

- They will vary in length from 15 to 30 seconds or so. A few women may find them lasting a bit longer.

- These contractions will continue no matter how you change your activity level.

- You will find that you gradually progress to needing to use all your concentration and are no longer able to talk and laugh during a contraction.

Physical Effects

- The cervix continues thinning out (effacement).
- The cervix will dilate to 4 or 5 centimeters.
- You may have a couple of loose bowel movements.

- You may lose your mucous plug.
- You may notice a bloody show.

Emotional Effects

- Excitement and joy are often primary emotions when you realize you are finally in labor.
- Don't be concerned to find that you are somewhat fearful, after all, this is going to be a big day, full of hard work and intense sensations.
- You will still be interested in conversation, though only between contractions.

Active Labor (First Stage): Active Phase

The active phase of labor will continue with contractions that grow longer stronger and closer together. This is the part of your experience that really warrants the label labor. It begins about the time you are 4 to 5 centimeters dilated and ends at about 9 centimeters. Keep in mind that these beginning and ending measurements are average; they will vary from woman to woman and from birth to birth.

Length

- The active phase of active labor can last anywhere from a couple of hours to 10 hours or more.

Contractions

- Each of these contractions has a definite beginning, peak, and end. Some women describe them as waves. The gripping sensation in your belly and back starts mildly and quickly grows stronger until it reaches a peak, then it grows weaker until it goes completely away.
- They will grow longer, stronger, and closer together.
- The timing of these contractions can vary widely from woman to woman. In general, contractions through this stage start at about 5 minutes apart and grow closer together until they are coming about every 2 minutes or so.
- They will vary in length from 30 to 60 seconds. A few women may find them lasting a bit longer.

357

- A few women will experience camel-back contractions, a second contraction beginning before the first entirely goes away. You don't have the usual 2 minutes of rest between contractions. You will probably need your entire support team to help you to deal with them.

- These contractions will continue no matter how you change your activity level.

Physical Effects

- The cervix continues thinning out (effacement).

- The cervix will dilate to 9 or more centimeters.

- Your body will be working very hard during this stage. Some women sweat, some may have cold hands or feet.

- Your water may break at any point. If it does, you may find your contractions increasing in intensity.

- You may notice a bit more bloody show. Some blood is normal now as your cervix stretches open and some of its tiny blood vessels break. If you are uncomfortable with the amount of blood, bring it to the attention of your care provider, nurse, or doula.

- Most women are no longer interested in eating anything.

- It is important to continue to get enough to drink to avoid dehydration.

Emotional Effects

- During this stage you will find yourself working so hard that everything outside your body almost ceases to exist.

- Some women want lots of support people around them now, however many women find too many people distracting and want only their doula and one primary support person (husband, mother, sister, friend) with them.

- You will find that you need lots of support from your team to help you deal with your labor.

- You will probably be concentrating so hard on your labor that you find conversation annoying.

- You will want your support people within reach at all times and may feel abandoned if left alone even to go to the bathroom.

Transition

As its name suggests, transition marks the period when your body completes its labor and prepares to move into birthing your baby. Transition is perhaps the most intense part of the labor process, both physically and emotionally. While it is a very trying time, you can take comfort in the knowledge that it is also the shortest phase of labor and that soon your dilation will be complete and you can begin pushing.

Length

Transition will last from ten minutes to an hour and encompass as few as three to as many as 25 contractions.

Contractions

- The contractions come closer together, perhaps one to two minutes apart.

- They will last from one minute to ninety seconds.

- Some may come in pairs with no rest period between them. These are called camelback contractions.

- These contractions will be the most intense in strength. They reach their peak quickly and maintain it for most of the contraction.

Physical Effects

- The cervix will dilate to 9 or more centimeters.

- Your body will be working very hard during this stage. Some women will tremble or shake.

- Some women may be nauseous and/or vomit.

- If your water hasn't broken yet, it may do so at any time.

Emotional Effects

- Transition is a difficult time emotionally. Many women during transition say, "I just can't do this anymore."

- Some women find themselves more drawn to the women in their support team at this point.

- You will find that you need lots of support from your team to help you deal with your labor.

- It is not unusual for your sense of time to slow down.

Second Stage (Birth): Latent Phase

The latent phase of second stage is the period that it takes your body to switch gears, moving from the dilating of your cervix to pushing your baby down the birth canal. It begins when your cervix is completely dilated and ends with the urge to push along with your contractions. It is a kind of rest period for you. After the intense sensations of the end of labor, you may find the lack of contraction activity disturbing. Don't worry though, you will have more contractions and they will end in the birth of your baby.

Length

- Some women skip this little rest period altogether and have the urge to push immediately. Some women have up to 30 minutes before they feel the urge to push.

Contractions

- The contractions become further apart since the work of dilating the cervix is completed. It is not unusual for there to be five or more minutes between contractions.

- For some women contractions may all but cease.

Physical Effects

- The cervix is completely dilated.

- The uterus is shifting gears from dilating contractions, to pushing contractions.

Emotional Effects

- Most women feel a good deal of relief at hearing the cervix is completely dilated and find themselves able to smile and converse for the first time in hours.

- Some women find themselves disoriented by the relative lack of activity.

Second Stage (Birth): Active Phase

The active phase of second stage is the long-awaited pushing. Although completely different in sensation from your labor so far, it is every bit as intense and just as much hard work.

Length

- Pushing the baby out can take as little as five minutes or as long as three hours.

Contractions

- Pushing contractions are usually five to ten minutes apart.
- They are accompanied for most women by an intense urge to push.
- Some women may feel little or no urge to push.
- You may be able to feel the baby's head moving down the vagina.

Physical Effects

- The baby's head is molding to fit through the pubic outlet, stretching the birth canal as it goes.
- You may expel some feces, urine, or gas.
- You may feel nauseous and/or vomit.

Emotional Effects

- Pushing the baby out will take a great deal of concentration and possibly some direction from your care provider, nurse, or doula.
- While most women start out pushing with a burst of enthusiasm and energy, some women find themselves becoming exhausted and discouraged if it drags on with little apparent progress.

Crowning and Birth

As your baby's head becomes visible it is called crowning. This is an extremely intense phase emotionally and physically. After all, we're talking about the actual birth of the baby!

Length

- From the first sight of the baby at the vaginal outlet to the birth of the baby, this stage can last from two to twenty minutes or so.

Contractions

- These pushing contractions may be a bit farther apart if you are especially tired. Otherwise they remain unchanged from pushing.

Physical Effects

- First the baby's head will emerge.

- Following a short pause to make sure the umbilical cord is not wrapped around the baby's neck; your care provider will gently ease the top shoulder out first, then the bottom shoulder. The rest of the baby's body should slip right out.

- You may feel an intense burning at the vaginal outlet, although many women do not.

- You may expel some feces, urine, or gas, though you will probably be unaware of it.

Emotional Effects

- You will be intensely focused on what you are doing. This is the time that many women find that they are conscious only of what is within a few inches of their bodies.

- You may need to be reminded that you are birthing your baby. Many women become so focused on the work that they forget what they are working so hard to accomplish.

- Many women, if they reach down and feel their baby's head emerging, experience a burst of energy and enthusiasm, finishing the birth immediately.

- If everyone attending you is focused on the emergence of the baby, you may feel a bit ignored.

- As your baby is born it you will be euphoric, proud, and amazed that you accomplished such an incredible feat!

Third Stage: Delivery of the Placenta

Although the baby has been born, you have a little more work to do. The placenta or afterbirth needs to be expelled.

Length

- The delivery of the placenta after the birth of the baby may take from five to thirty minutes.

Contractions

- Other than a cramping sensation, there will be no more contractions.

Physical Effects

- The placenta separates from the uterine wall and is expelled through the vagina.

- You may feel the uterus cramp, especially if the baby begins suckling immediately.

- You may feel an uncomfortable "full" sensation even though the baby is out, until the placenta is delivered.

- Many women notice no sensation at all until they are asked to bear down "one more time."

Emotional Effects

- The delivery of the afterbirth is truly an afterthought. Most women are so involved with their new baby that the delivery of the placenta is hardly noticed.

- You may feel a real sense of relief when the placenta is out. Now the birth is truly over.

- You may be annoyed at the interruption in your bonding.

- If the placenta is delayed, your caregiver may encourage its expulsion by having an assistant knead your belly to get the uterus to contract more effectively. This is called fundal massage and can be quite painful.

363

Section 36.9

Recovering from Delivery

This information was provided by KidsHealth, one of the largest resources online for medically reviewed health information written for parents, kids, and teens. For more articles like this one, visit www.KidsHealth.org, or www.TeensHealth.org. © 2001 The Nemours Center for Children's Health Media, a division of The Nemours Foundation.

Your baby's finally here, and you're thrilled—but you're also exhausted, uncomfortable, on an emotional roller coaster, and wondering whether you'll ever fit into your jeans again. Childbirth classes helped prepare you for giving birth, but not for this.

What to Expect in the First Few Weeks

After your baby arrives, you'll notice you've changed somewhat—both physically and emotionally. Physically, you might experience the following:

- **sore breasts**—Your breasts may be painfully engorged when your milk comes in, and your nipples may be sore.

- **constipation**—The first postpartum bowel movement is typically delayed to the third or fourth day after delivery, and sensitive hemorrhoids and sore muscles may make bowel movements painful.

- **episiotomy**—If your perineum (the area of skin between the vagina and the anus) was cut by your doctor or if it was torn during the birth, the stitches may make it painful to sit or walk for a little while during healing.

- **hemorrhoids**—Although common, hemorrhoids (swollen anal tissues) are frequently unexpected and initially unnoticed.

- **hot and cold flashes**—Your body's adjustment to new hormone and blood flow levels can wreak havoc on your internal thermostat.

- **urinary or fecal incontinence**—The stretching of your muscles during delivery can cause you to inadvertently pass urine when you cough, laugh, or strain or may make it difficult to control your bowel movements, especially if a lengthy labor preceded a vaginal delivery.

- **after pains**—The shrinking of your uterus can cause contractions that worsen when your baby nurses or when you take medication to reduce bleeding.

- **vaginal discharge (lochia)**—Heavier than your period and often containing clots (sometimes golf-ball sized), vaginal discharge gradually fades to white or yellow and stops within 2 months.

- **weight**—Your postpartum weight will probably be about 10 pounds (the weight of the baby, placenta, and amniotic fluid) below your full-term weight, before additional water weight drops off within the first week as your body regains its sodium balance.

Emotionally, you may be feeling:

- **baby blues**—About 80% of new moms experience irritability, sadness, crying, or anxiety, beginning within days or weeks postpartum. Like the more severe associated syndromes of postpartum depression and postpartum psychosis, these baby blues result from hormonal changes, exhaustion, unexpected birth experiences, adjustments to changing roles, and a sense of lack of control over your altered life as you adjust to your new baby.

- **postpartum depression (PPD)**—More serious than the baby blues, this condition is evident in 10% to 20% of new moms and may cause mood swings, anxiety, guilt, and persistent sadness. Your baby may be several months old before PPD strikes, and it's more common in women with a family history of depression.

- **postpartum psychosis**—Postpartum psychosis is a severe and fairly rare condition that makes it difficult to think clearly or function and may become life-threatening to you or your baby. It's common for women with postpartum psychosis to have thoughts about harming themselves or their babies. If you experience any such feelings, call your doctor immediately.

In addition, when it comes to sexual relations, you and your partner may be on completely different pages. He may be ready to pick up where you left off before baby's arrival, whereas you may not feel comfortable enough—physically or emotionally—and may be craving nothing more than a good night's sleep.

The Healing Process

It took your body months to prepare to give birth, and it takes time to recover. If you've had a cesarean section, it can take even longer because this major surgery requires a longer healing time. If unexpected, it may have also raised emotional issues. Pain is greatest the day after the surgery and should gradually subside. Take sponge baths for several days, and don't scratch the incision. If the incision becomes red and swollen, have your doctor check for an infection. Begin gentle exercises as soon as possible (abdominal tightening, bending and straightening your knees, walking—with assistance at first) to speed recovery and help avoid constipation. Drink eight to ten glasses of water daily. Expect vaginal discharge. Avoid stairs and lifting until you've healed, and don't drive until you can make sudden movements and wear a safety belt properly without discomfort.

Some other things to consider during the healing process include:

- **birth control**—You can become pregnant again before your first postpartum period. If you are exclusively breastfeeding (day and night, no solids, at least every 6 hours), have not had a period, and your baby is younger than 6 months old, you have about 98% protection. If you're not breastfeeding exclusively or want additional protection, discuss your options with your doctor. Many recommend starting low-dose oral contraceptives or injections about 6 weeks postpartum. These methods shouldn't affect milk production or your baby. Barrier methods (condoms, diaphragms, spermicidal jellies, and foams) affect breastfeeding less, but are also less effective than pills or shots.

- **breastfeeding**—You need adequate sleep, fluids, and nutrition. Drink a glass of water whenever your baby nurses. Until your milk supply is well established, avoid caffeine, which causes loss of fluid through urine and sometimes makes babies wakeful and fussy. Your clinic or hospital lactation specialist can advise you on how to deal with any breastfeeding problems. Relieve painful, clogged milk ducts with breast massage, frequent nursing, and warm moist packs applied throughout the day. If you develop a fever and your breast becomes tender and red, you may have an infection (mastitis) and need antibiotics. Continue nursing from both breasts. Drink plenty of fluids.

- **engorged breasts**—They resolve as your breastfeeding pattern becomes established or, if you can't or don't choose to breastfeed, when your body stops producing milk—usually within 3 days.

- **episiotomy care**—Continue sitz baths (sitting in just a few inches of warm water and covering the buttocks, up to the hips, in the bathtub). Squeeze the cheeks of your bottom together when you sit to avoid pulling painfully on the stitches. Use a squirt bottle to wash the area with water when you urinate; pat dry. After a bowel movement, wipe from front to back to avoid infection. Reduce swelling with ice packs.

- **exercise**—Resume as soon as possible to help restore your strength and prepregnancy body, increase your energy and sense of well-being, and reduce constipation. Begin slowly and increase gradually. Walking and swimming are excellent choices.

- **hemorrhoids and constipation**—Alternating warm sitz baths and cold packs help. Ask your doctor about a stool softener. Don't use laxatives, suppositories, or enemas without your doctor's approval. Increase your intake of fluids and fiber-rich fruits and vegetables.

- **sexual relations**—Your body needs time to heal. Doctors usually recommend waiting 4 to 6 weeks to reduce the risk of infection or increased bleeding. Fewer than 20% of couples resume sexual activity in the first month, but 90% do so by 4 months. Begin slowly, with kissing, cuddling, and other intimate activities. You'll probably notice reduced vaginal lubrication (this is due to hormones and usually temporary), so a water-based lubricant might be useful. Try to find positions that put less pressure on sore areas and are most comfortable for you. Tell your partner if you're sore or frightened about pain during sexual activity—talking it over can help both of you to feel less anxious and more secure about resuming your sex life.

- **urinary or fecal incontinence**—This usually resolves gradually as your body returns to its normal prepregnancy state. Encourage the process with Kegel exercises, which help strengthen the pelvic floor muscles. To find the correct muscles, pretend you're trying to stop urinating. Squeeze those muscles for a few

seconds, then relax (your doctor can check to be sure you're doing them correctly). Wear a sanitary pad for protection. If the
problem doesn't resolve in several months, tell your doctor.

What Else You Can Do to Help Yourself

You'll enjoy your new role—and it will be much easier—if you care
for both yourself and your new baby. For example:

- When your baby sleeps, take a nap. Get some extra rest for
  yourself!

- Set aside time each day to relax with a book or listen to music.

- Shower daily.

- Get plenty of exercise and fresh air—either with or without
  your baby, if you have someone who can babysit.

- Schedule regular time—even just 15 minutes a day—for you
  and your partner to be alone and talk.

- Make time each day to enjoy your baby, and encourage your
  partner to do so, too.

- Lower your housekeeping and gourmet meal standards—there's
  time for that later. If visitors stress you, restrict them temporarily.

- Talk with other new moms (perhaps from your birthing class)
  and create your own informal support group.

Getting Help from Others

Remember, Wonder Woman is fiction. Ask your partner, friends,
and family for help. Jot down small, helpful things people can do as
they occur to you. When people offer to help, check the list. For example:

- Ask friends or relatives to stop by and hold your baby while you
  take a walk or a bath.

- Hire a neighborhood teen—or a cleaning service—to clean once
  a week, if possible.

- Investigate hiring a doula, a supportive companion profession-
  ally trained to provide postpartum care.

When to Call Your Doctor

There are times when you should call your doctor about your postpartum health. Be sure to call if you:

- experience an unexplained fever of 100.4 degrees Fahrenheit (38 degrees Celsius) or above in the first 2 weeks

- soak more than one sanitary napkin an hour or if the bleeding level increases

- had a C-section or episiotomy and the incision becomes more red or swollen or drains pus

- have new pain, swelling, or tenderness in your legs

- have hot-to-the-touch, significantly reddened, sore breasts or any cracking or bleeding from the nipple or areola (the dark-colored area of the breast)

- find your vaginal discharge has become foul-smelling

- have painful urination or a sudden urge to urinate or inability to control urination

- have increasing pain in the vaginal area

- develop a cough or chest pain, nausea, or vomiting

- become depressed or experience hallucinations, suicidal thoughts, or any thoughts of harming your baby

Note: All information on KidsHealth is for educational purposes only. For specific medical advice, diagnoses, and treatment, consult your doctor.

Part Five

Menopause

Chapter 37

Aging Women

What are some ways to combat the signs of aging?

Regular exercises and a healthy diet will always contribute positively to your health. As you age, exercise tends to become more difficult yet more important. It is especially important to stretch regularly to keep your muscles relaxed, but active, and to keep your joints flexible. Regular exercise can improve some diseases and disabilities in older people who already have them. It can improve mood and relieve depression, too.

Does aging slow down your metabolism? Does that mean fewer calories are needed?

While it is true that older women need fewer than the FDA recommended 2,200 calories/day, no one should consume fewer than 1,500 calories per day. (Even in an attempt to lose weight.) As the body ages, there are also unique nutritional concerns. Cholesterol intake should be monitored due to an increased risk of cardiovascular disease (heart diseases and stroke.)

High blood pressure can be controlled through a low-fat and low-salt diet. Fruits and vegetables are known to combat the risk of cancer, and can help regulate your digestive system. In addition, postmenopausal

Excerpted from "Aging and Women Getting Older," U.S. Department of Health and Human Services, National Women's Health Information Center (NWHIC); published October 2000; updated August 2002. Available online at http://www.4woman.gov; accessed June 2003.

women should consult their doctor regarding calcium supplements to prevent osteoporosis. As always, see a physician for specific recommendations.

If I become forgetful as I age, does that mean I might be getting Alzheimer's disease?

No. It is natural to lose some mental acuity as you age. Think of your brain as a computer, with megabytes of information added each year, year after year. Unlike a computer, however, we can't delete useless information. So our minds can at times experience something that feels like overload, and it's easy to forget some of life's details. Serious memory loss, however, is more rare. As many as 1% of people over the age of 60 suffer from some form of dementia. Dementia is characterized significant loss of intellectual abilities such as memory capacity, severe enough to interfere with social or occupational functioning. Alzheimer's disease (AD) is the most common cause of dementia in older people. AD begins slowly. At first, the only symptom may be mild forgetfulness.

People with AD may have trouble remembering recent events, activities, or the names of familiar people or things. Simple math problems may become hard for these people to solve. Such difficulties may be a bother, but usually, they are not serious enough to cause alarm.

However, as the disease progresses, symptoms are more easily noticed and become serious enough to cause people with AD or their family members to seek medical help. For example, people with AD may forget how to do simple tasks like brushing their teeth or combing their hair. They can no longer think clearly; and they begin to have problems speaking, understanding, reading, or writing. Later on, people with AD may become anxious or aggressive, or wander away from home. Eventually, they may need total care.

There is no cure for AD. Doctors may prescribe certain medication in an attempt to slow the progression of the disease. People with AD should go to their doctor regularly. The doctor will check to see how the disease is progressing and treat any other illnesses that occur. The doctor and other health professionals also can offer help and support to patients and their families. Currently, there is ongoing research into preventing and curing Alzheimer's Disease.

Does aging necessarily mean bad eyesight?

No. Many older people have relatively good eyesight into their eighties and beyond. Growing older does not always mean you see poorly. But age brings changes that can weaken your eyes, making reading in particular more difficult. There are some easy things to try when these changes happen. You might add brighter lights in more places around the house—like at work counters, stairways, and favorite reading places. This may help you see better and can sometimes prevent accidents caused by weak eyesight. You might need prescription glasses for reading, or simple reading glasses bought at the drugstore might be enough. If you already have eyeglasses, you might need a stronger prescription.

Cataracts are common among older people. Cataracts are cloudy areas in part or all of the eye lens. The lens is usually clear and lets light through. Cataracts keep light from easily passing through the lens, and this causes loss of eyesight. Cataracts often form slowly and cause no pain, redness, or tearing in the eye. If a cataract becomes large or thick, it usually can be removed by surgery.

Glaucoma is another common eye disease. This is the result of too much fluid pressure inside the eye. It can lead to vision loss and blindness. The cause of glaucoma is unknown. African-American women over the age of forty are at particular risk for glaucoma, as are all women over 60. If treated early, glaucoma often can be controlled and blindness prevented. To find glaucoma, the eye doctor will look at your eyes through dilated pupils. Treatment may be prescription eye drops, oral medications, or surgery. Most people with glaucoma have no early symptoms or pain from increased pressure.

As always, it is important to see your doctor regularly to check on your eyesight and other related problems.

What can you do about hearing loss?

About one third of Americans between age 65 and 74 and one half of those age 85 and older have hearing problems. They may mistake words in a conversation, miss musical notes at a concert, or leave a ringing doorbell unanswered. Hearing problems can be small (missing certain sounds) or large (more serious deafness). However, you can get help. Special training, hearing aids, certain medicines, and surgery are some of the choices that help people with hearing problems. Older women often don't want to admit their hearing loss, which is unfortunate because it is treatable in most cases.

Does getting older mean not having a sex life?

Absolutely not. Women can enjoy sex well into their senior years. Women may notice changes in the shape and flexibility of the vagina, however. These changes do not usually mean a serious loss in the ability to enjoy sex. Most women will have a decrease in vaginal lubrication that affects sexual pleasure. A pharmacist, doctor, or nurse can suggest over-the-counter vaginal lubricants. Use of some over-the-counter medications as well as alcohol may dampen an older woman's sexual drive.

Sexuality is often a delicate balance of emotional as well as physical issues: How we feel emotionally may affect what we are able to do physically. For example, older men may fear that impotence will become a more frequent problem as they age. As a woman ages, she may become more anxious about her appearance. This emphasis on youthful physical beauty or sexual powers can interfere with a man or woman's ability to enjoy sex.

Older couples may have the same problems that affect people at any age. But they may also have added concerns of age, retirement and other lifestyle changes, and chronic illness. These problems can cause sexual difficulties. Talk openly with your doctor or see a therapist. These health professionals can often help. It is also important to discuss these issues and worries openly and non-judgmentally with your mate.

Are there any benefits to aging?

Aging women face many changes mentally, physically, and emotionally. Many of these changes offer women new opportunities in life and a new outlook. It is important to maintain an optimistic and active lifestyle. There are many aging societies, which help seniors remain active and involved. For example, the Older Women's League provides many activities and a social network for aging women. Check out the Administration on Aging website [http://www.aoa.gov] for further information and resources.

Chapter 38

Menopause Basics

What is menopause?

Menopause is a normal part of life. It is one step in a long, slow process of reproductive aging. For most women this process begins silently somewhere around age 40 when periods may start to be less regular. Declining levels of the hormones estrogen and progesterone cause changes in your periods. These hormones are important for keeping the vagina and uterus healthy as well as for normal menstrual cycles and for successful pregnancy. Estrogen also helps to keep bones healthy. It helps women keep good cholesterol levels in their blood.

Some types of surgery can bring on menopause. For instance, removal of your uterus (hysterectomy) will make your periods stop. When both ovaries are removed (oophorectomy), menopause symptoms may start right away, no matter what your age.

Hormones and change. A woman's body changes throughout her lifetime. Many of those changes are due to varying hormone levels that happen at different stages in life.

Puberty often starts when a girl is about 12 years old. Her body changes—breasts and pubic hair develop, monthly periods begin.

Menopausal transition, commonly called perimenopause, is the time when a woman's body is closer to menopause. At this time, a

Excerpted from "Menopause," National Institute on Aging, September 2002. Available online at http://www.nia.nih.gov; accessed July 2003.

woman's periods may become less regular, and she may start to feel menopause symptoms, such as hot flashes and night sweats. Perimenopause usually begins about 2 to 4 years before the last menstrual period. It lasts for about 1 year after your last period.

Menopause is marked by a woman's last menstrual period. You cannot know for sure what is your last period until you have been period free for 1 full year.

Postmenopause follows menopause and lasts the rest of your life. Pregnancy is no longer possible. There may be some symptoms, such as vaginal dryness, which may continue long after you have passed through menopause.

What are the signs of menopause?

Changing hormone levels can cause a variety of symptoms that may last from a few months to a few years or longer. Some women have slight discomfort or worse. Others have little or no trouble. If any of these changes bother you, check with your doctor. The most common symptoms are:

Changes in periods. One of the first signs may be a change in a woman's periods. Many women become less regular; some have a lighter flow than normal; others have a heavier flow and may bleed a lot for many days. Periods may come less than 3 weeks apart or last more than a week. There may be spotting between periods. Women who have had problems with heavy menstrual periods and cramps will find relief from these symptoms when menopause starts.

Hot flashes. A hot flash is a sudden feeling of heat in the upper part or all of your body. Your face and neck become flushed. Red blotches may appear on your chest, back, and arms. Heavy sweating and cold shivering can follow. Flashes can be as mild as a light blush or severe enough to wake you from a sound sleep (called night sweats). Most flashes last between 30 seconds and 5 minutes.

Problems with the vagina and bladder. The genital area can get drier and thinner as estrogen levels change. This dryness may make sexual intercourse painful. Vaginal infections can become more common. Some women have more urinary tract infections. Other problems can make it hard to hold urine long enough to get to the bathroom. Some women find that urine leaks during exercise, sneezing, coughing, laughing, or running.

Sex. Some women find that their feelings about sex change with menopause. Some have changes to the vagina, such as dryness, that makes sexual intercourse painful. Others feel freer and sexier after menopause—relieved that pregnancy is no longer a worry. Until you have had 1 full year without a period, you should still use birth control if you do not want to become pregnant. After menopause a woman can still get sexually transmitted diseases (STDs), such as HIV/AIDS or gonorrhea. If you are worried about STDs, make sure your partner uses a condom each time you have sex.

Sleep problems. Some women find they have a hard time getting a good night's sleep—they may not fall asleep easily or may wake too early. They may need to go to the bathroom in the middle of the night and then find they aren't able to fall back to sleep. Hot flashes also may cause some women to wake up.

Mood changes. There may be a relationship between changes in estrogen levels and a woman's mood. Shifts in mood may also be caused by stress, family changes such as children leaving home, or feeling tired. Depression is not a symptom of menopause.

Changes in your body. Some women find that their bodies change around the time of menopause. With age, waists thicken, muscle mass is lost, fat tissue may increase, skin may get thinner. Other women have memory problems, or joint and muscle stiffness and pain. With regular exercise and attention to diet, many of these changes may be eased or prevented.

What about heart and bones?

You may not even notice two important changes that happen with menopause.

- Loss of bone tissue can weaken your bones and cause osteoporosis.

- Heart disease risk may grow, due to age-related increases in weight, blood pressure, and cholesterol levels.

Osteoporosis. To maintain strong bones, the body is always breaking down old bone and replacing it with new healthy bone. For women, the loss of estrogen around the time of menopause causes more bone to be lost than is replaced. If too much bone is lost, bones become thin

379

and weak and can break easily. Many people do not know they have weak bones until they break a wrist, hip, or spine bone (vertebrae). Doctors can test bone density (bone densitometry) to find out if you are at risk of osteoporosis. You can lower your risk of bone loss and osteoporosis by making changes to your lifestyle—regular weight-bearing exercise and getting plenty of calcium and vitamin D can help. There are also drugs available that prevent bone loss. Talk to your doctor to find out what is best for you.

Heart Disease. Younger women have a lower risk of heart disease than do men of the same age. But after menopause, a woman's risk of heart disease is almost the same as a man's. In fact, heart disease is the major cause of death in women, killing more women than lung or breast cancer. It's important to know your blood pressure, and levels of cholesterol, HDL, triglycerides, and fasting blood glucose. You can lower your chance of heart disease by eating a healthy diet, not smoking, losing weight, and exercising regularly. There are also drugs that can help. Talk to your doctor to be sure you are doing everything possible to protect your heart.

How can I stay healthy throughout menopause?

To stay healthy you can make some changes in the way you live. For example:

- Don't smoke.

- Eat a healthy diet that is low in fat and cholesterol and moderate in total fat. Your diet should aim to be high in fiber and include fruits, vegetables, and whole-grain foods. It should also be well balanced in vitamins and minerals, including calcium.

- Lose weight if you are overweight.

- Take part in weight-bearing exercise, such as walking, jogging, running, or dancing, at least 3 days each week.

- Take medicine to lower your blood pressure if your doctor prescribes it for you.

- For vaginal discomfort, use a water-based vaginal lubricant (not petroleum jelly) or an estrogen cream.

- If you frequently feel an urgent need to urinate, ask your doctor about techniques such as pelvic muscle exercises, biofeedback, and bladder training that can help you improve muscle control.

- Be sure to get regular pelvic and breast exams, Pap tests, and mammograms. Contact your doctor right away if you notice a lump in your breast.

- If you are having hot flashes, keep a diary to track when they happen. You may be able to use this information to help find out what triggers them.

- Try these tips to help manage hot flashes: when a hot flash starts, go somewhere cool; if hot flashes wake you at night, try sleeping in a cool room; dress in layers that you can take off if you get too warm; use sheets and clothing that let your skin breathe; and have a cold drink (water or juice) at the beginning of a flash.

Chapter 39

Facts about Postmenopausal Hormone Therapy

Choosing whether or not to use postmenopausal hormone therapy can be one of the most important health decisions women face as they age. As with taking any treatment, the decision involves carefully weighing the risks and benefits involved.

But, until recently, the picture of those risks and benefits has been unclear. Studies gave conflicting results about the therapy's effects on breast cancer, heart disease, and other conditions.

In the summer of 2002, new findings emerged that have finally begun to fill in some of the picture's details. While much more remains to be learned, the findings offer women some guidance about the risks and benefits of using postmenopausal hormone therapy.

This chapter discusses those findings and gives you an overview of such topics as menopause, hormone therapy, and alternative treatments to the symptoms of menopause and various health risks that come in its wake. It also provides a list of sources you can contact for more information.

If you're on hormone therapy—whether short- or long-term use—you're bound to have a lot of concerns. This chapter will provide some information, but it's important to talk with your doctor or other health care provider about your health profile. Being informed is one of the best ways you can protect your health.

Excerpted from "Facts about Postmenopausal Hormone Therapy," National Heart, Lung, and Blood Institute, NIH Publication No. 02-5200, October 2002. Revised by David A. Cooke, M.D. on July 25, 2003.

Menopause and Hormone Therapy

As you age, significant internal changes take place that affect your production of the two female hormones, estrogen and progesterone. The hormones, which are important in regulating the menstrual cycle and having a successful pregnancy, are produced by the ovaries, two small, oval-shaped organs.

During the years just before menopause, known as perimenopause, your ovaries begin to shrink. Levels of estrogen and progesterone fluctuate as your ovaries try to keep up production of the hormones. You can have irregular menstrual cycles, along with unpredictable episodes of heavy bleeding during a period. Perimenopause usually lasts several years.

Eventually, your periods stop. Menopause marks the time of your last menstrual period. It is not considered the last until you have been period-free for 1 year without being ill, pregnant, breast-feeding, or using certain medicines, all of which also can cause menstrual cycles to cease. There should be no bleeding, even spotting, during that year. Natural menopause usually happens sometime between the ages of 45 and 54.

You also can undergo menopause as the result of surgery. A surgical procedure, called a hysterectomy, removes the uterus and sometimes the ovaries and fallopian tubes as well. You go through menopause if both of your ovaries are removed. Otherwise, the surgery does not affect menopause, which still occurs naturally.

Whether you go through menopause naturally or surgically, symptoms can result as your body tries to adjust to the drop in estrogen levels. These symptoms vary greatly—one woman may breeze through menopause with few symptoms, while another has difficulty. Symptoms may last for several months or years, or persist. The most common symptoms are hot flashes or flushes, sweats, and sleep disturbances. (A hot flash is a feeling of heat in your face and upper body, which may cause the skin to appear flushed or red as blood vessels expand. Hot flashes that occur with severe sweating during sleep are called night sweats.) But the drop in estrogen also can contribute to other symptoms, such as changes in the vaginal and urinary tracts, which can cause painful intercourse, urinary infections, and the need to urinate more often.

To relieve the symptoms of menopause, doctors may prescribe postmenopausal hormone therapy. This can involve the use of either estrogen alone or with another hormone called progesterone, or progestin in its synthetic form. The two hormones normally help to regulate a woman's menstrual cycle. Progestin is added to estrogen to prevent the overgrowth (or hyperplasia) of cells in the lining of the uterus. This overgrowth can lead to uterine cancer. If you haven't had a hysterectomy, you'll receive estrogen plus progestin therapy; if you have had a hysterectomy, you'll receive estrogen-only therapy. Hormones may be taken daily (continuous use) or on only certain days of the month (cyclic use).

They also can be taken in several ways, including orally, through a patch on the skin, as a cream or gel, or with an intrauterine device (IUD) or vaginal ring. How the therapy is taken can depend on its purpose. For instance, a vaginal estrogen ring or cream can ease vaginal dryness, urinary leakage, or vaginal or urinary infections, but does not relieve hot flashes.

Hormone therapy may cause side effects, such as bleeding, bloating, breast tenderness or enlargement, headaches, mood changes, and nausea. Further, side effects vary by how the hormone is taken. For instance, a patch may cause irritation at the site where it's applied.

Postmenopausal Use

Menopause may cause other changes that produce no symptoms yet affect your health. For instance, a woman's risk of developing heart disease begins to rise around menopause. After menopause, women's rate of bone loss increases. The increased rate can lead to osteoporosis, which may in turn increase the risk of bone fractures, usually after age 70.

Through the years, studies were finding evidence that estrogen might help with some of these postmenopausal health risks—especially heart disease and osteoporosis. With more than 40 million American women over age 50, the promise seemed great.

Although erroneously thought of in the past as a "man's disease," heart disease is the leading killer of American women. Women typically develop it about 10 years later than men.

Similarly, menopause is a time of increased bone loss. Bone is living tissue. Old bone is continuously being broken down and new bone formed in its place. With menopause, bone loss is greater and, if not enough new bone is made, the result can be weakened bones and osteoporosis, which increases the risk of breaks. One of every two women over age 50 will have an osteoporosis-related fracture during her life.

Many scientists believed these increased health risks were linked to the postmenopausal drop in estrogen produced by the ovaries and that replacing estrogen would help protect against the diseases.

The Women's Health Initiative

In 1991, the NHLBI and other units of the NIH launched the "Women's Health Initiative" (WHI), one of the largest studies of its kind ever undertaken in the United States. It consists of a set of clinical trials, an observational study, and a community prevention study, which altogether involve more than 161,000 healthy, postmenopausal women.

WHI's three clinical trials, conducted at the same U.S. centers, are designed to test the effects of postmenopausal hormone therapy, diet modification, and calcium and vitamin D supplements on heart disease, osteoporotic fractures, and colorectal cancer risk.

The postmenopausal hormone therapy clinical trial has two parts. The first involved 16,608 postmenopausal women with a uterus who took either estrogen plus progestin therapy or a placebo. The second involves 10,739 women who have had a hysterectomy and are taking estrogen alone or a placebo.

The women in the WHI estrogen plus progestin study were aged 50 to 79. They enrolled in the study between 1993 and 1998. Their health was carefully monitored by an independent panel, called the Data and Safety Monitoring Board (DSMB).

The study's main goal was to see if the therapy would help prevent heart disease and hip fractures. Another goal was to see if those possible benefits were greater than the possible risks from breast cancer, endometrial (or uterine) cancer, and blood clots.

The study was to have continued until 2005. However, it was stopped in July 2002 because the DSMB found an increased risk of breast cancer and that, overall, risks from use of the hormones outweighed and outnumbered the benefits. "Outnumbered" means that more women had adverse effects from the therapy than benefited from it.

These results show both risks and benefits from use of the estrogen plus progestin therapy. The key adverse effects were more cases of breast cancer, heart attacks, strokes, and blood clots. The main benefits were fewer hip and other fractures and cases of colorectal cancer.

Additionally, there was no increase in deaths from breast cancer or from other causes. Further, there was no increase in the risk of endometrial cancer.

- Breast cancer. The increased risk of breast cancer appeared after 4 years of hormone use. After 5.2 years, estrogen plus progestin resulted in a 26 percent increase in the risk of breast cancer—or 8 more breast cancers each year for every 10,000 women. Women who had used estrogen plus progestin before entering the study were more likely to develop breast cancer than others, indicating that the therapy may have a cumulative effect.

- Heart attack. For heart attack, the risk began to increase in the first year of estrogen plus progestin use and became more pronounced in the second year.

- Stroke. For the first time, estrogen plus progestin was shown to cause more strokes in healthy women. By the end of the study, the estrogen plus progestin group had 41 percent more strokes than the placebo group—or 8 more strokes each year for every 10,000 women.

- Blood clots. The risk of total blood clots was greatest during the first 2 years of hormone use—four times higher than that of placebo users. By the end of the study, it had decreased to two times greater—or 18 more women with blood clots each year for every 10,000 women.

- Fractures. Estrogen plus progestin reduced hip fractures by 34 percent—or 5 fewer hip fractures for every 10,000 women.

- Colorectal cancer. The therapy also lowered the risk of colorectal cancer by 37 percent—or 6 fewer colorectal cancers each year for every 10,000 women.

- Dementia. A substudy within the WHI trial looked at the effects of estrogen plus progestin on the development of Alzheimer's disease and other forms of dementia. The study found that estrogen plus progestin did not prevent dementia and actually increased risk.

The findings are important for several reasons: As a clinical trial, they establish a causal link between use of the particular hormone therapy and its effects on diseases. Further, the findings finally offer some firm guidance to the millions of American women who have a uterus and may consider taking the drugs—6 million already use a form of combination therapy. And, the results apply broadly—the study found no differences in risk by prior health status, age, or ethnicity. The findings do not apply to postmenopausal use of estrogen alone. That arm of the study, which used 0.625 mg per day of conjugated equine estrogen (Premarin), did not have the same increased breast cancer risk and continues.

However, an observational study, supported by the NIH's National Cancer Institute (NCI), recently found that estrogen-only therapy appeared to increase the risk of ovarian cancer. But other, similar studies have not found such an increased risk, and the possible relationship between estrogen use and ovarian cancer remains unclear. WHI participants were informed of these findings, and the results were reviewed for their significance to the study's continuation.

Putting It All Together

First, it's important to know that, because the study involved healthy women, only a small number of them had either a negative or positive effect from estrogen plus progestin therapy.

The percentages describe what would happen to a whole population—not to an individual woman. For example, the increased risk of breast cancer for the women in the WHI study who were taking the estrogen plus progestin therapy was less than a tenth of 1 percent each year.

But if you apply that increased risk to a large group of women and over several years, then the number of women affected becomes an important public health concern. As noted, about 6 million American women take estrogen plus progestin therapy. That would translate into nearly 6,000 more cases of breast cancer every year—and, if all of the women took the therapy for 5 years, that might result in 30,000 more cases of breast cancer.

Second, bear in mind that percentages aren't fate. Whether expressing risks or benefits, they do not mean you will develop a disease. Many factors affect that likelihood, including your lifestyle and other environmental factors, heredity, and your personal medical history.

Finally, realize that most treatments carry risks and benefits. No one can make a treatment choice for you. Talk with your doctor or other health care provider and decide what's best for your health and quality of life. Begin by finding out your personal risk profile for heart disease, stroke, breast cancer, osteoporosis, colorectal cancer, and other conditions. Discuss quality of life issues and alternatives to postmenopausal hormone therapy. Talk with your health care provider. Then weigh every factor carefully and choose the best option for your health and quality of life. And keep the dialogue going—your health status can change and so can your choice.

Advice about Postmenopausal Hormone Therapy

While many questions remain, the new WHI findings provide the basis for some advice about the use of postmenopausal hormone therapy. Here it is, along with advice for short-term hormone use to relieve menopausal symptoms:

Short-Term Estrogen Alone or Estrogen Plus Progestin Therapy

"Short-term" means the shortest time needed to manage menopausal symptoms. The benefits of such use could outweigh any risks for you. Most women use the hormone therapy for 2 to 3 years. However, some may require a longer period of treatment. Talk with your health care provider about your personal risks and needs.

Long-Term Estrogen Plus Progestin Therapy

Do not use estrogen plus progestin therapy to prevent heart disease. The new findings show that it doesn't work. In fact, the therapy increases the chance of a heart attack or stroke. And it increases the risk of breast cancer and blood clots.

To prevent osteoporosis, talk with your health care provider about what your personal risks and benefits would be from estrogen plus progestin therapy. Weigh any benefits against your risk of heart disease, stroke, and breast cancer. Ask about alternate approaches that are considered safe and effective in preventing osteoporosis and fractures, including oral bisphosphonates, being physically active, not smoking, and limiting how many alcoholic beverages you drink.

Long-Term Estrogen-Only Therapy

The WHI has not yet issued findings about the health risks and benefits of long-term use of estrogen-only therapy. Consult your health care provider about your personal health profile and needs.

General Advice

Whether or not you decide to use postmenopausal hormone therapy, you should keep your regular schedule of mammograms, and breast and clinical exams.

In addition to having regular mammograms, you should protect your health by having certain other tests done too. These include tests for high blood pressure, high blood cholesterol, high blood glucose (sugar), bone mineral density, and overweight.

If you stop taking hormone therapy and your menopausal symptoms return, consider alternative treatments. Be aware that some of these remedies have not been proved effective or safe.

Questions Remain

The new findings have provided some details about the dangers and benefits of postmenopausal hormone therapy, but many questions remain. The WHI is following women in the estrogen plus progestin trial to see if and when increased risks and benefits decline after use of the therapy ends. Also, in 2005, the WHI is expected to release key information about the effects of postmenopausal estrogen-only therapy.

Other WHI studies include:

- The observational study is examining other forms of hormone therapy, including other estrogens, progestins, and SERMs.

- The postmenopausal hormone therapy trial has been investigating hormones' effects on memory. While the estrogen plus progestin part of that study ended, the estrogen-only arm continues.

Additionally, scientists funded by the NHLBI, the National Cancer Institute, the National Institute on Aging, the National Institute of Arthritis and Musculoskeletal and Skin Diseases, the National Center for Complementary and Alternative Medicine, the National Institute of Mental Health, and other units of the NIH are supporting research on the effects of postmenopausal hormones and alternative therapies on the symptoms of menopause and conditions that occur after menopause. The research includes studies of: the effects of soy phytoestrogens on cardiovascular disease and osteoporosis, postmenopausal use of phytoestrogens on cardiovascular risk and health, black cohosh and antidepressants on hot flashes, botanical dietary supplements on women's health, plant estrogens on breast cancer, and estrogen on cognition.

Chapter 40

Alternative Therapies for Menopause Symptoms

Chapter Contents

Section 40.1

Alternatives to Hormone Replacement Therapy

"Alternative Therapies for Managing Menopausal Symptoms," National Institutes of Health, National Center for Complementary and Alternative Medicine, August 2, 2002. Available online at http://nccam.nci.nih.gov; accessed June 2003.

Deciding whether to use hormone replacement therapy (HRT) after menopause is a difficult decision many women face as they age. Research has shown that HRT is very effective for relieving menopausal symptoms such as hot flashes and vaginal dryness. It can also reduce the risk of osteoporosis. However, there are also known health risks and uncertainties about long-term use. Recent research has demonstrated that long-term use of estrogen in combination with progestin results in more risks than benefits.

On July 9, 2002, the National Heart, Lung, and Blood Institute (NHLBI) of the National Institutes of Health announced that they would stop a major clinical study of the type of postmenopausal hormone therapy in which estrogen is combined with progestin. The study, a part of the Women's Health Initiative, found increases in breast cancer, cardiovascular disease, stroke, and blood clots in study participants who were taking estrogen plus progestin compared to women taking placebo pills. There were noteworthy benefits of estrogen plus progestin, including fewer cases of hip fractures and colon cancer, but on balance the harm was greater than the benefit.

Many women may now be considering using alternatives to conventional HRT to relieve menopausal symptoms and to lower the risk of conditions such as osteoporosis and heart disease. According to a 1997 study conducted by the North American Menopause Society, more than 30 percent of women use acupuncture, natural estrogen(s), herbal supplements, or so-called plant estrogens (phytoestrogens).

At this time, there is not enough scientific evidence to determine whether these therapies are beneficial. In addition, we do not have sufficient information to show whether these therapies are as safe or safer than conventional drugs being used for menopausal symptoms, osteoporosis, or heart disease.

Botanical products containing or acting like estrogens may provide some of the benefits of estrogen in relieving menopausal symptoms. For example, studies have suggested that soy food products can benefit women with mild hot flashes. Some limited research provides conflicting results on the safety and effectiveness of herbal products—such as ginseng, black cohosh, and dong quai—that are marketed for menopausal symptoms. Currently, [National Center for Complementary and Alternative Medicine] NCCAM is funding research on several botanicals that have shown promise for reducing menopausal symptoms including black cohosh, red clover, hops, dong quai, flax seed, and dietary soy.

Through this research, we hope to learn more about the mechanism of action as well as the safety and effectiveness of these botanical products. Studies are needed to define the possible benefits of these botanical products in promoting bone, heart, and brain health, as well as the potential risks of increasing breast, endometrial, or other cancers in diverse populations of postmenopausal women.

Section 40.2

Black Cohosh and Menopause Symptoms

Excerpted from "Questions and Answers about Black Cohosh and the Symptoms of Menopause" by the National Center for Alternative and Complementary Medicine, Office of Dietary Supplements, updated October 21, 2002. Available online at http://ods.od.nih.gov; accessed August 2003.

What is black cohosh?

Black cohosh (known as both *Actaea racemosa* and *Cimicifuga racemosa*), a member of the buttercup family, is a perennial plant that is native to North America. Other common names include black snakeroot, bugbane, bugwort, rattleroot, rattletop, rattleweed, and macrotys. Insects avoid it, which accounts for some of these common names.

What are the historical uses of black cohosh?

Black cohosh was used in North American Indian medicine for malaise, gynecological disorders, kidney disorders, malaria, rheumatism, and sore throat. It was also used for colds, cough, constipation, hives, and backache and to induce lactation. In 19th-century America, black cohosh was a home remedy used for rheumatism and fever, as a diuretic, and to bring on menstruation.

What clinical studies have been done on black cohosh and its effect on menopausal symptoms?

Black cohosh is used primarily for hot flashes and other menopausal symptoms. A number of studies using various designs have been conducted to determine whether black cohosh affects menopausal symptoms. Few studies were placebo controlled, and most assessed symptoms by using the Kupperman index—a scale that combines measures of hot flashes, insomnia, and depression but not vaginal dryness.

Although some study results suggest that black cohosh may help relieve menopausal symptoms, other study results do not. Studies of black cohosh have yielded conflicting data, in part because of lack of rigor in study design and short study duration (6 months or less). In addition, interpretation of these studies is complicated by the fact that different amounts of black cohosh from different sources were used in the various studies and their outcome measures were different.

In 2001, the American College of Obstetricians and Gynecologists stated—primarily on the basis of consensus and expert opinion—that black cohosh may be helpful in the short term (6 months or less) for women with vasomotor symptoms of menopause.

What is the regulatory status of black cohosh in the United States?

In the United States, black cohosh is sold as a dietary supplement, and dietary supplements are regulated as foods, not drugs. Manufacturers do not have to provide the Food and Drug Administration (FDA) with evidence that dietary supplements are effective or safe before marketing. Because dietary supplements are not always tested for manufacturing consistency, the composition may vary considerably from lot to lot.

Can black cohosh be harmful?

Black cohosh can cause stomach discomfort and headaches. Clinical trials comparing estrogens with black cohosh preparations have shown a low incidence of adverse effects associated with black cohosh;

headaches, gastric complaints, heaviness in the legs, and weight problems were the main adverse effects noted.

Black cohosh usually has not been used for long periods, and published studies have followed women for only 6 months or less. Recently, a large study that followed postmenopausal women taking combined estrogen and progestin for an average of 5.2 years showed a small but significant increase in the risk of certain diseases, demonstrating the importance of long-term studies in revealing risks that may not be apparent in shorter studies. If black cohosh is estrogenic, long-term use may adversely affect uterine or breast tissue. No studies have been published on long-term safety in humans, particularly regarding abnormal stimulation of cells in the endometrium or breast.

There is a case report of neurological complications in a postterm baby after labor induction with a mixture of black cohosh and blue cohosh (*Caulophyllum thalictroides*) during a home birth.

Who should not take black cohosh?

The use of black cohosh during pregnancy has not been rigorously studied. Thus, it would be prudent for pregnant women not to take black cohosh unless they do so under the supervision of their health care provider.

Women with breast cancer may want to avoid black cohosh until its effects on breast tissue are understood.

Does black cohosh interact with any drugs or laboratory tests?

Although black cohosh has not been reported to interact with any drugs or to influence laboratory tests, this has not been rigorously studied.

Section 40.3

Antioxidant Vitamins and Hormone Therapy Fail to Benefit Menopausal Women with Heart Disease

"Study of Menopausal Women with Heart Disease Finds No Benefit, Potential for Harm from Hormone Therapy and Antioxidant Vitamins," National Institutes of Health, November 19, 2002. Available online at http://www.nih.gov; accessed August 2003.

A study sponsored by the National Heart, Lung, and Blood Institute (NHLBI) of the National Institutes of Health found that postmenopausal women with heart disease who took hormone therapy and high dose antioxidant vitamins—either alone or in combination with hormones—did not have fewer heart attacks, deaths, or progression of coronary disease. In fact, both treatments showed a potential for harm. Although the actual numbers of deaths in the study were small, participants taking both active hormones and vitamins had the highest death rate while participants on placebo versions of both treatments had the lowest death rate.

Furthermore, participants taking hormones and vitamins had either more or equal progression of their coronary disease compared to participants taking placebo versions of these treatments.

The results of the Women's Angiographic Vitamin and Estrogen (WAVE) trial were published in the November 20 [2002] issue of the *Journal of the American Medical Association* and presented November 20 [2002] at the American Heart Association's annual meeting in Chicago.

"This study adds to the growing body of evidence that hormone therapy is not helpful in the treatment—or in the prevention—of heart disease—and it provides new information on the absence of benefit from high-dose antioxidant vitamins," said NHLBI Director Claude Lenfant, M.D.

The hormone preparation taken by women with a uterus was the same as that used in the much larger Women's Health Initiative study, which was stopped in July 2002 due to an increased risk of breast cancer and because, overall, risks from use of the hormones outweighed and outnumbered the benefits. Unlike WAVE participants, most women in the WHI study did not have prior evidence of heart disease.

Chapter 41

Menopause and Bladder Control

Does menopause affect bladder control?

Yes. Some women have bladder control problems after they stop having periods (menopause or change of life). If you are going through menopause, talk to your health care team.

After your periods end, your body stops making the female hormone estrogen. Estrogen controls how your body matures, your monthly periods, and body changes during pregnancy and breast-feeding.

Estrogen also helps keep the lining of the bladder and the urethra plump and healthy.

Lack of estrogen causes the bladder control muscles to get weak. Your doctor may give you medicine to replace estrogen to prevent future bladder control problems.

What else causes bladder control problems in older women?

Sometimes bladder control problems are caused by other medical conditions. These problems include:

- infections
- heart problems
- medicines
- nerve damage from diabetes or stroke
- feeling depressed
- difficulty walking or moving

"Menopause and Bladder Control," National Institutes of Health, National Institute of Diabetes and Digestive and Kidney Diseases, NIH Pub. No. 02-4186, April 2002. Available online at http://www.niddk.nih.gov; accessed June 2003.

A very common kind of bladder control problem for older women is urge incontinence. This means the bladder muscles squeeze at the wrong time—or all the time—and cause leaks.

If you have this problem, your health care team can help you re-train yourself to go to the toilet on a schedule.

What should you do about bladder control after menopause?

Talk to your health care team. You may have stress or urge incontinence, but other things could also be happening. Medicines and exercises can restore bladder control in many cases. Your doctor will give you a checkup first.

What treatments can help you regain bladder control?

It depends on what kind of bladder control problem you have. Hormone medicines are only one treatment. Your health care team may also recommend some of the following:

- limiting caffeine
- exercising pelvic muscles
- training the bladder to hold more urine

If these simple treatments do not work, your health care team may have you try something different. These treatments might include:

- biofeedback
- electrical stimulation of pelvic muscles
- a device inserted in the vagina to hold up the bladder
- a device inserted directly into the urethra to block leakage
- surgery to lift a sagging bladder into a better position

What professionals can help you with bladder control?

Professionals who can help you with bladder control include:

- your primary care doctor
- a gynecologist: a women's doctor
- a urogynecologist: an expert in women's bladder problems
- a urologist: an expert in bladder problems
- a nurse or nurse practitioner
- a physical therapist

Part Six

Cancer in Women

Chapter 42

Lung Cancer: The Leading Cause of Cancer Death in Women

Introduction

Women with lung cancer now have more treatment choices and hope than ever before. Doctors keep finding ways to improve treatments for lung cancer and ways to help women with lung cancer have better lives. We are continually learning more about lung cancer, its prevention, detection, and treatment. This chapter will discuss all of these areas.

The information below discusses what we know about lung cancer in general, as well as its prevention and detection.

What Is Lung Cancer?

Lung cancer is cancer that begins in the lungs. It is the second most common cancer in women. There are two major types of lung cancer: small cell lung cancer and nonsmall cell lung cancer.

Approximately 80 percent of people with lung cancer have nonsmall cell cancer, while 20 percent have small cell lung cancer. The earlier that lung cancer is detected, the better the chance it will be cured. It is difficult, however, to detect lung cancer in its early stages.

The information in this chapter is reprinted with permission from CancerSource. For additional information on lung cancer and other cancers, visit the CancerSource website at www.cancersource.com. © 2003 CancerSource. All Rights Reserved. Published December 16, 2002.

The Anatomy of the Lung

The lungs are part of the body's respiratory system. The respiratory system is part of the body's system for breathing. The lungs are spongy organs shaped like cones. The left and right lung are similar, but are not exactly the same. The right lung is a little bit bigger than the left lung, and has three lobes, or sections. The left lung has just two lobes.

When we breathe, air comes in our nose and leaves out of our mouth. The air travels down the windpipe, or trachea. The windpipe is divided into two tubes, or bronchi. The bronchi carry the air into each of the lungs. The bronchi are divided into small tubes called bronchioles. At the end of each bronchiole are air sacs called alveoli. These small air sacs exchange oxygen for carbon dioxide. The lungs get oxygen when we take a breath, or inhale. When we breathe out, or exhale, the lungs get rid of the carbon dioxide.

Types of Lung Cancer

There are two main types of lung cancer: nonsmall cell lung cancer and small cell lung cancer. The doctor can determine what kind of cancer a woman has by looking at the cancer cells under a microscope. Nonsmall cell and small cell lung cancer grow and spread in different ways and therefore have different treatments.

Nonsmall cell lung cancer usually grows and spreads more slowly than small cell lung cancer. The three types of nonsmall cell lung cancer are adenocarcinoma (also called epidermoid carcinoma), squamous cell carcinoma (also called epidermoid carcinoma), and large cell carcinoma.

These types of nonsmall cell lung cancer are named after the cells where the cancer comes from. Table 42.1 gives details about the different types of nonsmall cell lung cancer.

Fewer people get small cell lung cancer. Small cell lung cancer, also called oat cell cancer, grows and spreads more quickly than nonsmall cell lung cancer. It often spreads to other parts of the body at an early stage.

Lung Cancer Statistics

Some people use statistics to try to figure out their chances of getting cancer or of being cured. Statistics show what happens with large groups of people. Because no two people are alike, statistics can't be used to know or predict what will happen to a particular person.

The following are some statistics about lung cancer:

- The American Cancer Society estimates that 80,100 women in the United States will be diagnosed with lung cancer this year.

- More women die from lung cancer each year than from breast cancer.

- Lung cancer is uncommon in people under age 40.

- Lung cancer makes up 12 percent of all cancer cases in women. It causes 25 percent of all cancer deaths in women.

- Cigarette smoking is the leading cause of lung cancer.

- Over 90 percent of lung cancer cases could be prevented if people did not smoke.

- Environmental tobacco smoke or secondhand smoke also contributes to lung cancer in non-smokers.

Lung Cancer Risk Factors

Certain factors can make one woman more likely to get lung cancer than another woman. These are called risk factors. Although such risk factors do exist, a woman who has one or more risk factors will

Table 42.1. Types of Nonsmall Cell Lung Cancer

Type of Nonsmall Cell Lung Cancer	Features	Where It Grows
Adenocarcinoma	Most common kind of nonsmall cell lung cancer; rarely shows symptoms in early stages	Grows in the outer edges of the lungs and in cells that coat the respiratory system with fat.
Squamous cell carcinoma	More slow-growing than adenocarcinoma or large cell carcinoma; develops more often in men; easier to find because the cancer cells are shed in the mucus and can be coughed up.	Found in cells lining the lungs. These cells have tiny hairs, called cilia, that move particles.
Large cell carcinoma	The least common of the three kinds of nonsmall cell lung cancer; may spread early to organs.	Found in other types of cells that make up linings of the organs.

not necessarily get lung cancer. In fact, a woman can have all the risk factors and still not get lung cancer, or a woman can have no known risk factors and still get the disease.

Doctors estimate that over 90 percent of lung cancer cases are related to smoking. However, a small percentage of people who get lung cancer do not have a history of smoking or being around secondhand smoke. So, not all smokers get lung cancer and not all lung cancer patients were smokers.

There is really no way to know for sure if a woman is going to get lung cancer. However, there are things that make some people more likely to get it. Many risk factors linked with lung cancer have to do with using tobacco. Many of these risk factors can be controlled. Risk factors for getting lung cancer include:

- **Cigarettes.** Smoking cigarettes causes lung cancer. Tobacco contains substances called carcinogens. Carcinogens harm cells in the lungs. After a while, these damaged cells may turn into cancer. The longer a woman smokes and the more cigarettes a woman smokes per day, the higher the chance that that woman will develop lung cancer.

- **Cigars and pipes.** Women who smoke cigars and pipes have a higher risk of developing lung cancer than women who don't smoke. If the woman has smoked for a long time, she has an even higher chance of developing lung cancer. A woman's risk of lung cancer also depends on how much she smokes every day.

- **Secondhand smoke.** If women are around smokers, they have a higher risk of getting lung cancer. For example, a non-smoker who lives with a heavy smoker has a higher risk of developing lung cancer than someone who does not spend time around a smoker. Being around secondhand smoke is called involuntary or passive smoking.

- **Radon.** Radon is a gas that is found in soil and rocks. You can't see, smell, or taste radon, but it can harm the lungs. Women who work in mines or live in houses with radon have a higher risk of developing lung cancer.

- **Asbestos.** Asbestos is a group of minerals used in shipbuilding, insulation, and some kinds of car repairs. If a woman breathes in tiny pieces of asbestos, they can get stuck in the lungs and harm the cells of the lungs. Women who are around asbestos have a higher chance of getting lung cancer. Their risk is much higher if they also smoke.

- **Pollution.** Women who breathe in a lot of air pollution over a long period of time have a higher risk of developing lung cancer.

- **Lung diseases.** Women who have lung diseases like tuberculosis (TB) have a greater chance of getting lung cancer. Lung cancer sometimes develops when there is scar tissue from TB in the lungs.

- **Medical history.** A woman who had lung cancer before has a higher chance of getting lung cancer again. If the woman quits smoking after having lung cancer, the chance of getting it again is reduced.

What can a woman do about risk factors? Since it is known that smoking tobacco causes most cases of lung cancer, a woman who smokes would benefit from quitting as soon as possible, even after being diagnosed with lung cancer. When a woman quits smoking, her risk of getting the disease declines over time. Non-smokers can benefit from never starting and from staying away from those who do smoke.

Smoking is known as a controllable risk factor. Quitting greatly reduces a woman's chances of getting lung cancer. In fact, quitting smoking can greatly reduce a woman's risk of many other cancers as well. These include cancers of the bladder, pancreas, larynx, mouth, esophagus, pharynx, and kidney. There are many ways to quit smoking. Women who would like to quit smoking should talk to their doctor about creating a plan to quit.

Lung Cancer Symptoms

Women with lung cancer may not notice signs of the disease in its early stages. In fact, many lung cancers are found through a chest x-ray taken for other reasons.

When early lung cancer does cause symptoms, they are often health problems that smokers have anyway. For example, some early signs of lung cancer include shortness of breath and the inability to exercise without feeling out of breath or having a cough.

Common symptoms of lung cancer in its later stages include: sudden shortness of breath; a cough that doesn't go away and gets worse over time; pneumonia or bronchitis occurring more than usual; constant chest pain; pain in the upper back that remains in one place and is constant for several days or weeks; shortness of breath, wheezing, or hoarseness; swelling of the neck and face; loss of appetite or weight loss; coughing up of blood; or fatigue.

These symptoms may be caused by lung cancer or by other, less serious conditions. It is important to check with a doctor to be sure.

Lung Cancer Diagnosis

In order to determine why a woman is having lung cancer-like symptoms, the doctor will find out the woman's medical history, smoking history, and family history of cancer, and other risk factors the woman has been exposed to. The doctor might also perform a physical exam, a chest x-ray, and other tests. If the doctor suspects the patient has lung cancer, he or she may perform a sputum cytology. In a sputum cytology, the doctor looks at cells from the mucus in the lungs. These exams may lead the doctor to decide that the woman doesn't need any more tests, and that she does not have lung cancer.

However, it is sometimes necessary to remove fluid or tissue from a suspicious area found in a lung to make a cancer diagnosis. This is called a biopsy. The kinds of biopsies done to find lung cancer, and some details about what will happen during each, are listed in Table 42.2.

Once the biopsy is completed, a pathologist—a doctor who looks at tissue samples in a lab—looks at the tissue under a microscope to check for cancer cells. It usually takes several days for the results of a woman's biopsy to come back. A biopsy is the only sure way to tell if a woman has cancer and what kind of cancer it is.

Patients are often overwhelmed with the information they receive from their doctor. It is important that they take the time to gather as much information as possible.

Tests and Second Opinions

A team of health care professionals, including a medical oncologist and an oncology nurse, will treat patients diagnosed with lung cancer. This health care team will answer any questions patients may have, and will help patients through each of the many steps they will take before, during, and after treatment. This health care team will also let patients know what tests are being done and the results of these tests, and will guide patients in making treatment decisions.

Treatment for lung cancer usually begins a few weeks after diagnosis. This gives patients time to talk with their doctor about treatment choices, to get a second opinion, to decide about treatment, and to prepare themselves and their loved ones.

Before treatment begins, special lab tests may be done to help the doctor find out more about the disease. These tests include: CAT or CT scans. During a CAT or CT scan, a computer creates pictures of the inside of the body from x-rays. These pictures help the doctor see where the cancer is in the chest, and whether it has spread to the liver or the adrenal glands on top of the kidneys.

- Radionuclide scanning. During radionuclide scanning, the patient will either swallow or get an injection of a radioactive substance. The doctor can then see on a special machine whether any areas look abnormal.

- Bone scan. A bone scan is one kind of radionuclide scanning. This test indicates whether cancer has spread to the bones.

- Mediastinoscopy/Mediastinotomy. During mediastinoscopy, a doctor makes a small incision in the patient's neck. The doctor then uses a lighted scope to look at the center of the chest and the lymph nodes. In mediastinotomy, the doctor makes the incision in the patient's chest instead. In either procedure, the doctor will use the scope to remove some tissue for inspection. The doctor can then determine whether the cancer has spread to the lymph nodes in the chest.

- Magnetic resonance imaging (MRI). MRIs are used to determine if cancer has spread to the chest or the brain.

Table 42.2. Types of Biopsies Used to Diagnose Lung Cancer

Name of Biopsy	What Is Performed
Bronchoscopy	The doctor places a thin, lighted tube called a bronchoscope into the patient's mouth or nose to look into the breathing passages and to take a tissue sample.
Needle biopsy	The doctor inserts a needle through the chest wall into the tumor to remove some tissue. Often, a CAT scan is done at the same time to help guide the placement of the needle.
Thoracentesis	The doctor uses a needle to take some fluid from around the lungs, if fluid is present.
Thoracotomy	This biopsy requires surgery and is done in a hospital. In this procedure, the surgeon looks for lung cancer in the chest.

- Positron emission tomography (PET) scan. A PET scan looks at tissues with increased metabolism, such as lymph nodes, that have cancer in them.

- Bone marrow biopsy. In small cell lung cancer, a bone marrow biopsy may be done to see if cancer cells are present. To perform this test, the doctor passes a needle through the skin into the hip bone.

- Pulmonary function test (PFT). This test involves breathing into a machine that measures lung function.

A woman with lung cancer will not always find it easy to decide which lung cancer treatment to have. Before starting any treatment, patients may want to talk to a second doctor about treatment options. Some insurance companies even encourage women diagnosed with lung cancer to get a second opinion. Patients should check with their health insurance providers to see if they will cover the cost of a second opinion. It is important to remember that taking time to make sure the best decision is made will not reduce the chance that a treatment will be successful. There are many ways to find a doctor who can give a second opinion.

Your doctor may be able to recommend a specialist, such as a surgeon, medical oncologist, or a radiation oncologist. These doctors usually work together at cancer centers or special centers for lung diseases.

The Cancer Information Service (1-800-4-CANCER) informs callers about treatment facilities, including cancer centers and other programs supported by the National Cancer Institute. Women can get the names of doctors from their local medical society, a nearby hospital, or a medical school, or local lung cancer advocacy groups, and other women who have had lung cancer.

The Directory of Medical Specialists lists doctors by state and specialty and gives information about their background. This resource can be found in most public libraries.

The Alliance for Lung Cancer Advocacy, Support, and Education (ALCASE) offers suggestions on finding lung cancer specialists (visit www.alcase.org or call 1-800-298-2436).

Reviewed by: Gail Wilkes, RN, MS, OCN, Oncology Nurse Specialist, Massachusetts General Hospital, Boston, Massachusetts; Teresa Knoop, RN, MSN, AOCN, Cancer Information Nurse Specialist, Vanderbilt-Ingram Cancer Center, Nashville, TN; Graeme Fisher, M.D., UMASS Medical Center, Worcester, MA.

Chapter 43

Skin Cancer: The Most Prevalent Cancer in Women

Chapter Contents

Section 43.1

Skin Cancer Overview

"(Healthy Living) Women's Health: Ages 40-49—Skin Cancer," January 2003. This information is reprinted with permission from the Cancer Research and Prevention Foundation. © 2003. For more information, call 800-227-2732, or visit their website at www.preventcancer.org.

Although you might not be spending as much time in the sun as you did in when you were a teenager, the effects of prior sun exposure may surface in your 40s.

Middle-aged women should continue to use sunscreen every day to help protect their skin from ultraviolet radiation.

The recommendations below offer guidance for protecting yourself against skin cancer and detecting precancerous growths before they spread.

What Is Skin Cancer?

Skin cancer develops when abnormal skin cells, which often form a group called a tumor, begin to grow out of control and invade other parts of the body—a process called metastasis. Benign tumors do not spread and are usually not harmful. Malignant tumors, however, spread from their sources and can grow into life-threatening cancers.

Types of Skin Cancer

Because they develop differently and carry different risks, skin cancers (also called carcinomas) are separated into two groups: melanoma and nonmelanoma cancers. Melanomas, which account for about 4 percent of skin cancers, start in the pigment-producing cells that are in the skin's outer layer (the epidermis). They are usually brown or black mole-like growths that appear most often on women's arms and lower legs.

When identified early, melanomas can be successfully removed most of the time. If neglected, however, melanomas are likely to metastasize and are deadly. Although melanomas are the least common, they are the most dangerous skin cancers.

Nonmelanoma skin cancers, mostly flesh-colored to reddish-brown nodules, primarily involve two types of cells: basal cells (lower epidermis) and squamous cells (upper epidermis). About 75 percent of skin cancers are basal cell carcinomas, which are sun-induced, slow-growing, and unlikely to metastasize. Squamous cell carcinomas are also caused by sun exposure and account for about 20 percent of skin cancers.

The development of squamous cell carcinomas around the anus and genital area has been associated with human papillomavirus (HPV), a sexually transmitted disease that is also linked to cervical cancer.

Although melanomas cause the most deaths, other types of skin cancers can also be fatal. The best way to start protecting yourself against all skin cancers is learning how to examine your body for suspicious skin changes that signal precancerous growths.

Skin cancer might seem like a disease that only affects only the elderly, but increased exposure to the sun and use of tanning beds have resulted in earlier onset of the disease. More middle-age women are developing skin cancer than ever before.

Stats and Facts about the Most Prevalent Cancer

- With skin cancer rates on the rise, more than 1 million Americans will be diagnosed with nonmelanomas in 2003, and about 54,200 will be diagnosed with melanoma.

- An estimated 9,800 people die from skin cancer this year—approximately 7,600 from melanoma and 2,200 from other skin cancers.

- Since 1981, the rate of incidence has slowed to a little less than 3 percent per year.

- Melanoma risk is more than 10 times higher for whites than African-Americans.

- Approximately 50 percent of all melanomas occur in people over the age of fifty (that means that half occur in youth and middle age).

- Men are twice as likely to develop basal cell carcinomas and are three times as likely to have squamous cell carcinomas.

What Is Your Risk?

While everyone should practice sun safety, certain people are at greater risk for developing skin cancer. Risk factors include:

411

- Light hair color and blue, gray, or green eyes
- Fair complexion and/or freckles
- Sun sensitivity (skin that burns easily)
- Taking prescription medications that increase sun sensitivity
- Family history (one or more close relatives with skin cancer)
- Several moles on your body
- Presence of a congenital mole (since birth)
- One or more large or irregularly pigmented lesions
- Suppressed immune system
- Exposure to certain chemicals, such as arsenic, and to radiation therapy
- Excessive exposure to the sun and repeated blistering sunburns before the age of 15

Prevention Tips: Minimizing Your Skin Cancer Risk

Avoid sun exposure from 10 a.m. to 4 p.m. During the middle of the day, the sun's UV rays are most intense. Try to minimize your midday sun exposure.

Always wear a waterproof, broadband sunscreen of SPF 15 or higher. Sunscreen offers some protection against the sun's harmful rays. If applied correctly, a sun protection factor (SPF) of 15 or higher should allow you to stay in the sun 15 times longer than you would normally be able to without burning. Sunscreen does not block all of the sun's radiation, however, and most people do not use sunscreen appropriately.

One mistake people make is having a false sense of sun invincibility. Wearing sunscreen helps protect against sun damage, but it does not give you a license to spend unlimited time in the sun. Some other common missteps include not using enough sunscreen, not using a waterproof formula, not reapplying frequently enough, and not using broadband protection.

To block more of the sun's rays, your sunscreen should include broadband protection. Broadband is a term that sunscreen manufacturers use to describe a product that offers protection from both UVA and UVB radiation emitted by the sun.

To completely cover your body, slather on one ounce of sunscreen. If you are visiting the shore or laying out by the pool, you should apply about an ounce—the amount of a full shot glass—of sunscreen to all exposed skin.

Apply sunscreen at least 20 minutes before going out in the sun. Since sunscreen takes at least 20 minutes to absorb into the skin, apply it prior to going outside to give it time to work.

Wear sunscreen every day, even overcast, cloudy days. When you're outside during daylight hours, UV rays can damage skin regardless of season, location, or weather. In the United States, exposure to sunlight is almost as intense in April as it is in August. Year-round protection is important whether you're headed to the pool or the ski slopes since surfaces such as water, snow and sand can reflect up to 85 percent of the sun's rays.

Protect your eyes and lips. Facial features, especially eyes and lips, are susceptible sites for skin cancer. To protect your eyes, wear sunglasses treated to absorb UV radiation and make sure they cover the area surrounding your eyes. For lips, use a lip balm that has an SPF of at least 15.

Wear clothing with a tight weave and a wide-brimmed hat. Clothes block the sun's rays even better than commercial sunscreen products do. Dark, tightly woven fabrics offer the better sun protection than light, thin, and loosely woven materials do. A wide-brimmed hat provides good coverage for your face, ears, neck and scalp. Although a cap is better than no hat at all, it doesn't shade your ears and neck.

If you have children, teach them to apply their own sunscreen (under your supervision). Teach your children that, by using sunscreen, they can be cancer-fighters. Remember that all of the prevention tips offered here not only apply to adults, but also apply to children.

Keep babies less than six months old out of the sun. Experts dissuade against using sunscreen on infants, who may react negatively to the chemicals. Instead of using sunscreen on infants, cover them well—using a hat or bonnet and sunglasses—if they must be in the sun.

Encourage your kids to play in the shade. When you take your kids to playgrounds, look for areas that include shade trees or covered areas so they can take a break from being in the sun.

Early Detection

Examine yourself. Once a month, give yourself a skin exam or ask your partner to examine your skin. If you are doing this yourself, use a hand mirror and a full-length mirror to look for the following signs and changes:

- A brown or black irregularly pigmented spot with uneven margins

- A slow-growing, raised, translucent, pearly nodule that may crust, ulcerate and possibly bleed without treatment. These are typically found on the face, neck, hands and trunk.

- A change in sensation, itchiness, tenderness, or pain from a mole

- A small, smooth, shiny, pale, or waxy lump on the skin

- A flat red spot, either scaly and crusty or smooth and shiny

- A new mole

Remember the **ABCD rule**: asymmetry, border irregularity, color that is not uniform and a diameter greater than 6 millimeters.

If you have children, examine their skin regularly, too. It is possible for children to develop skin cancer just like adults, and it's never too early to start forming good habits!

See a Professional

Your risk of developing skin cancer increases as you age. Starting when you turn 40, you should be examined by a health care professional every year for a skin cancer checkup.

If you discover a suspicious growth while conducting your monthly self-examination, however, get a clinician to inspect the area as soon as possible. Early detection can allow you to catch abnormal skin growths before they have a chance to spread.

Section 43.2

Questions and Answers about Sun Exposure

Excerpted from "Choose Your Cover Q&A," Centers for Disease Control and Prevention, National Center for Chronic Disease Prevention and Health Promotion, November 15, 2001. Available online at http://www.cdc.gov; accessed May 2003.

When do I need to protect myself from sun exposure?

Protection from sun exposure is important all year round, not just during the summer or at the beach. Any time the sun's ultraviolet (UV) rays are able to reach the earth, you need to protect yourself from excessive sun exposure. UV rays can cause skin damage during any season or temperature.

Relatively speaking, the hours between 10 a.m. and 4 p.m. during daylight savings time (9 a.m. to 3 p.m. during standard time) are the most hazardous for UV exposure in the continental United States. UV radiation is the greatest during the late spring and early summer in North America.

Remember: UV rays reach you on cloudy and hazy days, as well as on bright and sunny days. UV rays will also reflect off any surface like water, cement, sand, and snow.

How can I protect myself from the sun's UV rays?

When possible, avoid outdoor activities during midday, when the sun's rays are strongest. This usually means the hours between 10 a.m. and 4 p.m. You can also wear protective clothing, such as a wide-brimmed hat, long-sleeved shirt, and long pants.

For eye protection, wear wraparound sunglasses that provide 100 percent UV ray protection. And always wear a broad-spectrum (protection against both UVA and UVB rays) sunscreen and lipscreen with at least SPF 15. Remember to reapply as indicated by the manufacturer's directions.

Also, check the sunscreen's expiration date. Sunscreen without an expiration date has a shelf life of no more than three years. Exposure to extreme temperatures can shorten the expiration date or shelf life of sunscreen.

Does it matter what kind of sunscreen I use?

Sunscreens come in a variety of forms such as lotions, gels, and sprays, so there are plenty of different options. There are also sunscreens made for specific purposes, such as the scalp, sensitive skin, and for use on babies. Regardless of the type of sunscreen you choose, be sure that you use one that blocks both UVA and UVB rays and that it offers at least SPF 15.

What kinds of clothing best protect my skin from UV rays?

Clothing that covers your skin protects against the sun's UV rays. Loose-fitting long-sleeved shirts and long pants made from tightly woven fabric offer the best protection. A wet T-shirt offers you much less UV protection than does a dry one.

If wearing this type of clothing isn't practical, at least try to wear a T-shirt or a beach cover-up. Keep in mind, however, that a typical T-shirt actually has an SPF rating substantially lower than the recommended SPF 15, so double-up on protection by using sunscreen with at least SPF 15 (and UVA and UVB protection) and staying in the shade when you can.

Will a hat help protect my skin? Are there recommended styles for the best protection?

Hats can help shield your skin from the sun's UV rays. Choose a hat that provides shade for all of your head and neck. For the most protection, wear a hat with a brim all the way around that shades your face, ears, and the back of your neck. If you choose to wear a baseball cap, you should also protect your ears and the back of your neck by wearing clothing that covers those areas, using sunscreen with at least SPF 15, or by staying in the shade.

Chapter 44

Thyroid Cancer Affects Women Twice as Often as Men

What is the thyroid?

The thyroid gland is located on the anterior aspect (front) of the neck. It can be felt just below the thyroid cartilage, or Adam's apple. It is a butterfly shaped organ that stretches across the midline of the neck just below the Adam's apple, with its wings spreading superiorly (towards the head) on either side of the Adam's apple. These wings are called the lobes of the thyroid, with the portion extending across midline called the isthmus. As an endocrine gland, the thyroid gland produces and secretes thyroid hormones into the bloodstream. The thyroid does this as a response to a hormone produced by the pituitary gland called thyroid stimulating hormone, or TSH. When the thyroid gland is turned on by TSH, it increases its uptake of iodine, which is required to make thyroid hormone, and manufactures and secretes thyroid hormones. These thyroid hormones are very important for many functions ranging from the regulation of our metabolic rate to helping to maintain the function of our heart to regulation of body temperature. An increase in the production (hyperthyroid) or a decrease in the production (hypothyroid) of thyroid hormone can be easily managed, though can cause serious problems if not properly treated. The principal cells of the thyroid are called follicular cells, and are mainly responsible for the production of thyroid hormone.

417

What is thyroid cancer?

The definition of a tumor is a mass of abnormally growing cells. Tumors can be either benign or malignant. Benign tumors have uncontrolled cell growth, but without any invasion into normal tissues and without any spread. A malignant tumor is called cancer when these tumor cells gain the propensity to invade tissues and spread locally as well as to distant parts of the body. In this sense, thyroid cancer occurs when cells of the thyroid gland grow uncontrollably to form tumors that can invade the tissues of the neck, spread to the surrounding lymph nodes, or to the bloodstream and then to other parts of the body. The most common types of cancers of the thyroid gland are derived from the cells responsible for thyroid hormone production. The general term for cancers that come from glandular tissue is adenocarcinoma.

In the thyroid, the most common types of cancer are papillary adenocarcinoma of the thyroid (75% to 80%) and follicular adenocarcinoma of the thyroid (about 15%). Papillary thyroid cancer takes on a folded appearance under the microscope, which eases its diagnosis. Follicular thyroid cancer may closely resemble normal thyroid tissue, but as a malignancy, has a propensity to divide uncontrollably and invade and spread. The next most common type of cancer of the thyroid is called medullary thyroid cancer (5%), which is derived from the parafollicular cells of the thyroid. This is often associated with a familial genetic predisposition to develop certain types of cancers (see below). The other major type of thyroid cancer often described is called anaplastic thyroid cancer (2%). This cancer usually affects older people and is very aggressive. Other types of cancers, such as lymphomas (cancer of the lymph gland cells), sarcomas (cancer of soft tissues such as muscle or cartilage cells), or metastases (cancers from other sites that have spread to the thyroid gland) are also seen in the thyroid gland.

Am I at risk for thyroid cancer?

Thyroid cancer is fairly common, as it is found at autopsy in approximately 5% of people with no known thyroid disease. However, death due to thyroid cancer is uncommon, explained by the fact that thyroid cancer is usually an indolent disease, tending to remain localized to the thyroid gland for many years. Most cases of thyroid cancer are sporadic; meaning there is no obvious predisposition or risk factor for development. However, it is more common in women, occurring in a 3:1 ratio. This has prompted studies into the investigation of estrogen as a possible risk factor for thyroid cancer, though this has never been proven. Studies have also shown a preponderance of certain types of thyroid cancer in regions with a high incidence of goiters (enlarged thyroid glands), which occur as a result of a lack of dietary iodine. This is further supported by the decrease of thyroid cancers in population given supplemental iodine.

The most firmly established risk factor for the development of thyroid cancer is exposure to ionizing radiation to the neck region. This is supported by the high incidence of thyroid cancer seen in many populations exposed to radiation.

Notably, this includes patients with Graves disease (a hyperthyroid condition) treated with radiation, Hodgkin disease patients treated with radiation, survivors of atomic blasts at Nagasaki and Hiroshima, and survivors of the Chernobyl explosion. In fact, thyroid cancer is one of the most common cancers noted in populations exposed to large doses of radiation through accident or war.

A notable genetic predisposition is associated with medullary thyroid cancer, which is associated with a syndrome called multiple endocrine neoplasia (MEN) type 2 syndrome. Patients with MEN type 2 (Sippler's syndrome) have a strong familial history of medullary thyroid cancers and a type of adrenal cancer, called pheochromocytoma.

How can I prevent thyroid cancer?

As most cases of thyroid cancers are sporadic and not associated with any risk factors, there is usually no method to prevent the development of thyroid cancer. Careful examination of the thyroid and consideration of screening for patients at high risk could be considered, though the general prevention of thyroid cancers is impossible.

What screening tests are available?

Ultrasound testing has been proven to detect thyroid nodules—benign or malignant—of sizes of less than 1 cm. However, using ultrasound for mass screening is not likely to be efficacious because of the incidences and natural history of thyroid cancer. Notably, the majority of thyroid cancers are papillary thyroid cancer, which are historically very indolent cancers. Therefore, the small tumors that ultrasound has the ability to detect are likely to be very small papillary thyroid cancers, which are unlikely to affect the survival of most patients—akin to very early stage indolent prostate cancers and non-melanoma skin cancers. Hence, the early detection of thyroid cancers is generally through careful physical examination of the neck. Palpation of the neck will detect most clinically significant thyroid cancers.

Obviously, the story can be quite different in patients diagnosed with MEN type 2 and the subsequent high risk of medullary thyroid cancer. The present recommendation for patients with the genetic mutation associated with MEN type 2 is to undergo a prophylactic total thyroidectomy (complete removal of the thyroid) to prevent the development of a possibly aggressive medullary thyroid cancer.

What are the signs of thyroid cancer?

By far, the most common presentation of thyroid cancer is a solitary nodule on the thyroid, which can be felt on physical exam. As the thyroid gland is a fairly superficial organ in the neck, a thyroid nodule could be noticed early, at which time medical attention should be sought. By no means is every thyroid nodule a thyroid cancer. In fact, most represent hyperplasia (benign growth of the thyroid) of the thyroid gland.

Less commonly, thyroid cancer can present as multiple nodules in the thyroid or a large mass in the neck. The large mass can be located either in the region of the thyroid, representing the primary thyroid cancer, or in a separate region of the neck, representing a spread of cancer to the lymph nodes. Thyroid tumors can also at times present as hoarseness or with symptoms of tracheal or esophageal compression, such as shortness of breath, air hunger, problems or pain with swallowing, or neck pain.

How is thyroid cancer diagnosed?

Any thyroid nodule deserves attention. Once a thyroid nodule is noted, the next steps are all designed to determine if the nodule represents a benign growth or malignant tumor. The most common etiology behind a thyroid nodule is a small portion of benign functioning thyroid tissue, which must be differentiated from a thyroid cancer. Obviously a careful physical exam should be done by a physician, with attention to the examination of the neck to attempt to detect enlarged lymph nodes. Other laboratory tests are also usually done to determine the function of the thyroid gland. Tests that indicate an overfunctioning gland point more toward the nodule being composed of benign functional tissue.

After a diagnosis is made, further work-up is done to determine if there was spread of disease to the local lymph nodes and distant areas of the body including the lungs and bones. Hence, this includes a CT scan of the neck to evaluate lymph nodes and an MRI of the neck to evaluate muscle or tracheal involvement. Some also recommend a bone scan and chest x-ray, as thyroid cancer can (rarely) metastasize to the bones and lungs.

What are the treatments for thyroid cancer?

The treatment of thyroid cancer can involve an approach combining surgery, radioactive iodine and radiation therapy, depending on the stage and type of thyroid cancer. Surgery always plays the central role, with the removal of the cancer being key. Usually the surgical procedure is a total thyroidectomy (the removal of the entire thyroid gland) or a near total thyroidectomy (leaving only a small remnant of thyroid tissue with parathyroid glands, which are attached to the thyroid). These more extensive surgical procedures have been shown to be more efficacious than more conservative surgeries, such as the removal of a single lobe of the thyroid gland (lobectomy). An exception to this philosophy can be in patients with small, Stage I papillary thyroid cancers, where a lobectomy may be appropriate. However, if the thyroid gland is not completely removed at the first surgical procedure, the patient is always at risk for recurrence in the portion of the thyroid left behind. Secondary operations to remove the remaining portion of the thyroid gland can be performed to attempt to salvage a cure in these patients, though the complication rates in these "completion thyroidectomies" may be high.

A controversy in the surgical treatment of thyroid cancer is how to address the lymph nodes of the neck. When lymph nodes are felt on physical exam or found by ultrasound, they are obviously removed. However, the role of a prophylactic removal of the lymph nodes of the neck when they are not obviously involved is unclear. The lymph nodes very close to the thyroid gland are usually dissected without much difficulty and therefore should be removed. However, most would agree that radical neck dissections to remove a majority of the lymph nodes of the neck are not indicated unless lymph nodes are known to be involved.

In more advanced cases of thyroid cancers, surgical treatment is not enough, and patients require various adjuvant therapies. The first and simplest is the use of supplemental thyroid hormone following surgery. Patients with near total or total thyroidectomies are likely to be hypothyroid anyway, hence requiring supplemental thyroid hormone regardless of the state of the cancer. The standard of care is therefore to use this supplemental thyroid hormone in order to keep the remaining thyroid gland (or remaining thyroid cancer) asleep or inactive through a feedback system. In other words, if the body detects that there is a sufficient amount of thyroid hormone already present (through supplementation), it will not produce signals to turn on the thyroid to create hormone itself. This can be quite successful in keeping residual thyroid cancers dormant.

As thyroid tissue (and often thyroid cancers) preferentially take up iodine into their cells as part of normal functioning, the use of radioactive iodine (RAI) can be used to kill any remaining cancer cells. The iodine is simply taken up into the cell and the radiation within the radioactive iodine itself is released locally, delivering a lethal dose of radiation to the cancer cells.

Indications for RAI include tumors with high risk features such as sizes of >1.5 cm, invasion of the cancer through the thyroid capsule or into the soft tissues of the neck, spread to the lymph nodes or more distantly, or recurrent disease (thyroid cancer that has come back). RAI can be a very effective therapy in many cases, though there are thyroid tumors that do not take up iodine, rendering RAI useless.

Radiation therapy can also be used in the adjuvant setting, if it is felt that the patient has a high risk of recurrence following surgery alone. It is often used in patients with papillary, follicular, or medullary thyroid cancer with high risk features, such as incomplete resection or spread outside the thyroid gland to soft tissues of the neck or to regional lymph nodes that do not take up RAI. It is also used in all cases of anaplastic thyroid cancer to attempt to halt this aggressive disease. In practice, the most common indications for radiation therapy are when the thyroid cancer is adherent to the trachea, has mediastinal lymph node involvement, or does not take up RAI. In these cases, radiation therapy has been proven to decrease the risk of local recurrences.

Chemotherapy has not classically been used in the treatment of thyroid cancer. However, chemotherapy drugs such as adriamycin, cisplatin, and etoposide have been used in anaplastic thyroid cancers or disease that has progressed through RAI or radiation therapy.

The vast majority of patients with thyroid cancer are curable using these modalities. However, further research is needed in patients who do not respond to conventional therapy.

Chapter 45

Breast Cancer

Chapter Contents

423

Section 45.1

What You Need to Know about Breast Cancer

Excerpted from "What You Need To Know About™ Breast Cancer," National Cancer Institute, NIH Pub. No. 00-1556; published November 20, 2000; updated March 2003. Available online at http://www.cancer.gov; accessed August 2003.

Introduction

Other than skin cancer, breast cancer is the most common type of cancer among women in the United States. In 2003, an estimated 211,000 women will be diagnosed with breast cancer.

Research has led to progress against breast cancer—better treatments, a lower chance of death from the disease, and improved quality of life. Through research, knowledge about breast cancer keeps increasing. Scientists are learning more about what causes breast cancer and are exploring new ways to prevent, detect, diagnose, and treat this disease.

The Breasts

Each breast has 15 to 20 sections called lobes. Within each lobe are many smaller lobules. Lobules end in dozens of tiny bulbs that can produce milk. The lobes, lobules, and bulbs are all linked by thin tubes called ducts. These ducts lead to the nipple in the center of a dark area of skin called the areola. Fat surrounds the lobules and ducts. There are no muscles in the breast, but muscles lie under each breast and cover the ribs.

Each breast also contains blood vessels and lymph vessels. The lymph vessels carry colorless fluid called lymph, and lead to small bean-shaped organs called lymph nodes. Clusters of lymph nodes are found near the breast in the axilla (under the arm), above the collarbone, and in the chest. Lymph nodes are also found in many other parts of the body.

Recognizing Symptoms

Early breast cancer usually does not cause pain. In fact, when breast cancer first develops, there may be no symptoms at all. But as the cancer grows, it can cause changes that women should watch for:

- A lump or thickening in or near the breast or in the underarm area

- A change in the size or shape of the breast

- Nipple discharge or tenderness, or the nipple pulled back (inverted) into the breast

- Ridges or pitting of the breast (the skin looks like the skin of an orange)

- A change in the way the skin of the breast, areola, or nipple looks or feels (for example, warm, swollen, red, or scaly)

A woman should see her doctor about any symptoms like these. Most often, they are not cancer, but it's important to check with the doctor so that any problems can be diagnosed and treated as early as possible.

Diagnosing Breast Cancer

To help find the cause of any sign or symptom, a doctor does a careful physical exam and asks about personal and family medical history. In addition, the doctor may do one or more breast exams:

- Clinical breast exam. The doctor can tell a lot about a lump by carefully feeling it and the tissue around it. Benign lumps often feel different from cancerous ones. The doctor can examine the size and texture of the lump and determine whether the lump moves easily.

- Mammography. X-rays of the breast can give the doctor important information about a breast lump.

- Ultrasonography. Using high-frequency sound waves, ultrasonography can often show whether a lump is a fluid-filled cyst (not cancer) or a solid mass (which may or may not be cancer). This exam may be used along with mammography.

425

Based on these exams, the doctor may decide that no further tests are needed and no treatment is necessary. In such cases, the doctor may need to check the woman regularly to watch for any changes.

Often, fluid or tissue must be removed from the breast so the doctor can make a diagnosis—this procedure is called a biopsy. A woman's doctor may refer her for further evaluation to a surgeon or other health care professional who has experience with breast diseases.

When Cancer Is Found

The most common type of breast cancer is ductal carcinoma. It begins in the lining of the ducts. Another type, called lobular carcinoma, arises in the lobules. When cancer is found, the pathologist can tell what kind of cancer it is (whether it began in a duct or a lobule) and whether it is invasive (has invaded nearby tissues in the breast).

Special lab tests of the tissue help the doctor learn more about the cancer. For example, hormone receptor tests (estrogen and progesterone receptor tests) can help determine whether hormones help the cancer to grow. If test results show that hormones do affect the cancer's growth (a positive test result), the cancer is likely to respond to hormonal therapy. This therapy deprives the cancer cells of estrogen.

Other tests are sometimes done to help the doctor predict whether the cancer is likely to progress. For example, the doctor may order x-rays and lab tests. Sometimes a sample of breast tissue is checked for a gene (the human epidermal growth factor receptor-2 or HER-2 gene) that is associated with a higher risk that the breast cancer will come back. The doctor may also order special exams of the bones, liver, or lungs because breast cancer may spread to these areas.

Treatment Choices

A woman's treatment options depend on a number of factors. These factors include her age and menopausal status; her general health; the size and location of the tumor and the stage of the cancer; the results of lab tests; and the size of her breast. Certain features of the tumor cells (such as whether they depend on hormones to grow) are also considered.

In most cases, the most important factor is the stage of the disease. The stage is based on the size of the tumor and whether the cancer has spread. The following are brief descriptions of the stages of breast cancer and the treatments most often used for each stage. (Other treatments may sometimes be appropriate.)

Stage 0

Stage 0 is sometimes called noninvasive carcinoma or carcinoma in situ.

Lobular carcinoma in situ (LCIS) refers to abnormal cells in the lining of a lobule. These abnormal cells seldom become invasive cancer. However, their presence is a sign that a woman has an increased risk of developing breast cancer. This risk of cancer is increased for both breasts. Some women with LCIS may take a drug called tamoxifen, which can reduce the risk of developing breast cancer. Others may take part in studies of other promising new preventive treatments. Some women may choose not to have treatment, but to return to the doctor regularly for checkups. And, occasionally, women with LCIS may decide to have surgery to remove both breasts to try to prevent cancer from developing. (In most cases, removal of underarm lymph nodes is not necessary.)

Ductal carcinoma in situ (DCIS) refers to abnormal cells in the lining of a duct. DCIS is also called intraductal carcinoma. The abnormal cells have not spread beyond the duct to invade the surrounding breast tissue. However, women with DCIS are at an increased risk of getting invasive breast cancer. Some women with DCIS have breast-sparing surgery followed by radiation therapy. Or they may choose to have a mastectomy, with or without breast reconstruction (plastic surgery) to rebuild the breast. Underarm lymph nodes are not usually removed. Also, women with DCIS may want to talk with their doctor about tamoxifen to reduce the risk of developing invasive breast cancer.

Stage I and Stage II

Stage I and stage II are early stages of breast cancer in which the cancer has spread beyond the lobe or duct and invaded nearby tissue. Stage I means that the tumor is no more than about an inch across and cancer cells have not spread beyond the breast. Stage II means one of the following: the tumor in the breast is less than 1 inch across and the cancer has spread to the lymph nodes under the arm; or the tumor is between 1 and 2 inches (with or without spread to the lymph nodes under the arm); or the tumor is larger than 2 inches but has not spread to the lymph nodes under the arm.

Women with early stage breast cancer may have breast-sparing surgery followed by radiation therapy to the breast, or they may have a mastectomy, with or without breast reconstruction to rebuild the breast.

427

These approaches are equally effective in treating early stage breast cancer. (Sometimes radiation therapy is also given after mastectomy.)

The choice of breast-sparing surgery or mastectomy depends mostly on the size and location of the tumor, the size of the woman's breast, certain features of the cancer, and how the woman feels about preserving her breast. With either approach, lymph nodes under the arm usually are removed.

Many women with stage I and most with stage II breast cancer have chemotherapy and/or hormonal therapy after primary treatment with surgery or surgery and radiation therapy. This added treatment is called adjuvant therapy. If the systemic therapy is given to shrink the tumor before surgery, this is called neoadjuvant therapy. Systemic treatment is given to try to destroy any remaining cancer cells and prevent the cancer from recurring, or coming back, in the breast or elsewhere.

Stage III

Stage III is also called locally advanced cancer. In this stage, the tumor in the breast is large (more than 2 inches across) and the cancer has spread to the underarm lymph nodes; or the cancer is extensive in the underarm lymph nodes; or the cancer has spread to lymph nodes near the breastbone or to other tissues near the breast.

Inflammatory breast cancer is a type of locally advanced breast cancer. In this type of cancer the breast looks red and swollen (or inflamed) because cancer cells block the lymph vessels in the skin of the breast.

Patients with stage III breast cancer usually have both local treatment to remove or destroy the cancer in the breast and systemic treatment to stop the disease from spreading. The local treatment may be surgery and/or radiation therapy to the breast and underarm. The systemic treatment may be chemotherapy, hormonal therapy, or both. Systemic therapy may be given before local therapy to shrink the tumor or afterward to prevent the disease from recurring in the breast or elsewhere.

Stage IV

Stage IV is metastatic cancer. The cancer has spread beyond the breast and underarm lymph nodes to other parts of the body.

Women who have stage IV breast cancer receive chemotherapy and/ or hormonal therapy to destroy cancer cells and control the disease. They may have surgery or radiation therapy to control the cancer in the breast. Radiation may also be useful to control tumors in other parts of the body.

Recurrent Cancer

Recurrent cancer means the disease has come back in spite of the initial treatment. Even when a tumor in the breast seems to have been completely removed or destroyed, the disease sometimes returns because undetected cancer cells remained somewhere in the body after treatment.

Most recurrences appear within the first 2 or 3 years after treatment, but breast cancer can recur many years later. Cancer that returns only in the area of the surgery is called a local recurrence. If the disease returns in another part of the body, the distant recurrence is called metastatic breast cancer. The patient may have one type of treatment or a combination of treatments for recurrent cancer.

Section 45.2

Breast Cancer: Better Treatments Save More Lives

Excerpted from "Breast Cancer: Better Treatments Save More Lives," by Carol Lewis, *FDA Consumer*, U.S. Food and Drug Administration. The full text is available online at www.fda.gov. Published August 1999; updated and revised June 2000.

Every three minutes a woman in the United States learns she has breast cancer. It is the most common cancer among women, next to skin cancers, and is second only to lung cancer in cancer deaths in women. Only 5 to 10 percent of breast cancers occur in women with a clearly defined genetic predisposition for the disease. The overall risk for developing breast cancer increases as a woman gets older.

Although treatment is initially successful for many women, the American Cancer Society (ACS) says that breast cancer will return in about 50 percent of these cases. New drugs, new treatment regimens, and better diagnostic techniques have improved the outlook for many, and are responsible, according to ACS, for breast cancer death rates going down.

Breast Cancer Treatments

Breast cancer can be treated with surgery, radiation, and drugs (chemotherapy and hormonal therapy). Doctors may use one of these or a combination, depending on factors such as the type and location of the cancer, whether the disease has spread, and the patient's overall health.

Most women with breast cancer will have some type of surgery, depending on the stage of the breast cancer. The least invasive, lumpectomy (breast-conserving surgery), removes only the cancerous tissue and a surrounding margin of normal tissue. Removal of the entire breast is a mastectomy. A modified radical mastectomy includes the entire breast and some of the underarm lymph nodes. The very disfiguring radical mastectomy, in which the breast, lymph nodes, and chest wall muscles under the breast are removed, is rarely performed today because doctors believe that a modified radical mastectomy is just as effective.

While removing underarm lymph nodes after surgery is important in order to determine if the cancer has spread, this procedure may add chronic arm swelling and restricted shoulder motion to the discomforts of the overall treatment. But a new method, sentinel node biopsy, still under investigation, allows physicians to pinpoint the first lymph node into which a tumor drains (the sentinel node), and remove only the nodes most likely to contain cancer cells.

Radiation therapy is treatment with high-energy rays or particles given to destroy cancer. In almost all cases, lumpectomy is followed by six to seven weeks of radiation, an integral part of breast-conserving treatment. Although radiation therapy damages both normal cells and cancerous cells, most of the normal cells are able to repair themselves and function properly.

Radiation therapy can cause side effects such as swelling and heaviness in the breast, sunburn-like skin changes in the treated area, and lymphedema (swelling of the arm due to fluid buildup) if the underarm lymph nodes were treated after a node dissection.

Drug Options Expand

Drugs are used to reach cancer cells that may have spread beyond the breast—in many cases even if no cancer is detected in the lymph nodes after surgery.

While doctors once believed that the spread of breast cancer could be controlled with extensive surgery, they now believe that cancer cells may break away from the primary tumor and spread through the bloodstream, even in the earliest stages of the disease. These cells cannot be felt by examination or seen on x-rays or other imaging methods, and they cause no symptoms. But they can establish new tumors in other organs or the bones. The goal of drug treatment, even if there's no detectable cancer after surgery, is to kill these hidden cells. This treatment, known as adjuvant therapy, is not needed by every patient. Doctors will make recommendations regarding specific types of therapy based on the stage of the breast cancer.

FDA has approved several new drugs and new uses for older drugs in recent years that improve the chances of successfully treating breast cancer. These drugs include:

Herceptin: About 30 percent of women with breast cancer have an excess of a protein called HER2, which makes tumors grow quickly. A genetically engineered drug, Herceptin (trastuzumab), binds to HER2 and kills the excess cancer cells, theoretically leaving healthy cells alone.

Selection of patients who are most likely to benefit from Herceptin is important because of the possible serious risks from the drug, including weakening of the heart muscle that can lead to congestive heart failure. It is not known whether Herceptin has beneficial effects in women with normal levels of the HER2 protein.

Nolvadex: A drug that has been used as a breast cancer treatment for more than 20 years, Nolvadex (tamoxifen citrate) was approved by FDA in October 1998 for breast cancer risk reduction in high-risk women.

Doctors know that estrogen promotes the growth of breast cancer cells. Tamoxifen interferes with the activity of estrogen by slowing or stopping the growth of cancer cells already present in the body. As adjuvant therapy, tamoxifen has been shown to help prevent both the original breast cancer from returning, and also the development of new cancers in the other breast.

Due to potentially serious side effects, including endometrial (lining of the uterus) cancer and blood clots in major veins and the lungs, the American Society of Clinical Oncology recommends that patients talk with their regular health care providers to determine whether individual medical circumstances and histories are appropriate for considering use of tamoxifen.

431

Xeloda: Xeloda (capecitabine), made by Hoffmann-La Roche, Nutley, N.J., was approved by FDA in April 1998 for the treatment of breast cancer that has spread to other parts of the body (metastasized) and is resistant to both paclitaxel and an anthracycline-containing regimen. Xeloda does not kill the cancer cells directly. Instead, once the drug enters the cancer cells, it is metabolized to 5-fluorouracil (5-FU), a drug routinely used for breast cancer.

Taxotere: In May 1996, FDA gave accelerated approval to Taxotere (docetaxel) to treat patients whose locally advanced or metastasized breast cancer has progressed despite treatment with other drugs.

Others: In addition to these newer drugs, combinations of the anticancer drugs Cytoxan (cyclophosphamide) and Adriamycin (doxorubicin), with or without Adrucil (fluorouracil), may be used to treat breast cancer.

Chemotherapy (drug treatment) is given in cycles, with each period of treatment followed by a recovery period. The total course of chemotherapy can last three to six months, depending on the drugs and how far the cancer has spread.

In addition to the drugs actually battling the disease, there also is help for patients in severe pain from cancer. FDA approved Actiq (oral transmucosal fentanyl citrate) in November 1998 as a treatment specifically for cancer patients with severe pain that breaks through their regular narcotic therapy. A narcotic more potent than morphine, Actiq is in the form of a flavored sugar lozenge that dissolves slowly in the mouth. Actiq is approved for patients already taking at least 60 milligrams of morphine per day for their underlying persistent cancer pain.

Carol Lewis is a staff writer for *FDA Consumer*.

Section 45.3

Breast Cancer Risk after Stopping Hormone Therapy

"Study Confirms Breast Cancer Risk in Continuous Combined Hormone Therapy Risk Begins to Return to Normal After Women Stop Taking Hormones," National Institutes of Health, November 29, 2002.

Researchers confirmed that a daily, combined dose of estrogen and progestin increases breast cancer risk in postmenopausal women, but added that this risk begins to return to normal about six months after women stop taking the hormones.

The analysis was part of the National Institute of Child Health and Human Development (NICHD) Women's Contraceptive and Reproductive Experiences Study and appears in the December 2002 *Obstetrics & Gynecology*. The majority of the study's funding was provided by the NICHD. The Centers for Disease Control and Prevention in Atlanta contributed additional staff and computer support for the study. The National Cancer Institute also provided additional funding.

The NIH Women's Health Initiative (WHI) trial was the first large clinical trial to assess the risks and benefits of continuous combined hormone therapy. Last July, researchers stopped the WHI trial because the risk of breast cancer and heart disease from combined hormone replacement therapy outweighed its potential benefits.

In this form of therapy, women take a combination of the hormones estrogen and progestin. Essentially, the hormone estrogen relieves such symptoms of menopause as hot flashes, night sweats, sleeplessness, and vaginal dryness. When taken alone, however, estrogen also increases a woman's risk for cancer of the uterine lining, or endometrium. Combining estrogen with progestin virtually eliminates the risk of endometrial cancer.

The analysis also found that an alternate form of hormone therapy, which involves taking the hormones separately, on different days of the month, may not increase breast cancer risk in this group of women. The alternate form of therapy, sequential estrogen-progestin therapy, includes a number of regimens in which patients take the hormone

433

progestin only for 5 to 14 days per month. Earlier studies have indicated, however, that sequential estrogen-progestin therapy may increase the risk for cancer of the uterine lining, or endometrium. The increase in endometrial cancer from sequential estrogen-progestin therapy is thought to be less than the risk from taking estrogen alone.

Estrogen alone may be prescribed to women whose uterus has been surgically removed, as these women no longer have a risk of endometrial cancer. The NICHD study did not find any additional risk of breast cancer in women who took estrogen alone. A recent study by the NCI found, however, that women taking estrogen alone may be at increased risk for cancer of the ovary.

A separate WHI study of estrogen alone in women who had a hysterectomy before joining the WHI hormone program continues unchanged because, at this point, researchers are uncertain of the balance of risks and benefits of estrogen.

Chapter 46

Gynecological Cancers

Chapter Contents

Section 46.1

What You Need to Know about Cancer of the Uterus

Excerpted from "What You Need To Know About™ Cancer of the Uterus," National Cancer Institute, July 30, 2001, updated September 16, 2002. Available online at http://www.cancer.gov; accessed June 2003.

The Uterus

The uterus is part of a woman's reproductive system. It is the hollow, pear-shaped organ where a baby grows. The uterus is in the pelvis between the bladder and the rectum.

The narrow, lower portion of the uterus is the cervix. The broad, middle part of the uterus is the body, or corpus. The dome-shaped top of the uterus is the fundus. The fallopian tubes extend from either side of the top of the uterus to the ovaries.

The wall of the uterus has two layers of tissue. The inner layer, or lining, is the endometrium. The outer layer is muscle tissue called the myometrium.

In women of childbearing age, the lining of the uterus grows and thickens each month to prepare for pregnancy. If a woman does not become pregnant, the thick, bloody lining flows out of the body through the vagina. This flow is called menstruation.

Benign Conditions of the Uterus

Fibroids are common benign tumors that grow in the muscle of the uterus. They occur mainly in women in their forties. Women may have many fibroids at the same time. Fibroids do not develop into cancer. As a woman reaches menopause, fibroids are likely to become smaller, and sometimes they disappear.

Endometriosis is another benign condition that affects the uterus. It is most common in women in their thirties and forties, especially in women who have never been pregnant. It occurs when endometrial tissue begins to grow on the outside of the uterus and on nearby organs. This condition may cause painful menstrual periods, abnormal vaginal bleeding, and sometimes loss of fertility (ability to get pregnant), but it does not cause cancer. Women with endometriosis may be treated with hormones or surgery.

Endometrial hyperplasia is an increase in the number of cells in the lining of the uterus. It is not cancer. Sometimes it develops into cancer. Heavy menstrual periods, bleeding between periods, and bleeding after menopause are common symptoms of hyperplasia. It is most common after age 40.

Malignant Tumors

Malignant tumors are cancer. They are generally more serious and may be life threatening. Cancer cells can invade and damage nearby tissues and organs. Also, cancer cells can break away from a malignant tumor and enter the bloodstream or lymphatic system. That is how cancer cells spread from the original (primary) tumor to form new tumors in other organs. The spread of cancer is called metastasis.

When uterine cancer spreads (metastasizes) outside the uterus, cancer cells are often found in nearby lymph nodes, nerves, or blood vessels. If the cancer has reached the lymph nodes, cancer cells may have spread to other lymph nodes and other organs, such as the lungs, liver, and bones.

When cancer spreads from its original place to another part of the body, the new tumor has the same kind of abnormal cells and the same name as the primary tumor. For example, if cancer of the uterus spreads to the lungs, the cancer cells in the lungs are actually uterine cancer cells. The disease is metastatic uterine cancer, not lung cancer. It is treated as uterine cancer, not lung cancer. Doctors sometimes call the new tumor distant disease.

The most common type of cancer of the uterus begins in the lining (endometrium). It is called endometrial cancer, uterine cancer, or cancer of the uterus. In this chapter, we will use the terms uterine cancer or cancer of the uterus to refer to cancer that begins in the endometrium.

A different type of cancer, uterine sarcoma, develops in the muscle (myometrium). Cancer that begins in the cervix is also a different type of cancer. This chapter does not deal with uterine sarcoma or with cancer of the cervix.

Symptoms

Uterine cancer usually occurs after menopause. But it may also occur around the time that menopause begins. Abnormal vaginal bleeding is the most common symptom of uterine cancer. Bleeding may start as a watery, blood-streaked flow that gradually contains more blood. Women should not assume that abnormal vaginal bleeding is part of menopause.

A woman should see her doctor if she has any of the following symptoms:

- Unusual vaginal bleeding or discharge
- Difficult or painful urination
- Pain during intercourse
- Pain in the pelvic area

These symptoms can be caused by cancer or other less serious conditions. Most often they are not cancer, but only a doctor can tell for sure.

Diagnosis

If a woman has symptoms that suggest uterine cancer, her doctor may check general signs of health and may order blood and urine tests. The doctor also may perform one or more of the exams or tests described on the next pages.

- Pelvic exam—A woman has a pelvic exam to check the vagina, uterus, bladder, and rectum. The doctor feels these organs for any lumps or changes in their shape or size. To see the upper part of the vagina and the cervix, the doctor inserts an instrument called a speculum into the vagina.

- Pap test—The doctor collects cells from the cervix and upper vagina. A medical laboratory checks for abnormal cells. Although the Pap test can detect cancer of the cervix, cells from inside the uterus usually do not show up on a Pap test. This is why the doctor collects samples of cells from inside the uterus in a procedure called a biopsy.

- Transvaginal ultrasound—The doctor inserts an instrument into the vagina. The instrument aims high-frequency sound waves at the uterus. The pattern of the echoes they produce creates a picture. If the endometrium looks too thick, the doctor can do a biopsy.

- Biopsy—The doctor removes a sample of tissue from the uterine lining. This usually can be done in the doctor's office. In some cases, however, a woman may need to have a dilation and curettage (D&C). A D&C is usually done as same-day surgery with anesthesia in a hospital. A pathologist examines the tissue to check for cancer cells, hyperplasia, and other conditions. For a short time after the biopsy, some women have cramps and vaginal bleeding.

Staging

If uterine cancer is diagnosed, the doctor needs to know the stage, or extent, of the disease to plan the best treatment. Staging is a careful attempt to find out whether the cancer has spread, and if so, to what parts of the body.

The doctor may order blood and urine tests and chest x-rays. The woman also may have other x-rays, CT scans, an ultrasound test, magnetic resonance imaging (MRI), sigmoidoscopy, or colonoscopy.

In most cases, the most reliable way to stage this disease is to remove the uterus (hysterectomy). After the uterus has been removed, the surgeon can look for obvious signs that the cancer has invaded the muscle of the uterus. The surgeon also can check the lymph nodes and other organs in the pelvic area for signs of cancer. A pathologist uses a microscope to examine the uterus and other tissues removed by the surgeon.

These are the main features of each stage of the disease:

- Stage I—The cancer is only in the body of the uterus. It is not in the cervix.

- Stage II—The cancer has spread from the body of the uterus to the cervix.

- Stage III—The cancer has spread outside the uterus, but not outside the pelvis (and not to the bladder or rectum). Lymph nodes in the pelvis may contain cancer cells.

- Stage IV—The cancer has spread into the bladder or rectum. Or it has spread beyond the pelvis to other body parts.

Methods of Treatment

Women with uterine cancer have many treatment options. Most women with uterine cancer are treated with surgery. Some have radiation therapy. A smaller number of women may be treated with hormonal therapy. Some patients receive a combination of therapies.

The doctor is the best person to describe the treatment choices and discuss the expected results of treatment. A woman may want to talk with her doctor about taking part in a clinical trial, a research study of new treatment methods. Clinical trials are an important option for women with all stages of uterine cancer.

Most women with uterine cancer have surgery to remove the uterus (hysterectomy) through an incision in the abdomen. The doctor also removes both fallopian tubes and both ovaries. (This procedure is called a bilateral salpingo-oophorectomy.)

The doctor may also remove the lymph nodes near the tumor to see if they contain cancer. If cancer cells have reached the lymph nodes, it may mean that the disease has spread to other parts of the body. If cancer cells have not spread beyond the endometrium, the woman may not need to have any other treatment. The length of the hospital stay may vary from several days to a week.

In radiation therapy, high-energy rays are used to kill cancer cells. Like surgery, radiation therapy is a local therapy. It affects cancer cells only in the treated area.

Some women with Stage I, II, or III uterine cancer need both radiation therapy and surgery. They may have radiation before surgery to shrink the tumor or after surgery to destroy any cancer cells that remain in the area. Also, the doctor may suggest radiation treatments for the small number of women who cannot have surgery.

Doctors use two types of radiation therapy to treat uterine cancer:

- External radiation: In external radiation therapy, a large machine outside the body is used to aim radiation at the tumor area. The woman is usually an outpatient in a hospital or clinic and receives external radiation 5 days a week for several weeks. This schedule helps protect healthy cells and tissue by spreading out the total dose of radiation. No radioactive materials are put into the body for external radiation therapy.

- Internal radiation: In internal radiation therapy, tiny tubes containing a radioactive substance are inserted through the vagina and left in place for a few days. The woman stays in the hospital during this treatment. To protect others from radiation exposure, the patient may not be able to have visitors or may have visitors only for a short period of time while the implant is in place. Once the implant is removed, the woman has no radioactivity in her body.

Some patients need both external and internal radiation therapies.

Hormonal therapy involves substances that prevent cancer cells from getting or using the hormones they may need to grow. Hormones can attach to hormone receptors, causing changes in uterine tissue. Before therapy begins, the doctor may request a hormone receptor test. This special lab test of uterine tissue helps the doctor learn if estrogen and progesterone receptors are present. If the tissue has receptors, the woman is more likely to respond to hormonal therapy.

Hormonal therapy is called a systemic therapy because it can affect cancer cells throughout the body. Usually, hormonal therapy is a type of progesterone taken as a pill.

The doctor may use hormonal therapy for women with uterine cancer who are unable to have surgery or radiation therapy. Also, the doctor may give hormonal therapy to women with uterine cancer that has spread to the lungs or other distant sites. It is also given to women with uterine cancer that has come back.

Section 46.2

Endometrial Cancer

PDQ® Cancer Information Summary. National Cancer Institute; Bethesda, MD. Excerpted from Endometrial Cancer (PDQ®): Treatment—Patient. Updated 06/2003. Available at: http://cancer.gov. Accessed July 31, 2003.

General Information about Endometrial Cancer

Endometrial cancer is a disease in which malignant (cancer) cells form in the tissues of the endometrium.

The endometrium is the lining of the uterus. The uterus is a hollow, muscular organ in a woman's pelvis. The uterus is where a fetus grows. In most nonpregnant women, the uterus is about 3 inches long.

Cancer of the endometrium is different from cancer of the muscle of the uterus, which is called sarcoma of the uterus.

Taking tamoxifen for breast cancer or taking estrogen alone (without progesterone) can affect the risk of developing endometrial cancer.

Endometrial cancer may develop in breast cancer patients who have been treated with tamoxifen. A patient taking this drug should have a pelvic examination every year and report any vaginal bleeding (other than menstrual bleeding) as soon as possible. Women taking estrogen (a hormone that can affect the growth of some cancers) alone have an increased risk of developing endometrial cancer. Taking estrogen in combination with progesterone (another hormone) does not increase a woman's risk of this cancer.

Possible signs of endometrial cancer include unusual vaginal discharge or pain in the pelvis.

A woman should see her doctor if any of the following problems occur:

- Bleeding or discharge not related to menstruation (periods)
- Difficult or painful urination
- Pain during sexual intercourse
- Pain in the pelvic area

Tests that examine the endometrium are used to detect (find) and diagnose endometrial cancer.

Because endometrial cancer begins inside the uterus, it does not usually show up in the results of a Pap test. For this reason, a sample of endometrial tissue must be removed and examined under a microscope to look for cancer cells. One of the following procedures may be used:

- Endometrial biopsy: A procedure in which a thin flexible tube is inserted through the cervix into the uterus. The tube is used to gently scrape small amounts of tissue from the lining of the uterus. The tissue samples of the endometrium are then sucked out through the tube.

- Dilatation and curettage (D&C): A procedure in which the cervix is dilated so that a surgical instrument can be inserted into the uterus to remove larger samples of tissue.

Certain factors affect treatment options and prognosis (chance of recovery).

The treatment options and prognosis (chance of recovery) depend on the stage of the cancer (whether it is in the endometrium only, involves the whole uterus, or has spread to other places in the body), the type of cancer, the size of the tumor, and the patient's general health. The chance of recovery may also depend on how the cancer cells look under a microscope and whether they are affected by progesterone.

442

Stages of Endometrial Cancer

Endometrial cancer is highly curable.

After endometrial cancer has been diagnosed, tests are done to find out if cancer cells have spread within the uterus or to other parts of the body.

The process used to find out whether the cancer has spread within the uterus or to other parts of the body is called staging. The information gathered from the staging process determines the stage of the disease. It is important to know the stage in order to plan the best treatment. Certain tests and procedures are used in the staging process. A hysterectomy (an operation in which the uterus is removed) will usually be done to help find out how far the cancer has spread.

The following stages are used for endometrial cancer:

Stage I

In stage I, cancer is found in the uterus only. Cancer is not found in the cervix (the canal between the uterus and the vagina). Stage I is divided into stages IA, IB, and IC, based on how far the disease has spread from the endometrium into the muscles of the uterus.

Stage II

In stage II, cancer has spread from the uterus to the cervix, but not beyond the cervix. Stage II is divided into stages IIA and IIB, based on how far the disease has spread into the cervix.

Stage III

In stage III, cancer has spread beyond the uterus and cervix, but has not spread beyond the pelvis. Stage III is divided into stages IIIA, IIIB, and IIIC, based on whether cancer has spread to the connective tissue holding the uterus in place, the ovaries, fallopian tubes, vagina, and lymph nodes in the pelvis. (Lymph nodes are small, bean-shaped structures that are found throughout the body. They filter substances in a fluid called lymph and help fight infection and disease.)

Stage IV

In stage IV, cancer has spread beyond the pelvis. Stage IV is divided into stages IVA and IVB, based on whether cancer has spread to the lining of the bladder (the sac that holds urine), to the bowel, or to lymph nodes or other parts of the body beyond the pelvis.

Recurrent Endometrial Cancer

Recurrent endometrial cancer is cancer that has recurred (come back) after it has been treated. The cancer may come back in the pelvis, in lymph nodes in the abdomen, or in other parts of the body.

Treatment Option Overview

Different types of treatment are available for patients with endometrial cancer. Some treatments are standard (the currently used treatment), and some are being tested in clinical trials. Before starting treatment, patients may want to think about taking part in a clinical trial. A treatment clinical trial is a research study meant to help improve current treatments or obtain information on new treatments for patients with cancer. When clinical trials show that a new treatment is better than the standard treatment, the new treatment may become the standard treatment.

Clinical trials are taking place in many parts of the country. Information about ongoing clinical trials is available from the NCI Cancer.gov website. Choosing the most appropriate cancer treatment is a decision that ideally involves the patient, family, and health care team.

Three types of standard treatment are used:

Surgery

Surgery (removing the cancer in an operation) is the most common treatment for endometrial cancer. The following surgical procedures may be used:

- Hysterectomy and bilateral salpingo-oophorectomy: This surgery involves removing the uterus, fallopian tubes, and ovaries through an incision in the abdomen. Pelvic lymph nodes may also be removed to see if they contain cancer cells.

- Radical hysterectomy: This surgery involves removing the cervix, uterus, fallopian tubes, ovaries, and part of the vagina. Lymph nodes in the area may also be removed.

Even if the doctor removes all the cancer that can be seen at the time of the operation, some patients may be offered radiation therapy or hormone treatment. Treatment given after the surgery to increase the chances of a cure is called adjuvant therapy.

Chemotherapy

Chemotherapy is the use of drugs to kill cancer cells. Chemotherapy may be taken by mouth, or it may be put into the body by inserting a needle into a vein or muscle. Either type of chemotherapy is called systemic treatment because the drugs enter the bloodstream, travel through the body, and can kill cancer cells throughout the body.

Radiation Therapy

Radiation therapy is the use of x-rays or other types of radiation to kill cancer cells and shrink tumors. Radiation therapy may use external radiation (using a machine outside the body) or internal radiation. Internal radiation involves putting radioisotopes (materials that produce radiation) through thin plastic tubes into the area where cancer cells are found. Endometrial cancer is treated with internal and external radiation therapy. Radiation may be used alone or in addition to surgery, chemotherapy, or both.

Hormone Therapy

Hormones are chemicals produced by glands in the body and circulated in the bloodstream. Estrogen and progesterone are hormones that affect the way some cancers grow. If tests show that the cancer cells have estrogen and progesterone receptors (molecules found in some cancer cells to which estrogen and progesterone will attach), hormone therapy is used to block the way these hormones help the cancer grow. This may be done by using drugs that block the way the hormones work or by surgically removing organs that make hormones, such as the ovaries.

Other types of treatment are being tested in clinical trials.

Section 46.3

Ovarian Cancer

"What You Need To Know About™ Ovarian Cancer," National Cancer Institute, NIH Publication No. 00-1561, June 16, 2000; updated September 16, 2002. Available online at http://www.cancer.gov; accessed August 2003.

The Ovaries

The ovaries are a pair of organs in the female reproductive system. They are located in the pelvis, one on each side of the uterus (the hollow, pear-shaped organ where a baby grows).

Each ovary is about the size and shape of an almond. The ovaries have two functions: they produce eggs and female hormones (chemicals that control the way certain cells or organs function).

Every month, during the menstrual cycle, an egg is released from one ovary in a process called ovulation. The egg travels from the ovary through the fallopian tube to the uterus.

The ovaries are also the main source of the female hormones estrogen and progesterone. These hormones influence the development of a woman's breasts, body shape, and body hair. They also regulate the menstrual cycle and pregnancy.

Understanding Ovarian Cancer

Cancer is a group of many related diseases that begin in cells, the body's basic unit of life. To understand cancer, it is helpful to know about normal cells and what happens when they become cancerous.

The body is made up of many types of cells. Normally, cells grow, divide, and produce more cells when the body needs them. This orderly process helps to keep the body healthy.

Sometimes, however, cells keep dividing when new cells are not needed. These extra cells form a mass of tissue, called a growth or tumor. Tumors can be benign or malignant.

- Benign tumors are not cancer. They often can be removed and, in most cases, they do not come back. Cells in benign tumors do not spread to other parts of the body. Most important, benign tumors are rarely a threat to life.

- Ovarian cysts are a different type of growth. They are fluid-filled sacs that form on the surface of an ovary. They are not cancer. Cysts often go away without treatment. If a cyst does not go away, the doctor may suggest removing it, especially if it seems to be growing.

- Malignant tumors are cancer. Cells in these tumors are abnormal and divide without control or order. They can invade and damage nearby tissues and organs. Cancer cells can also spread (metastasize) from their original site to other parts of the body.

A malignant tumor that begins in the ovaries is called ovarian cancer. There are several types of ovarian cancer. Ovarian cancer that begins on the surface of the ovary (epithelial carcinoma) is the most common type. This is the type of cancer discussed in this chapter. Ovarian cancer that begins in the egg-producing cells (germ cell tumors) and cancer that begins in the supportive tissue surrounding the ovaries (stromal tumors) are rare and are not discussed in this chapter.

Ovarian cancer cells can break away from the ovary and spread to other tissues and organs in a process called shedding. When ovarian cancer sheds, it tends to seed (form new tumors) on the peritoneum (the large membrane that lines the abdomen) and on the diaphragm (the thin muscle that separates the chest from the abdomen). Fluid may collect in the abdomen. This condition is known as ascites. It may make a woman feel bloated, or her abdomen may look swollen.

Ovarian cancer cells can also enter the bloodstream or lymphatic system (the tissues and organs that produce and store cells that fight infection and disease). Once in the bloodstream or lymphatic system, the cancer cells can travel and form new tumors in other parts of the body.

Detecting Ovarian Cancer

The sooner ovarian cancer is found and treated, the better a woman's chance for recovery. But ovarian cancer is hard to detect early. Many times, women with ovarian cancer have no symptoms or just mild symptoms until the disease is in an advanced stage. Scientists are studying ways to detect ovarian cancer before symptoms develop. They are exploring the usefulness of measuring the level of CA-125, a substance called a tumor marker, which is often found in higher-than-normal amounts in the blood of women with ovarian cancer. They also are evaluating transvaginal ultrasound, a test that may help detect the disease early.

A large-scale study, known as the PLCO (Prostate, Lung, Colorectal, and Ovarian) Cancer Screening Trial, is currently evaluating the usefulness of a blood test for the tumor marker known as CA-125 and a test called transvaginal ultrasound for ovarian cancer screening.

Recognizing Symptoms

Ovarian cancer often shows no obvious signs or symptoms until late in its development. Signs and symptoms of ovarian cancer may include:

- General abdominal discomfort and/or pain (gas, indigestion, pressure, swelling, bloating, cramps)

- Nausea, diarrhea, constipation, or frequent urination

- Loss of appetite

- Feeling of fullness even after a light meal

- Weight gain or loss with no known reason

- Abnormal bleeding from the vagina

These symptoms may be caused by ovarian cancer or by other, less serious conditions. It is important to check with a doctor about any of these symptoms.

To help find the cause of symptoms, a doctor evaluates a woman's medical history. The doctor also performs a physical exam and orders diagnostic tests. Some exams and tests that may be useful are described below:

- Pelvic exam includes feeling the uterus, vagina, ovaries, fallopian tubes, bladder, and rectum to find any abnormality in their shape or size. (A Pap test, a good test for cancer of the cervix, is often done along with the pelvic exam, but it is not a reliable way to find or diagnose ovarian cancer.)

- Ultrasound refers to the use of high-frequency sound waves. These waves, which cannot be heard by humans, are aimed at the ovaries. The pattern of the echoes they produce creates a picture called a sonogram. Healthy tissues, fluid-filled cysts, and tumors look different on this picture.CA-125 assay is a blood test used to measure the level of CA-125, a tumor marker that is often found in higher-than-normal amounts in the blood of women with ovarian cancer.

- Lower GI series, or barium enema, is a series of x-rays of the colon and rectum. The pictures are taken after the patient is given an enema with a white, chalky solution containing barium. The barium outlines the colon and rectum on the x-ray, making tumors or other abnormal areas easier to see.

- CT (or CAT) scan is a series of detailed pictures of areas inside the body created by a computer linked to an x-ray machine.

- Biopsy is the removal of tissue for examination under a microscope. A pathologist studies the tissue to make a diagnosis. To obtain the tissue, the surgeon performs a laparotomy (an operation to open the abdomen). If cancer is suspected, the surgeon performs an oophorectomy (removal of the entire ovary). This is important because, if cancer is present, removing just a sample of tissue by cutting through the outer layer of the ovary could allow cancer cells to escape and cause the disease to spread.

If the diagnosis is ovarian cancer, the doctor will want to learn the stage (or extent) of disease. Staging is a careful attempt to find out whether the cancer has spread and, if so, to what parts of the body. Staging may involve surgery, x-rays and other imaging procedures, and lab tests. Knowing the stage of the disease helps the doctor plan treatment.

Treatment for Ovarian Cancer

Treatment depends on a number of factors, including the stage of the disease and the general health of the patient. Patients are often treated by a team of specialists. The team may include a gynecologist, a gynecologic oncologist, a medical oncologist, and/or a radiation oncologist. Many different treatments and combinations of treatments are used to treat ovarian cancer.

Surgery is the usual initial treatment for women diagnosed with ovarian cancer. The ovaries, the fallopian tubes, the uterus, and the cervix are usually removed. This operation is called a hysterectomy with bilateral salpingo-oophorectomy. Often, the surgeon also removes the omentum (the thin tissue covering the stomach and large intestine) and lymph nodes (small organs located along the channels of the lymphatic system) in the abdomen.

449

Staging during surgery (to find out whether the cancer has spread) generally involves removing lymph nodes, samples of tissue from the diaphragm and other organs in the abdomen, and fluid from the abdomen. If the cancer has spread, the surgeon usually removes as much of the cancer as possible in a procedure called tumor debulking. Tumor debulking reduces the amount of cancer that will have to be treated later with chemotherapy or radiation therapy.

Chemotherapy is the use of drugs to kill cancer cells. Chemotherapy may be given to destroy any cancerous cells that may remain in the body after surgery, to control tumor growth, or to relieve symptoms of the disease.

Most drugs used to treat ovarian cancer are given by injection into a vein (intravenously, or IV). The drugs can be injected directly into a vein or given through a catheter, a thin tube. The catheter is placed into a large vein and remains there as long as it is needed. Some anticancer drugs are taken by mouth. Whether they are given intravenously or by mouth, the drugs enter the bloodstream and circulate throughout the body.

Another way to give chemotherapy is to put the drug directly into the abdomen through a catheter. With this method, called intraperitoneal chemotherapy, most of the drug remains in the abdomen.

After chemotherapy is completed, second-look surgery may be performed to examine the abdomen directly. The surgeon may remove fluid and tissue samples to see whether the anticancer drugs have been successful.

Radiation therapy, also called radiotherapy, involves the use of high-energy rays to kill cancer cells. Radiation therapy affects the cancer cells only in the treated area.

The radiation may come from a machine (external radiation). Some women receive a treatment called intraperitoneal radiation therapy in which radioactive liquid is put directly into the abdomen through a catheter.

Clinical trials (research studies) to evaluate new ways to treat cancer are an important treatment option for many women with ovarian cancer. In some studies, all patients receive the new treatment. In others, doctors compare different therapies by giving the promising new treatment to one group of patients and the usual (standard) therapy to another group. Through research, doctors learn new, more effective ways to treat cancer.

Section 46.4

Cervical Cancer

Excerpted from "Cervical Cancer," U.S. Department of Health and Human Services, National Women's Health Information Center (NWHIC); June 2001. Available online at http://www.4woman.gov; accessed August 2003.

What is cervical cancer?

Cancer of the cervix, a very common kind of cancer in women, is a disease in which cancer (malignant) cells are found in the tissues of the cervix.

The cervix is the opening of the uterus (womb). It connects the uterus to the vagina (the birth canal). Cancer of the cervix usually grows slowly over a period of time. Before cancer cells are found on the cervix, the tissues of the cervix go through changes in which abnormal cells begin to appear (a condition called dysplasia). Later, cancer starts to grow and spread more deeply into the cervix and to surrounding areas.

What are the symptoms of cervical cancer?

There are no real symptoms of the early stages of cervical cancer. That is why is it is so important that your doctor does a series of tests regularly to look for it. The first of these is a Pap smear, which is done by using a piece of cotton, a brush, or a small wooden stick to gently scrape the outside of the cervix to pick up some cells that can be examined under a microscope. You may feel some pressure, but you usually do not feel pain. Most cervical cancers can be caught early with regular screening.

What if abnormal cells are seen on my Pap smear?

Results from five to 10% of Pap smears performed each year on women in the United States are reported as abnormal.

If the Pap test abnormality is unclear or minor, the doctor may repeat the test to ensure accuracy. If the Pap test shows a significant abnormality, the doctor may then perform a test called a colposcopy.

451

For this test, the doctor uses a magnifying instrument to view the tissue surrounding the vagina and cervix to check for any abnormalities. A Schiller test may also be performed. For this test, the doctor coats the cervix with an iodine solution. Healthy cells turn brown and abnormal cells turn white or yellow. Both of these procedures can be done in the doctor's office.

Finally, the doctor may also remove a small amount of cervical tissue for examination. This procedure is called a biopsy and is the only sure way to know whether the abnormal cells indicate cancer.

What kind of attention do each type of cell abnormalities require?

All doctors agree that women who show HSIL cells on their Pap tests should receive a colposcopy and, if necessary, a biopsy. Most doctors either perform immediate colposcopy and, if necessary, biopsy, as for women with high grade lesions. Since low-grade cell changes in many women tend to go back to normal on their own, other doctors choose to wait and repeat the Pap smear every four to six months, then perform colposcopy if the abnormality is still present.

What are the treatments for cervical cancer?

Treatments for cancer of the cervix depend on the stage of disease, the size of the tumor, and a woman's age, overall physical condition, and desire to have children. Treatment for cervical cancer during pregnancy may be delayed, depending on the stage of the cancer and how many months of pregnancy remain. There are three kinds of treatment for women with cancer of the cervix:

- surgery—removing the cancer in an operation
- radiation therapy—using high-dose x-rays or other high-energy rays to kill cancer cells
- chemotherapy—using drugs to kill cancer cells

The National Cancer Institute recommends that doctors should strongly consider giving chemotherapy at the same time as radiation therapy for women with invasive cervical cancer. Five major studies showed that chemotherapy that includes the drug cisplatin, when given at the same time as radiation therapy, prolongs survival in women with this disease. Up to now, surgery or radiation alone has been considered standard treatment for this form of cancer.

Section 46.5

Vulvar and Vaginal Cancer

American College of Obstetricians and Gynecologists.
Cancer of the Vulva and Vagina. (Patient Education Pamphlet
No. AP149). Washington, DC. © ACOG 2001.

Cancer of the vulva or in the vagina is rare, but it can occur.

What Is Precancer and Cancer?

Sometimes, cells develop abnormally and begin to grow out of control. These cells can be benign (not cancer), precancer, or malignant (cancer). The precancer cells can turn into cancer if they are not treated.

It is vital to find cancer as early as possible so that it can be removed or treated.

Types of Vulvar and Vaginal Cancer

Most cancers of the vulva and vagina are a type of skin cancer. In their earliest form, they are precancer.

Rarely, other types of cancer develop on the vulva or vagina.

Who Is at Risk?

Women of any age can have cancer of the vulva or vagina.

Some vulvar and vaginal cancers may be linked to a virus called human papillomavirus (HPV). About 10 percent of women with vulvar cancer and HPV also have another cancer on the cervix or vagina.

Vaginal Cancer: You may be at risk for vaginal cancer if you were born between 1938 and 1971 and your mother took DES when she was pregnant with you.

Vulvar Cancer: Vulvar cancers most often occur in white women older than 60 years. Risk factors for vulvar cancer include smoking and taking steroids or other drugs that weaken the immune system.

Symptoms

Cancers of the vulva and vagina may have early warning signs.

Vulva: The most common symptom of vulvar cancer is itching of the vulva. Other symptoms include: burning, pain, or other discomfort; a sore on the vulva; and changes in skin color.

Vagina: The most common symptom of cancer of the vagina is bleeding after sexual intercourse.

Diagnosis

Office tests can diagnose cancer of the vulva or vagina in most cases. If you have symptoms, your doctor will do an exam. Your doctor may do a biopsy to obtain a tissue sample for further study.

Treatment

The type of treatment you receive depends on your condition.

Precancer

If precancer is found, surgery is the most common treatment. Your doctor will remove only as much tissue as needed to treat you.

Cancer

Vagina: In most cases, radiation therapy is used to treat cancer of the vagina. Chemotherapy rarely is used in treating vaginal cancer.

Vulva: Vulvar cancers may require removal of lymph nodes in the groin. It also may require more surgery.

The type of treatment you receive depends on the stage of cancer.

After Your Treatment

After your treatment, you will need frequent followup exams for a few years.

Finally

Precancer and cancer of the vulva and vagina give early warning signs in most cases. Report any change on the vulvar skin or in your vaginal discharge to your doctor. If found early, cancers in this area have a very high cure rate.

Section 46.6

Gynecologic Cancer and Sexuality

Because of the physical changes in the body, gynecologic cancers may affect how a woman feels about her self, her relationships, and her comfort with sexual intimacy. These are very real and natural feelings. Comfort with sexual intimacy becomes an issue for many women who receive cancer treatment.

Be aware of how you are feeling and find ways to discuss your feelings with your partner, doctor, nurse, friend, another patient with gynecologic cancer, or a counselor. It is important to understand and address concerns so that they do not have a long-term effect on you and people close to you.

Will I be able to have sexual relations with my partner?

Following treatment most patients find that they are able to resume sexual relations with their partner. Often patients prefer to wait for the immediate effects of cancer therapy to subside before returning to normal sexual activity. During this period many couples maintain intimacy through touching, stroking, cuddling, and other outercourse activities.

Once you resume intercourse, you may find that your usual sexual techniques or positions are not comfortable. Experimenting either alone or with your partner can help you discover new methods. You have to find what works for you and your partner. Be patient, and don't give up. It can take time to regain sexual arousal and satisfaction.

It's important to let your partner know how you feel and what they can do to help.

Will my sexual desire change?

It is possible that you and your partner may need to have less sexual activity for a while and to find different ways of expressing intimacy. There are many physical reasons for a decrease in sexual desire. The presence of pain can lead to a decrease in sexual desire. Treatment can reduce hormone levels that can lead to a decrease in desire. Other reasons include nausea or fatigue related to chemotherapy.

Emotional issues can be a factor as well. Because of the physical change in your body, your feelings about yourself may change which may lead to a loss of desire. Becoming more comfortable with yourself and accepting of your physical changes is key. Remember that you as a person have not changed. Recognizing how you and your partner are feeling, and accepting these feelings, is part of the process of recovery. Many of the factors that contribute to a personal change in sexual desire resolve over time.

What are the immediate effects of gynecologic cancer therapy?

Everyone experiences some inflammation in the pelvis after surgery or radiation therapy. Muscles, nerves, and organs may all be affected. Irritation of the pelvis may cause every day activities such as urinating, having bowel movements, or walking to become painful. Women often find intercourse uncomfortable after treatment.

Radiation treatment may cause a decrease in vaginal lubrication, creating a need for externally applied lubricants, such as Astroglide, Silken Secret or Replens. Removal or radiation of ovaries can decrease the production of estrogen (a female sex hormone). The loss of estrogen can cause shrinking, thinning, and loss of elasticity of the vagina, vaginal dryness, hot flashes, urinary tract infections, mood swings, fatigue, and irritability. Talk to your doctor about the possibility of hormone replacement therapy.

Once cancer therapy has ended, inflammation gradually subsides. Medications can be helpful in controlling discomfort until this occurs. The immediate effects of therapy may last up to three months and should diminish with time. If you continue to experience discomfort or other symptoms beyond this period, please tell your doctor.

What if intercourse is painful?

A discussion with your physician can help to find out the reasons for the pain and help you manage it. Painful intercourse may occur for a number of reasons. The vaginal lining may be thin or lack lubrication. Radiation therapy can cause the vagina to contract (shrink), limiting penetration during intercourse. The vaginal wall may be close to the bowel causing pain with some sexual positions.

Can I have children?

You should talk to your doctor or nurse if you are concerned about having children. If normal conception is not possible, you might be a candidate for assisted reproductive techniques.

Will I feel depressed?

Depression can occur as a result of your cancer experience. Your feelings about yourself and your life can change significantly during the experience. Depression can be treated with counseling and/or medication to help you regain a sense of control and enjoyment in your life. It is important to tell your doctor or nurse about how you feel so they can help you.

How will my partner feel?

Gynecologic cancer brings on many stresses for both you and your partner. Studies have shown that partners care most about their loved one being with them and a part of their lives. It is very important to talk with your partner. It is also important to acknowledge feelings you may have about the changes in your body. Just as you want your partner to understand and accept the changes you are experiencing, you will need to assure your partner that you accept their fears, concerns, and feelings. This takes communication and work, but it can be done.

Chapter 47

Risk Factors Associated with Gynecological Cancers

Chapter Contents

Section 47.1

Oral Contraceptives and Cancer Risk

National Cancer Institute, Cancer Information Service, February 12, 2003. Available online at http://cis.nci.nih.gov; accessed August 2003.

Oral contraceptives (OCs) first became available to American women in the early 1960s. The convenience, effectiveness, and reversibility of action of birth control pills (popularly known as the pill) have made them the most popular form of birth control in the United States. However, concerns have been raised about the role that hormones play in a number of cancers, and how hormone-based OCs might contribute to their development.

This chapter addresses only what is known about OC use and the risk of developing cancer. It does not deal with the role of hormones in postmenopausal hormone therapy or the most serious side effect of OC use—the increased risk of cardiovascular disease for certain groups of women.

Breast Cancer

A woman's risk of developing breast cancer depends on several factors, some of which are related to her natural hormones. Hormonal factors that increase the risk of breast cancer include conditions that allow high levels of hormones to persist for long periods of time, such as early age at first menstruation (before age 12), late age at menopause (after age 55), having children after age 30, and not having children at all. A woman's risk of breast cancer increases with the amount of time she is exposed to hormones.

Because many of the risk factors for breast cancer are related to natural hormones, and because OCs work by manipulating these hormones, there has been some concern about the possible effects of medicines such as OCs on breast cancer risk, especially if women take them for many years.

Sufficient time has elapsed since the introduction of OCs to allow investigators to study large numbers of women who took birth control pills for many years, beginning at a young age, and to follow them as they became older. Two major studies are described below.

Women's CARE Study

The Women's Contraceptive and Reproductive Experience (Women's CARE) study examined the use of OCs as a risk factor for breast cancer in women ages 35 to 64. The results, which were published in 2002, indicated that current or former use of OCs among women ages 35 to 64 did not significantly increase the risk of breast cancer.

Collaborative Group on Hormonal Factors in Breast Cancer Study

A 1996 analysis of worldwide epidemiologic data found that women who were current or recent users of birth control pills had a slightly elevated risk of developing breast cancer. However, 10 years or more after they stopped using OCs, their risk of developing breast cancer returned to the same level as if they had never used birth control pills.

OCs and Collaborative Analyses of Breast Cancer in Younger Women

Although in general there does not appear to be an association between OC use and most breast cancers, OC use may increase the risk of early-onset breast cancer (breast cancer that is diagnosed before age 40). Data from collaborative analyses have suggested that OC use is most strongly related to breast cancer in younger women. These findings indicate that OCs may promote the growth of newly developing tumors.

Ovarian and Endometrial Cancers

Studies have consistently shown that using OCs reduces the risk of ovarian cancer. Researchers estimate that the risk is reduced by 5 to 10 percent for each additional year of use. Several hypotheses have been offered to explain how oral contraceptives might protect against ovarian cancer, such as a reduction in the number of ovulations a woman has during her lifetime, but the exact mechanism is still not known.

Researchers have also found that OC users have a reduced risk of endometrial cancer. Findings from the CASH study and other reports show that combination OC use can protect against the development

461

of endometrial cancer. The level of risk reduction is greater in women who have used OCs for a longer time, and the protection apparently persists after women have stopped taking OCs.

The reduction in risk of ovarian and endometrial cancers from OC use does not apply to the sequential type of pill, in which each monthly cycle contains 16 estrogen pills followed by 5 estrogen-plus-progesterone pills. (Sequential OCs were taken off the market in 1976, so few women have been exposed to them.) Researchers believe OCs reduce ovarian and endometrial cancer risk only when the estrogen content of birth control pills is balanced by progestogen in the same pill.

Cancer of the Cervix

There is some evidence that long-term use of OCs may increase the risk of cancer of the cervix (the narrow, lower portion of the uterus). The results of studies conducted by National Cancer Institute scientists and other researchers support a relationship between extended use of the pill (5 or more years) and a slightly increased risk of cervical cancer. However, the exact nature of the association between OC use and risk of cervical cancer remains unclear.

Human Papillomavirus

The two major risk factors mentioned above that contribute to the development of cervical cancer are also risk factors that contribute to the development of human papillomavirus (HPV) infection in the cervix. Of the more than 100 types of HPV, over 30 types can be passed from one person to another through sexual contact. HPV is one of the most common sexually transmitted diseases. Certain HPVs, particularly HPV type 16, are known to cause cervical cancer. Compared to non-OC users, women who use OCs may be less likely to use barrier methods of contraception (such as condoms). Because condoms are partially effective in preventing HPV infection, OC users who do not use condoms may be at increased risk of becoming infected with HPV. Therefore, the increased risk of cervical cancer that some studies found to be caused by prolonged OC use may actually be the result of HPV infection.

OC product labels have been revised to inform women of the possible risk of cervical cancer. The product labels also warn that birth control pills do not protect against human immunodeficiency virus (HIV) and other sexually transmitted diseases such as HPV, chlamydia, and genital herpes.

Liver Tumors

There is some evidence that OCs may increase the risk of certain malignant (cancerous) liver tumors. However, the risk is difficult to evaluate because of different patterns of OC use and because these tumors are rare in American women (the incidence is approximately 2 cases per 100,000 women). A benign (noncancerous) tumor of the liver called hepatic adenoma has also been found to occur, although rarely, among OC users. These tumors do not spread, but they may rupture and cause internal bleeding.

Section 47.2

Fertility Drugs as a Risk Factor for Ovarian Cancer

National Cancer Institute, Cancer Information Service, February 1, 2000. Available online at http://cis.nci.nih.gov; accessed August 2003.

In recent decades, an increasing number of women have been treated for infertility with drugs. The possibility that the use of fertility drugs may increase the risk of ovarian cancer has prompted researchers to conduct studies to determine the long-term effects of such drugs. The results of these studies have been conflicting. Some studies have identified certain fertility drugs as increasing a woman's risk for ovarian cancer, while others have not shown any increased risk from fertility drugs.

There are several theories about factors that may increase a woman's risk of ovarian cancer. Two theories in particular have prompted researchers to examine fertility drugs as a risk factor. One theory is that an increased number of uninterrupted ovulations in a woman's lifetime increases her chance of developing ovarian cancer. This theory may explain why events that interrupt the constant cycle of ovulations, such as pregnancy, breastfeeding, and oral contraceptive use, are associated with a decreased risk of ovarian cancer. Another theory is that increased levels of certain hormones associated with ovulation (such as human chorionic gonadotropin or HCG) increase the risk of ovarian cancer. Fertility drugs can increase both the number of ovulations and the levels of hormones associated with ovulation.

An evaluation of previous studies of women who had ovarian cancer found that infertile women who used fertility drugs but still never became pregnant had a significantly increased risk of ovarian cancer compared with women who had no history of infertility. Infertile women who used fertility drugs and became pregnant did not have a significantly increased risk for ovarian cancer. Another study found that use of the fertility drug clomiphene citrate for more than a year may increase the risk of developing ovarian tumors of low malignant potential. This type of tumor responds better to treatment than epithelial ovarian cancer, the most common type of ovarian cancer.

These studies and other recent research raise questions about whether infertile women who take fertility drugs and do not become pregnant, and women who take certain fertility drugs for extended periods of time, may be at increased risk of developing ovarian cancer. However, these links have not been proven, and more research is needed. Research is also being conducted to explore the relationship between infertility and ovarian cancer.

Women who have taken fertility drugs and who are concerned about their risk of developing ovarian cancer should discuss their previous treatment with these drugs with a gynecologist. At this time, however, there are no screening tests that are consistently accurate enough to detect ovarian cancer at an early stage when there are no symptoms. Research to identify better methods of diagnosing ovarian cancer and to evaluate currently available tests is under way.

For information about fertility drugs, write to the U.S. Food and Drug Administration, HFI-40, Rockville, MD 20857, call 1-888-INFO-FDA (1-888-463-6332), or visit the FDA website at http://www.fda.gov on the Internet.

Section 47.3

Increased Risk of Ovarian Cancer Is Linked to Estrogen Replacement Therapy

"Increased Risk of Ovarian Cancer Is Linked to Estrogen Replacement Therapy," National Institutes of Health, National Cancer Institute, July 16, 2002. Available online at http://www.cancer.gov; accessed August 2003.

Researchers from the National Cancer Institute (NCI) have found that women in a large study who used estrogen replacement therapy after menopause were at increased risk for ovarian cancer. The report was published in the July 17, 2002, issue of *JAMA* [*Journal of the American Medical Association*].

Estrogen is a natural hormone produced primarily by the ovaries. After menopause, the ovaries produce lower levels of the hormones estrogen and progesterone. By the time natural menopause is complete—usually between ages 45 and 55—hormone output decreases significantly. As early as the 1940s, women began using estrogens in high doses to counteract some of the short-term discomforts of menopause (hot flashes, vaginal drying and thinning, and urinary tract incontinence and infections).

However, after it became clear in the 1970's that women who took estrogen alone had a six to eight times higher risk of developing endometrial cancer (cancer of the lining of the uterus), doctors began prescribing progestin along with much lower doses of estrogen. Progestin is a synthetic form of the natural hormone progesterone. The addition of progestin to estrogen therapy reduces the increased risk of endometrial cancer associated with using estrogen alone.

Past studies suggested that postmenopausal hormone treatments might be effective in preventing or reducing some of the negative long-term effects of aging, such as heart disease and osteoporosis. However, the results from a large multi-center clinical trial, also published in the July 17 issue of *JAMA* (*JAMA* 2002;288:321-333), showed increases in breast cancer, coronary heart disease, stroke, and blood clots in the lungs and legs for women on estrogen-progestin therapy for an average of 5.2 years. The trial, part of the Women's Health Initiative

(WHI), also found fewer cases of hip fractures and colon cancer among women taking the combined therapy. However, because overall the harm was greater than the benefit, the trial was stopped last week, three years ahead of schedule. The WHI randomized trial for estrogen alone in women who have had their uterus removed is continuing.

Every year, about 23,000 U.S. women are diagnosed with ovarian cancer and 14,000 women die from the disease. A woman's lifetime risk of developing ovarian cancer is 1.7 percent. This means that in a group of 100 women followed from birth to age 85, fewer than two would get ovarian cancer. In comparison, about 13 women would get breast cancer (lifetime risk is 13.3 percent), fewer than three women would develop uterine cancer (lifetime risk is 2.7 percent), and between 16 and 32 women would develop osteoporosis.

Section 47.4

Human Papillomaviruses and Cancer

Excerpted from "Human Papillomaviruses and Cancer," National Institutes of Health, National Cancer Institute, January 2001. Available online at http://www.cancer.gov; accessed August 2003.

Human papillomaviruses (HPVs) are a group of more than 100 types of viruses. They are called papillomaviruses because certain types may cause warts, or papillomas, which are benign (noncancerous) tumors. The HPVs that cause the common warts which grow on hands and feet are different from those that cause growths in the mouth and genital area. Some types of HPVs are associated with certain types of cancer.

Of the more than 100 types of HPVs, over 30 types can be passed from one person to another through sexual contact. HPV infection is one of the most common sexually transmitted diseases (STDs). Some types of HPVs may cause warts to appear on or around the genitals or anus. Genital warts (technically known as *Condylomata acuminatum*) are most commonly associated with two HPV types, numbers 6 and 11. Warts may appear within several weeks after sexual contact with a person who has HPV, or they may take months or years to appear; or they may never appear. HPVs may also cause flat, abnormal growths in the genital area and on the cervix (the lower part of the uterus that extends into the vagina). HPV infections often do not cause any symptoms.

HPVs and Cancer Risk

HPVs are now recognized as the major cause of cervical cancer. Studies also suggest that HPVs may play a role in cancers of the anus, vulva, vagina, and penis, and some cancers of the oropharynx (the middle part of the throat that includes the soft palate, the base of the tongue, and the tonsils).

Some types of HPVs are referred to as low-risk viruses because they rarely develop into cancer; these include HPV–6 and HPV–11. HPV viruses that can lead to the development of cancer are referred to as high-risk. Both high-risk and low-risk types of HPVs can cause the growth of abnormal cells, but generally only the high-risk types of HPVs may lead to cancer. Sexually transmitted, high-risk HPVs have been linked with cancer in both men and women; they include HPV types 16, 18, 31, 33, 35, 39, 45, 51, 52, 56, 58, 59, 68, and 69. These high-risk types of HPVs cause growths that are usually flat and nearly invisible, as compared with the warts caused by HPV–6 and HPV–11. It is important to note, however, that the majority of HPV infections go away on their own and do not cause any abnormal growths.

Risk Factors for HPV and Cervical Cancer

Behaviors such as beginning sexual intercourse at an early age (especially age 16 or younger) and having many sexual partners increase the chance that a woman will develop an HPV infection in the cervix. Most HPV infections go away on their own without causing any type of abnormality.

It is important to note that infection with high-risk HPV types may increase the chance that mild abnormalities will progress to more severe abnormalities or cervical cancer. Still, of the women who do develop abnormal cell changes with high-risk types of HPV, only a small percentage will develop cervical cancer if the abnormal cells are not removed.

Studies suggest that whether a woman develops cervical cancer depends on a variety of factors acting together with high-risk HPVs. The factors that may increase the risk of cancer in women with HPV infection include smoking, having many children, and human immunodeficiency virus (HIV) infection.

Part Seven

Other Leading Causes of Death and Disability among Women

Chapter 48

Leading Causes of Death and Disease among Women

This chapter touches upon a few of the diseases and conditions that adversely affect women. Our aim is to highlight several of the alarming gaps in knowledge which make effective prevention, treatment, and cure impossible. Our goal is to bring much needed attention and resources to women's health research.

- Women account for 52% of the U.S. population.

- Women make three fourths of the health care decisions in American households and spend almost two of every three health care dollars, approximately $500 billion annually.

- Over 59% of physician visits are made by women, 59% of prescription drugs are purchased by women, and 75% of nursing home residents over the age of 75 are women.

Cardiovascular Disease

- Heart disease is the number one killer of U.S. women (58% of all deaths); death rates are highest for women of color.

- Among Native American women age 18 and older, 61.4 percent have one or more cardiovascular disease risk factors-hypertension, current cigarette smoking, high blood cholesterol, obesity, or diabetes.

"Women's Health Fact Sheet" reprinted with permission of the Society for Women's Health Research (http://www.womancando.org), June 1999.

- Women who are diagnosed with heart disease are typically ten years older and sicker than men with the same condition; a marked increase in incidence is observed after menopause.

- Heart disease in women often goes undetected and untreated until the disease has become severe. As a result, 39% of women who have heart attacks die within one year compared to 31% of men.

- Hypertension—a major risk factor in cardiovascular disease—is two to three times more common in women than men and highest among African-American women. Drugs to treat hypertension have been tested primarily on white male populations.

Lung Cancer

- Lung cancer is the number one cancer killer of American women today.

- If current trends continue, the death rate among women from smoking-related diseases will exceed that of men by early next century. Teenage women now smoke at higher rates than their male counterparts.

- Smoking lowers a woman's estrogen level and increases her risk for early menopause, pregnancy complications, and having a low-birth-weight baby.

- Studies show doctors are more apt to give stop-smoking messages to male patients than to women, although such advice greatly increases the likelihood of quitting.

Breast Cancer

- Options for breast cancer treatment—surgery, radiation and/or chemotherapy—have not appreciably changed over the last 30 years.

- In 1996, approximately 184,300 new cases of invasive breast cancer are expected to be diagnosed, and 44,300 women are expected to die from this disease.

- 1 in 8 women in the United States will develop breast cancer during her lifetime.

- Although heart disease is the leading cause of death in women in the United States, breast cancer is the leading cause of death in women between the ages of 40 and 55.

- Hispanic women are the only racial/ethnic group for which the mortality rate for breast cancer is higher than for lung cancer.

Ovarian, Cervical, and Uterine Cancers

- There is no early detection method for ovarian cancer. Yet, there is a 90% survival rate even after 5 years when detected in Stage I (cancer confined to the ovary).

- In 1995, 26,600 new cases of ovarian cancer were expected to be diagnosed; 14,500 women are expected to have died in 1995 from this form of cancer. Women of color die from ovarian cancer at disproportionate rates.

- Nearly one third of all American women will have had hysterectomies by age 60; this is the highest rate in the world. Ovaries do not usually need to be removed, but doctors, lacking alternatives, often remove them to prevent ovarian cancer.

- Cervical cancer mortality rate of Native American women is twice that of all racial/ethnic groups in the US.

Violence against Women

- One-quarter of all women in the United States will be abused at some point in their lives.

- A recent study found that 92% of women who were physically abused by their partners did not discuss these incidents with their physicians; 57% did not discuss the incidents with anyone.

- Twenty-three percent of pregnant women seeking prenatal care are battered.

Osteoporosis

- Osteoporosis, a debilitating disease characterized by loss of bone mass, is a major public health threat for 20 million American women.

- Osteoporosis is prevalent in more than one fifth of Asian American and Pacific Islander women.

- In 1990, of the 7 million women over age 75, nearly 2 million were limited in their ability to carry out major life activities. The cause of this disability was often osteoporosis.

- Each day about $38 million is spent on osteoporosis and related fractures.

- A woman's risk of hip fracture, often related to osteoporosis, is equal to her combined risk of breast, uterine, and ovarian cancer.

Menopause

- Menopause, unlike menstruation, is often viewed by the medical profession as a disease rather than as a natural part of aging.

- There is little research data available for women seeking non-pharmacologic techniques and alternative methods for the management of symptoms associated with menopause. Data on pharmacologic treatments is only marginally more available and is often conflicting.

Mental Illness

- About one fourth of all women suffer from depression at some point in their lives.

- Elderly Hispanic women living in rural community are twice as likely to be depressed as the peers in other ethnic groups.

- Asian American women over the age of 65 have the highest depression and female suicide mortality rate among all racial/ethnic groups.

- Depression afflicts twice as many women as men, and only 3 in 10 depressed persons get any form of treatment. Without treatment, the frequency and severity of symptoms tend to increase over the years.

- More than 3 million people will have a panic disorder, in which one experiences brief episodes of intense fear accompanied by a variety of physical symptoms as a response to ordinary, non-threatening situations, at some time in their lives. Women are affected twice as frequently as men.

Eating Disorders

- Eating disorders, including anorexia and bulimia, are about 10 times as common in women as in men.

- Anorexia, in which a person starves oneself to control his or her weight, has the highest mortality rate—7 to 24%—of any psychiatric disorder.

Sexually Transmitted Diseases

- More than 12 million new cases of STDs (other than AIDS) are diagnosed each year in the United States.

- Women account for about half of these new cases of STDs. Since women are more susceptible to infection and are less likely to experience symptoms, women tend to suffer more frequent and severe long-term consequences than men.

- Chlamydia is currently the most common sexually transmitted disease and shows no symptoms in approximately 75% of chlamydia infection cases. Left untreated in women, chlamydia can cause urinary tract infections, pelvic inflammatory disease, and even sterility.

AIDS

- Women are one of the fastest-growing demographic groups affected by HIV infection.

- 63 percent of all reported AIDS cases were among African-American women.

- Of all AIDS cases in the United States, the proportion of women diagnosed with AIDS has increased from 7% in 1985 to 18% in 1994.

- AIDS is now the fourth leading cause of death among women ages 24 to 44 in the United States.

Chapter 49

Women and Cardiovascular Disease

Chapter Contents

477

Section 49.1

Women and Heart Disease

"Heart Disease in Women" excerpted from U.S. Department of Health and Human Services, Health Resources and Services Administration, Maternal and Child Health Bureau, *Women's Health USA 2002*, Rockville, Maryland: U.S. Department of Health and Human Services, 2002. "Three Keys to Surviving a Heart Attack," "Heart Attack Warning Signs," and "What You Can Do," are excerpted from "Women and Heart Disease," by Catherine Houck, U.S. Department of Health and Human Services, National Women's Health Information Center (NWHIC), February 2003. Available online at http://www.4woman.gov; accessed July 2003.

Heart Disease in Women

Heart disease is the leading cause of death for both males and females in the U.S. and a chronic condition that affects millions of American adults. According to the National Health Interview Survey (NHIS), the prevalence of heart disease in both men and women climbs significantly with increasing age. In 1995, the rate of heart disease was approximately three times higher among women aged 45 to 64 than among those under 45, and nearly seven times higher in women aged 65-74 than among those under 45. For women 75 years and older, the disease rate reached 318.0 per 1,000 persons in 1995, or nine times higher than the rate in women under 45 years.

High blood pressure, obesity, and smoking are significant risk factors for developing heart disease. Health professionals recommend modifying behaviors such as smoking, diet, and exercise to prevent onset or further progression of the disease.

Three Keys to Surviving a Heart Attack

- Know the symptoms.

- Get treatment within 60 minutes after symptoms begin. "If we get you within an hour, we can often stop a heart attack in its tracks," says Rose Marie Robertson, M.D., director of the Vanderbilt Women's Heart Institute. "The longer you wait, the greater your risk of dying or having serious heart damage." Yet only one in five heart attack patients gets to a hospital within that crucial hour. The average is two and a half hours.

- Dial 911. Don't drive to the ER. In an ambulance, emergency workers can begin treatment immediately. If your heart stops, they can often revive you. And in most cases, you get treated faster when you arrive by ambulance.

Heart Attack Warning Signs

Some heart attacks are sudden and intense where no one doubts what's happening. But most heart attacks start slowly, with mild pain or discomfort. Often people affected aren't sure what's wrong and wait too long before getting help. Here are signs that can mean a heart attack is happening:

- Chest discomfort. Most heart attacks involve discomfort in the center of the chest that lasts more than a few minutes or that goes away and comes back. It can feel like uncomfortable pressure, squeezing, fullness, or pain.

- Discomfort in other areas of the upper body. Symptoms can include pain or discomfort in one or both arms, the back, neck, jaw or stomach.

- Shortness of breath. This feeling often comes along with chest discomfort. But it can also occur before the chest discomfort.

- Other signs may include breaking out in a cold sweat, nausea, or lightheadedness.

What You Can Do

Certain lifestyle changes can have a dramatic impact on your risk for heart disease, especially since one simple change, such as building more physical activity into your daily life, can often improve cholesterol, blood pressure and blood glucose numbers at the same time.

- If you smoke, quit. Even secondhand smoke raises your chances of developing heart disease.

- Lose excess weight if you're overweight.

- Be physically active on a regular basis. Eat a heart-healthy diet low in saturated fat and dietary cholesterol, and abundant in fruits, vegetables, whole grains, lean protein and lowfat dairy products.

- Get your omega-3s. American Heart Association dietary guidelines call for healthy adults to eat at least two servings of fish per week, preferably fish that is high in heart-healthy omega-3 fatty acids, such as salmon, albacore tuna and mackerel. People with existing cardiovascular disease are advised to get at least 1 gram of omega-3s every day, either from fish or omega-3 supplements.

- Try controlling blood pressure through dietary choices.

If the changes above don't work or if other factors put you at increased risk for heart disease, you may be a candidate for anti-hypertensive, cholesterol-lowering or diabetes medication. Keep in mind, however, that medication works best when it's used in combination with the lifestyle changes above.

Section 49.2

A Woman's Guide to Diagnosis and Testing for Heart Disease

"How Do I Know I Have Heart Disease?: A Woman's Guide to Diagnosis and Testing" © 2002 WomenHeart: the National Coalition for Women with Heart Disease. Reprinted with permission. For additional information, visit www.womenheart.org.

Heart disease affects your heart's blood vessels, muscle, and electrical system, and is the leading cause of death among American women. The most common form of heart disease is coronary artery disease, in which fat-like deposits called plaque build up and clog the arteries to your heart and prevent sufficient blood circulation. Coronary artery disease can lead to heart attack, angina (chest pain), and heart failure (when the heart can't pump as much blood as the body needs). Knowing your risks and how well your heart is working are the first steps toward preventing these complications, and even an early death.

Know Your Risk Factors

Certain factors increase your risk for heart disease. It's important to know your risk factors and discuss them with your healthcare provider. Some you can't control—your age, family medical history, and race. But you can prevent or reduce others by eating healthy foods, getting regular exercise, controlling your blood pressure and cholesterol levels, not smoking, and taking medicines as your healthcare provider prescribes.

Listen to Your Body

Common heart disease symptoms include shortness of breath, fatigue, and chest discomfort or pain that can spread to the arms, neck, back, or jaw. Many of these symptoms occur during periods of physical activity or stress. Tell your healthcare provider about any worrisome or annoying symptoms you experience, especially those that are new. However, many women with heart disease experience no symptoms at all, which is why regular checkups are so important.

Visit Your Healthcare Provider

If you think you are at risk for heart disease or are experiencing symptoms, visit your healthcare provider to talk about your concerns. You'll be asked specific questions about your symptoms (how long you have had them and when and how often they occur), as well as your risk factors and past health history.

Your healthcare provider will evaluate your heart health by checking your heart rate and rhythm and your blood pressure. Then, he or she will look, feel, and listen with a stethoscope to your heart, lungs, and blood vessels for signs of heart failure, heart valve problems, and evidence of blockages in the arteries. If your healthcare provider thinks there is cause for concern, he or she will recommend further exams or refer you to a cardiologist (heart specialist).

Diagnostic Tests

It's important that you know what tests are available to diagnose heart disease and how these tests work, how reliable they are in women, what they show, and when they should be performed. If your healthcare provider does not suggest any of the following tests for you, ask why.

Blood Tests

Blood tests measure different components in your bloodstream to show your healthcare provider how healthy your blood and heart are.

Lipid profile measures your LDL (bad) and HDL (good) cholesterol and triglycerides. It should be performed by age 20, and repeated every five years if your levels are in a healthy range, and more frequently if they are not.

Blood sugar (glucose) detects the presence of diabetes and glucose intolerance (pre-diabetes). Both are powerful heart disease risks for women.

Complete blood count, thyroid studies, arterial blood gases, and other tests help diagnose other conditions that may be the cause of your symptoms.

Electrocardiography

An electrocardiogram (EKG or ECG) measures your heart's electrical activity by placing small electrodes on your chest, either while you are lying down or during stress. An EKG records your heart's rate and rhythm and can detect evidence of a heart attack or inadequate blood supply to the heart. It can sometimes miss a heart problem, especially if you are not having any symptoms when you have the test. Further testing may be necessary.

Chest X-Ray

A chest x-ray uses a small amount of radiation to take a picture of your heart and lungs. Chest x-rays show the size and shape of the heart, any fluid present, abnormalities in the lungs, and the major blood vessels in the chest. This test exposes you to a very small amount of radiation, so tell your healthcare provider if you think you might be pregnant.

Stress Tests

Stress tests help to diagnose blockages in your coronary arteries by seeing if you develop symptoms or other abnormalities as your heart works harder under stress. Standard EKG exercise stress tests can be less accurate in women due to the rise and fall of menstrual hormones and other factors, so nuclear or echo imaging is often added to improve results. However, even these may be affected by a woman's breast tissue and obesity.

Exercise stress tests monitor your heart while you either walk on a treadmill or pedal a stationary bike. Your blood pressure, EKG, and any problems you might experience are recorded and observed during the test.

Pharmacologic stress tests use a drug, such as adenosine, to reproduce the effects of exercise on the heart. This is a safe alternative for many women who are not able to perform the required level of exercise due to older age, arthritis, or excess weight.

Nuclear Imaging

A nuclear scan, also called myocardial perfusion imaging or MPI, involves injecting a liquid called a tracer into your bloodstream, which then flows to your heart. While you lie on an exam table, a special camera moves over your chest and takes pictures of your heart. MPI is combined with exercise or pharmacologic stress tests to measure the blood flow to the heart. If there is a significant blockage of a coronary artery, the heart muscle may not get enough blood supply. The resulting images can show damage to the heart muscle and blood flow problems. Since this test exposes you to a very small amount of radiation, tell your healthcare provider if you think you might be pregnant.

Echocardiography

During an echocardiogram a small device called a transducer is moved around your chest and takes moving pictures of your heart using ultrasound waves. It gives detailed information about the heart muscle, valves, chambers, and major blood vessels around the heart, and it measures pressures within the heart and lungs.

Magnetic Resonance Imaging (MRI)

Magnetic resonance imaging uses strong magnets to detect energy signals from your heart. As you lie on a small bed and move through a circular MRI chamber, very clear 3-D images of your heart are produced. MRI images can also diagnose coronary artery disease during stress tests. Currently, MRI is used mostly as an investigational tool, but advances in technology may make it more practical and affordable in the future.

Electron Beam Computed Tomography (EBCT)

Sometimes called an ultra-fast CT or a heart scan, EBCT detects coronary calcium, a marker for coronary artery disease. While you lie on a special x-ray table, electron beams scan your heart to produce a 3-D picture. A dye is sometimes used to examine the large arteries and veins around your heart and other structures. EBCT is often used to detect early signs of plaque in women with several risk factors or symptoms, and can help your healthcare provider decide on further treatment. Since it exposes you to a very small amount of radiation, tell your healthcare provider if you think you might be pregnant.

Angiography

Angiography involves inserting a long, thin tube, called a catheter, through your arm or leg artery to your heart. A dye is then sent through the catheter into your coronary arteries. The healthcare provider observes the movement of the dye through your heart and blood vessels, noting the exact location and severity of any blockages. Angiograms are relatively expensive, invasive into your body, and carry a slight risk of complications. This procedure is generally recommended for women with severe symptoms, who do not respond to treatment, or whose noninvasive tests are inconclusive.

Section 49.3

Preventing and Controlling High Blood Pressure

Excerpted from the National Institutes of Health, National Heart, Lung, and Blood Institute's brochure "The Healthy Heart Handbook for Women," NIH No. 03-2720. Revised February 2003. Available online at http://www.nhlbi.nih.gov; accessed August 2003.

What Is Blood Pressure?

Blood pressure is the amount of force exerted by the blood against the walls of the arteries. Everyone has to have some blood pressure, so that blood can get to all of the body's organs.

Usually, blood pressure is expressed as two numbers, such as 120/80, and is measured in millimeters of mercury (mmHg). The first number is the systolic blood pressure, the force when the heart beats. The second number, or diastolic blood pressure, is the pressure that exists in the arteries between heartbeats.

Because blood pressure changes often, your health care provider should check it on several different days before deciding whether your blood pressure is too high. Blood pressure is considered high when it stays above normal levels over a period of time.

Your blood pressure category is determined by the higher number of either your systolic or your diastolic measurement. For example, if your systolic number is 125 but your diastolic number is 88, your category is high normal blood pressure.

Understanding Risk

But numbers don't tell the whole story. For example, if you have high normal blood pressure, you are still at increased risk for a heart attack, stroke, or heart failure. Also, if your systolic blood pressure (first number) is 140 or higher, you are more likely to develop cardiovascular and kidney diseases even if your diastolic blood pressure (second number) is not too high. Starting around age 55, women are more likely to develop high systolic blood pressure. High systolic blood pressure is high blood pressure. If you have this condition, you will need to take steps to control it. High blood pressure can be controlled in two ways: by changing your lifestyle and by taking medication.

Changing Your Lifestyle

If your blood pressure is not too high, you may be able to control it entirely by losing weight if you are overweight, getting regular physical activity, cutting down on alcohol, and changing your eating habits.

Table 49.1. Blood Pressure: How High Is High?

	Systolic	Diastolic
Optimal (ideal) blood pressure	Less than 120	Less than 80
Normal blood pressure	120-129	80-84
High normal blood pressure	130-139	85-89
High blood pressure	140 or above	90 or above

A special eating plan called the DASH diet can help you lower your blood pressure. DASH stands for Dietary Approaches to Stop Hypertension. The DASH diet emphasizes fruits, vegetables, whole-grain foods, and low-fat dairy products. It is rich in magnesium, potassium, and calcium, as well as protein and fiber. It's low in saturated and total fat and cholesterol, and limits red meat, sweets, and sugar-containing beverages. If you follow the DASH diet and also consume less sodium, you are likely to reduce your blood pressure even more.

Sodium is a substance that affects blood pressure. It is the main ingredient in salt and is found in many processed foods, such as soups, convenience meals, some breads and cereals, and salted snacks.

Taking Medication

If your blood pressure remains high even after you make lifestyle changes, your doctor will probably prescribe medicine. Lifestyle changes will help the medicine work more effectively. In fact, if you are successful with the changes you make in your daily habits, then you may be able to gradually reduce how much medication you take.

Taking medicine to lower blood pressure can reduce your risk of stroke, heart attack, congestive heart failure, and kidney disease. If you take a drug and notice any uncomfortable side effects, ask your doctor about changing the dosage or switching to another type of medicine.

A recent study found diuretics (water pills) work better than newer drugs to treat hypertension and to prevent some forms of heart disease. If you're starting treatment for high blood pressure, try a diuretic first. If you need more than one drug, ask your doctor about making one a diuretic. And, if you're already on treatment, ask about switching to or adding a diuretic.

Diuretics work for most people, but if you need a different drug, other medications are very effective. So talk with your doctor about your total health needs.

A reminder: It is important to take blood pressure medication exactly as your doctor has prescribed it. Before you leave your physician's office, make sure you understand the amount of medicine you are supposed to take each day, and the specific times of day you should be taking it.

Chapter 50

Women and Obesity

Obesity plays a significant role in causing poor health in women, negatively affecting quality of life and shortening quantity of life. More than half of adult U.S. women are overweight, and more than one third are obese. The life expectancy of women in the U.S. is approaching 80 years of age, and more women than ever are expected to turn 65 in the second decade of the new millennium. Prevention and early treatment of obesity are crucial to ensuring a healthy population of women of all age.

Prevalence

For women, ages 20 to 74, 62 percent are overweight (Body Mass Index [BMI] of 25 or more) and about half of that population (34 percent) is obese (BMI of 30 or more). The increase in overweight, obesity, and severe obesity (BMI of 40 or more) prevalence among U.S. women over the last decade is shown in Table 50.1.

Socioeconomic Status (SES)

- Obesity appears to have a strong inverse relationship with SES (obesity increases as income level decreases) among women in developed societies such as the U.S.[1]

- Low-income women in minority populations appear most likely to be overweight.[2]

Table 50.1. Increase in Overweight, Obesity, and Severe Obesity Prevalence (%) Among U.S. Women

Weight Category	1988 to 1994	1999 to 2000
Overweight (BMI ≥ 25)	51.2	62
Obesity (BMI ≥ 30)	26	34
Severe Obesity (BMI ≥ 40)	4	6.3

Note: Ages 20 to 74 for overweight and obesity prevalence and ages 20 and older for severe obesity. Source: CDC, National Center for Health Statistics, National Health and Nutrition Examination Survey. Health, United States (Table 70) 2002. Flegal et. al. 2002;288:1723–7.

Table 50.2. Increase in Overweight Prevalence with Age among U.S. Women (1999 to 2000)

Age (Years)	Prevalence (%)
20 to 39	54.3
40 to 59	66.1
60 and older	68.1

Source: CDC, National Center for Health Statistics, National Health and Nutrition Examination Survey. Flegal et. al. *JAMA*. 2002;288:1723–7.

Table 50.3. Increase in Obesity Prevalence (%) among Women by Age Group

Age (Years)	1988 to 1994	1999 to 2000
20 to 29	14.6	23.3
30 to 39	25.8	32.5
40 to 49	26.9	35.4
50 to 59	35.6	41.2
60 to 69	29.8	42.5
70 to 79	25	31.9
80 and older	15.1	19.5

Source: CDC, National Center for Health Statistics, National Health and Nutrition Examination Survey. Flegal et. al. *JAMA*. 2002;288:1723-7.

Age

- As shown in Table 50.2, women are more likely to become over-weight (BMI of 25 or more) as they become older.

- Obesity (BMI of 30 or more) has increased among U.S. women of all age groups over the last decade. See Table 50.3.

- Middle-age women are at a particularly high risk of becoming obese. The prevalence of obesity among middle-age women (ages 35 to 64) has increased at a minimum of 2 percentage points per year over a 40-year time period from 1960 to 2000. Table 50.4 indicates prevalence changes in obesity (BMI of 30 or more) be-tween 1960 and 2000 for U.S. women in various middle-age groups.

Table 50.4. Increase in Obesity Prevalence (%) among Middle-Age Women over a 40-Year Time Period

Age (Years)	1960 to 1962	1999 to 2000	Percentage Point Change
35 to 44	14.7	33.9	19.2
45 to 54	20.3	38.1	17.8
55 to 64	24.4	43.1	18.7

Source: CDC, National Center for Health Statistics, National Health and Nutrition Examination Survey. Health, United States (Table 70) 2002.

Table 50.5. Increase in Overweight and Obesity Prevalence (%) among Women by Racial/Ethnic Group

Racial/Ethnic Group	Overweight (BMI ≥ 25)	Obesity (BMI ≥ 30)
Black (non-Hispanic)	78	50.8
Mexican American	71.8	40.1
White (non-Hispanic)	57.5	30.6

Source: CDC, National Center for Health Statistics, National Health and Nutrition Examination Survey. Health, United States (Table 70) 2002.

Race

- Among U.S. adults, black (non-Hispanic) women have the highest prevalence of overweight (78 percent) and obesity (50.8 percent).

- Table 50.5 shows the discrepancy in overweight and obesity prevalence among U.S. women (ages 20 to 74) by racial/ethnic group.

Mortality

- A direct association has been found between body weight and deaths for all causes in women, ages 30 to 55.[3]

- When BMI exceeds 30, the relative risk of death related to obesity increases by 50 percent.[4]

Health Effects

- There are many obesity-related conditions, which uniquely or mostly affect women, including those detailed below.

Arthritis

- Women with obesity have almost four times the risk of osteoarthritis as non-obese women.[5]

- A stronger association between osteoarthritis and obesity has been observed in women than in men.[6]

Birth Defects

- Maternal obesity (BMI $\geq$ 29) has been associated with an increased incidence of neural tube defects (NTD) in several studies, although varied results have been found in this area.

- Folate intake, which decreases the risk of NTDs, was found in one study to have a reduced effect with higher prepregnancy weight.[7]

Breast Cancer

- After menopause, women with obesity have a higher risk of developing breast cancer. In addition, weight gain after menopause may also increase breast cancer risk.[8,9]

- Women who gain about 45 pound or more after age 18 are twice as likely to develop breast cancer after menopause than women with no weight gain.[9,10]

- Before menopause, high BMI has been associated with a decreased risk of breast cancer. However, a recent study found an increased risk of the most lethal form of breast cancer, called inflammatory breast cancer (IBC), in women with BMI as low as 26.7 regardless of menopausal status.[11]

- Before menopause, women who are overweight and have breast cancer appear to have a shorter life span than women with lower BMI.[12]

Endometrial Cancer (EC)

- Women with obesity have three to four times the risk of EC than women with lower BMI. An estimated 34 to 56 percent of EC risk has been attributed to overweight.[13,14]

- Body size is a risk factor for EC regardless of where fat is distributed in the body. Women with obesity and diabetes have a 3-fold increase in risk for EC above the risk of obesity along.[15]

Cardiovascular Disease (CVD)

- In middle and old age groups, heavier weight is associated with CVD and its risk factors, particularly for women.[16]

Gallbladder Disease

- Obesity is the best-established predictor of gallbladder disease in women.[17]

- Women with obesity have at least twice the risk of gallstone disease than women of normal weight.[18]

Infertility

- Obesity has been found to affect ovulation, response to fertility treatment, pregnancy rates, and pregnancy outcome.[19]

- Infertile women with obesity who lose weight have shown improvement in becoming pregnant and reaching full term.[19]

Obstetric and Gynecological Complications

- In addition to infertility, excess body fat can lead to complications such as menstrual abnormality, miscarriage and difficulties in performing assisted reproduction.[20]

- The frequency of menstrual disturbance in women with severe obesity is three times greater than for normal-weight women.[20]

- High prepregnancy weight is associated with an increased risk of pregnancy hypertension, gestational diabetes, urinary infection, Cesarean section delivery, and toxemia.[20]

- Women with obesity are 13 times more likely to have overdue births, longer labors, induced labor, and blood loss.[21]

- Complications after childbirth, related to obesity, include an increased risk of wound and endometrial infection, endometritis, and urinary tract infection.[21]

Urinary Stress Incontinence

- Obesity is a well-documented risk factor for the involuntary loss of urine as well as urgency.[22]

- Obesity has been found to be a strong risk factor for women of several urinary symptoms after childbirth.[22]

Stigma and Discrimination

- Women with obesity appear to have much more prejudice and discrimination directed against them than men with obesity.[23]

- Obesity contributes to unemployment for women. After undergoing obesity surgery, a drop in unemployment rate from 84 to 64 percent was reported for women in one study.[24]

- Women with obesity face significant barriers in establishing and maintaining social relationships in a society that emphasizes thinness as physical attractiveness.[25]

- Women with obesity have reported attending fewer years of college and receiving less financial support for higher education than women who are non-obese.[25]

References

1. Sarlio-Lahteenkorva S, Stunkard A, Rissanen A. Psychosocial factors and quality of life in obesity. *Int J Obes.* 1995;19(Suppl 6):S1–S5.

2. Kumanyika SK. Special issues regarding obesity in minority populations. *Ann Inter Med.* 1993;119(7 Pt 2):650–654.

3. Manson JE, Willett WC, Stampfer MJ, Colditz GA, Hunter DJ, Hankinson SE, Hennekens CH, Speizer FE. Body weight and mortality among women. *N Engl J Med.* 1995;333(11):677–685.

4. Bray G. Health hazards of obesity, endocrinology and metabolism clinics of North America. *Endocrinol Metab Clin North Am.* 1996;25(4):907–919.

5. Felson DT. Weight and osteoarthritis. *Am J Clin Nutr.* 1996;63 (Suppl):430S–432S.

6. Felson DT. Obesity and knee osteoarthritis: The Framingham Study. *Ann Int Med.* 1988;109:18–24.

7. Werler MM, Louik C, Shapiro S, Mitchell AA. Prepregnant weight in relation to risk of neural tube defects. *JAMA.* 1996;275(14):1089–1092.

8. Carroll KK. Obesity as a risk factor for certain types of cancer. *Lipids.* 1998;33(11)1055–1059.

9. Huang Z, Hankinson SE, Colditz GA, Stampfer MJ, Hunter DJ, Manson JE, Hennekens CH, Rosner B, Speizer FE, Willett WC. Dual effects of weight and weight gain on breast cancer risk. *JAMA.* 1997;278(17):1407–1411.

10. Bonn D. How weight gain affects breast cancer risk clarified. *Lancet.* 1997;350:1371.

11. Chang S, Buzdar AU, Hursting SD. Inflammatory breast cancer and body mass index. *J Clin Oncol.* 1998;16(12):3731–3735.

12. Ballard-Barbash R, Swanson CA. Body weight: estimation of risk for breast and endometrial cancers. *Am J Clin Nutr.* 1996;63(Suppl):437S–442S.

13. National Institutes of Health, National Heart, Lung, and Blood Institute. Clinical Guidelines on the Identification, Evaluation, and Treatment of Overweight and Obesity in Adults: The Evidence Report; 1998.

14. Shoff SM, Newcomb PA. Diabetes, body size, and risk of endometrial cancer. *Am J Epidemiology.* 1998;148:234–40.

15. Folsom AR, Kaye SA, Potter JD, Prineas RJ. Association of incident carcinoma on the endometrium with body weight and

fat distribution in older women: early findings of the Iowa Women's Health Study. *Can Res.* 1989;49(23):6828–6831.

16. Harris TB, Savage PJ, Tell GS, Haan M, Kumanyika S, Lynch JC. Carrying the burden of cardiovascular risk in old age: associations of weight and weight change with prevalent cardiovascular disease, risk factors, and health status in the Cardiovascular Health Study. *Am J Clin Nutr.* 1997;66(4):837–844.

17. Sahi T, Paffenbarger RS Jr, Hsieh CC, Lee IM. Body mass index, cigarette smoking, and other characteristics as predictors of self-reported, physician-diagnosed gallbladder disease in male college alumni. *Am J Epidemiol.* 1998;147(7):644–651.

18. Everhart JE. Contributions of obesity and weight loss to gallstone disease. *Ann Intern Med.* 19934;119:1029–1035.

19. Clark AM, Thornley B. Tomlinson L, Galletley C, Norman RJ. Weight loss in obese infertile women results in improvement in reproductive outcome for all forms of fertility treatment. *Hum Reprod.* 1998;13(6):1502–5.

20. Norman RJ, Clark AM. Obesity and reproductive disorders: a review. *Reprod Fertil Dev.* 1998;10:55–63.

21. Morin KH. Perinatal outcomes of obese women: a review of the literature. *JOGNN.* 1998;27(4):431–440.

22. Rasmussen KL, Krue S, Johansson LE, Knudsen HJ, Agger AO. Obesity as a predictor of postpartum urinary symptoms. *Acta Obstet Gynecol Scand.* 1997;76(4):359-362.

23. Rand CS, Macgregor AM. Morbidly obese patients' perception of social discrimination before and after surgery for obesity. *South Med J.* 1990:83(12):1390–1395.

24. Van Gemert WG, Adang EM, Greve JW, Soeters, PB. Quality of life assessment of morbidly obese patients: effects of weight-reducing surgery. *Am J Clin Nutr.* 1998;67(2):197–201.

25. Miller CT, Rothblum ED, Felicio D, Brand P. Compensating for stigma: obese and non-obese women's reaction to being visible. *Pers Soc Psych Bulletin.* 1995;21(10):1093–1106.

Chapter 51

Women and Diabetes

Chapter Contents

Section 51.1

Diabetes as a Women's Health Problem

Diabetes can be diagnosed in females of any age, and the number of cases in both male and female patients is on the rise. Diabetes presents different challenges at different stages of a woman's life. Younger diabetic women may be more prone to recurrent yeast infections, nursing mothers may face new challenges avoiding low blood sugar (hypoglycemia), and women past menopause may face seriously increased risks of heart disease, stroke, or reduced mental sharpness. Therefore, diabetic women are urged to learn all they can about their condition at each stage of life and to make healthy lifestyle changes that have been recommended by their physician.

Women who do not have diabetes are strongly encouraged to take precautions against the development of the disease by avoiding sugary snacks with low fiber content (e.g., white bread), achieving and maintaining a healthy weight, and getting regular exercise.

Why Are Young Girls Developing Adult-Onset Diabetes?

Previously seen only in adults, adult-onset or Type II diabetes is now being diagnosed in both girls and boys as a result of the dramatic increase in the number of overweight American youths. According to the American Heart Association, almost five million children between the ages of 6 and 17 are considered obese (more than 20 percent over their ideal body weight), with many more classified as overweight. Obesity in children is rapidly becoming a national crisis in the United States. Experts predict that if children continue to gain weight as they have been since 1964, then about 1 in 3 children are currently at risk of being overweight or are already overweight now.

What Complications Are Possible for Diabetic Teenage Girls?

It is often difficult for teenagers to control their diabetes by handling daily insulin injections and finger-prick glucose tests during the school day. In addition, beginning insulin therapy is associated with weight gain, which may impact a teen's body image and self-esteem. In an unwise attempt at weight control, some individuals purposefully take less insulin that what is prescribed, so that food would be flushed from the body instead of being absorbed. This strategy can develop into eating disorders and overall risk to health. Parents are encouraged to monitor their diabetic daughters for any changes in behavior.

Recurrent yeast infections are one possible sign of diabetes. Teenage diabetic girls may develop yeast infections more often than their peers—a trend that often continues throughout diabetic women's lives. High blood sugar levels supply more nourishment to yeast, causing it to grow and multiply. Other risk factors for a yeast infection include the following:

- Taking a round of antibiotics or steroids to reduce infection or inflammation

- Wearing tight jeans, spandex, or other tight-fitting clothing around the vaginal area

- Wearing underwear made of synthetic materials instead of cotton or other natural fibers

- Douching

Anyone with recurrent yeast infections is encouraged to speak to her physician.

What Should Diabetic Women Know about Breastfeeding?

It is imperative for pregnant diabetic women to control their diabetes in order to deliver a healthy baby. The high sugar levels resulting from uncontrolled diabetes have been associated with birth defects and an unusually heavy baby, which usually means a more difficult delivery for both mother and infant. Studies have shown that diabetic women are more likely to have a cesarean birth than women without diabetes.

Diabetic mothers who choose to breastfeed will likely be told by their physician about the additional strain that this will put on their bodies. For instance, breastfeeding requires the consumption of about 500 additional calories each day by the nursing mother. As a result, diabetic mothers are encouraged to speak with their physician about changes that need to be made in either their diet or their insulin dosage in order to avoid episodes of low blood sugar (hypoglycemia).

What Should Diabetic Women Know about Heart Disease?

More than seven percent of American women have been diagnosed with diabetes. African-American women are more likely to develop diabetes than White Americans or African-American men. Diabetes is a risk factor for both heart disease and stroke. The increased risk may be due to the diabetics' higher likelihood of developing blood clots. These blood clots could block the blood flow through a coronary artery (which supplies oxygen-rich blood to the heart); if the artery has already been narrowed by coronary artery disease, then a heart attack could result. Alternatively, the blood clots could block the blood flow through a cerebral artery (which supplies oxygen-rich blood to the brain); if the artery has been previously narrowed by carotid artery disease, then a stroke could result.

Many lives have been saved as a result of information from the Framingham Heart Disease Epidemiology Study, which identified diabetes as a heart disease risk factor. However, the rate of cardiovascular deaths among diabetic women has continued to increase. A 1999 report published in the *Journal of the American Medical Association* revealed important statistics about how death rates from heart disease have changed in recent years. These data are summarized in Table 51.1.

Table 51.1. Changes in Death Rates from Heart Disease.

Group of People	Changes in Death Rates from Heart Disease in Recent Years
Nondiabetic Men	Down over 36 percent
Diabetic Men	Down over 13 percent
Nondiabetic Women	Down over 26 percent
Diabetic Women	Up over 22 percent

Studies are investigating why diabetic women appear to be at such high risk for heart disease. There seems to be linked to more cardio-vascular risk factors in diabetic women than diabetic men. These risk factors include low HDL ("good") cholesterol levels and being over-weight.

It remains, though, that diabetics can do much on their own to control their condition, such as adopting and staying on healthy exercise programs and heart-healthy diets.

After Menopause, What Should Women Know about Diabetes?

After menopause, women who are not taking hormone replacement therapy (HRT) may notice some sexual changes as a result of their body's new hormonal balance. For example, they may experience a decreased desire for sex, particularly if sex has become painful due to a lack of vaginal moisture or lubrication. Postmenopausal diabetics are at greater risk of uncomfortable sexual changes because diabetes tends to reduce the oxygen-rich blood flow that travels to areas such as the vagina. As a result, there tends to be less moisture, less elasticity, and greater risk of vaginal infections (e.g., yeast infections). HRT is one option for relieving some of these concerns, and women are urged to speak with their physician about the risks and benefits of this treatment.

Earlier studies suggested that hormone replacement therapy (HRT) provided an added benefit in postmenopausal women by protecting them against heart disease. Current research has found differently. The Women's Health Initiative, which enrolled over 16,000 women, was terminated earlier than anticipated when it was shown that the risks of HRT outweighed its benefits. HRT involves the replacement of estrogen that is lost during menopause. For women who still have their uterus, estrogen is typically taken in combination with progesterone for protection from uterine cancer (women who have had a hysterectomy can take estrogen without progesterone).

HRT can relieve some symptoms of menopause (e.g., hot flashes), and has also shown to reduce the risks of osteoporosis. It seemed plausible, therefore, to extend estrogen-progesterone HRT to the possible protection from heart disease. However, after about five years, the study, which was to end in 2005, was terminated.

Researchers found that HRT consisting of estrogen and progesterone increased the risks of heart attack, stroke, breast cancer, blood clots, and overall cardiovascular disease (*Journal of the American Medical Association*; July 17, 2002). The estrogen-only part of the Women's Health Initiative continues, and no conclusions have yet been drawn about its long-term health outcomes.

What Are Some General Health Tips for Diabetic Women?

Some general health tips for women with diabetes are:

- Unless you choose not to drink, moderate alcohol use may be good for your heart. Studies have suggested that women with type 2 diabetes could be able to cut their risk of heart disease by approximately 50 percent by having a drink or two per day. However, moderation is the key. Heavy alcohol use has been linked to breast cancer in some research studies.

- Discuss with your physician the risks and benefits of cholesterol reducing drugs. Studies of diabetics taking statins, for example, found significantly less risk of heart attack or need for procedures such as balloon angioplasty or bypass surgery. This risk reduction was true even for those whose cholesterol levels had not been high to begin with.

- Speak with your physician before taking birth control pills while breastfeeding. Although the progestin only birth control pills do not interfere with nursing (because they contain no estrogen), these pills can be harmful for women who had gestational diabetes while pregnant. Such patients may be significantly more likely to develop diabetes later in life.

- See your OB/GYN if you are experiencing unusually heavy or irregular periods, missing periods, or having trouble getting pregnant. These may be symptoms of polycystic ovarian syndrome, which appears to be more common among women who are diabetic than women without diabetes.

Diabetes and Cancer

Studies have shown higher mortality rates from breast cancer among obese diabetic women. There has also been a noted increased risk for developing colorectal cancer among women with type 2 diabetes; this may be due to the role of insulin in promoting the growth of colon cancer cells.

About HeartCenterOnline

HeartCenterOnline is a cardiovascular specialized health care website providing tools to help patients and their families better understand the complex nature of heart-related conditions, treatments, and preventive care. The website includes a library of physician-edited patient education information, interactive health-tracking tools, and an online cardiovascular community for patients, their families and other site visitors.

HeartCenterOnline
1 South Ocean Boulevard
Suite 201
Boca Raton, FL 33432
Fax: (561) 620-9799
Website: http://www.heartcenteronline.com

Section 51.2

Diet Strategies for Women with Diabetes

If you're a woman with diabetes, have you ever cut back on your insulin—perhaps just a little—because you've discovered that you can lose a few pounds in a few days' time by doing so? And then, when you go back to using your normal amount of insulin, are you dismayed to discover that you gain the weight back—and perhaps more—in equally rapid fashion? Over time, have you come to blame the insulin for your weight gain problems, so you take less insulin than you should—even though you're blood sugars run higher as a result?

Over 40 women with diabetes, many of whom admitted to having let this familiar thought process influence their diabetes program, came together at Joslin's second Women and Diabetes symposium. The day-long symposium attracted nearly 100 women with diabetes who heard talks on topics ranging from the interrelationship of diabetes, menopause, and heart disease, to a session on having a healthy pregnancy if you have diabetes. One of the most popular sessions, however, was entitled "Living on the Edge." Presented by Joslin dietitian Karen Chalmers, M.S., R.D., C.D.E., who is the Director of Nutrition Services at Joslin, the session examined the balancing act women with diabetes encounter as they try to keep blood sugars in a safe range—and their weight down too.

"Most of the women at the session on insulin and weight gain were between 20 and 55 years old or so," notes Chalmers in an interview after the symposium. "Some were on intensive insulin therapy, but others were doing insulin manipulation to lose weight. This is a fairly common kind of problem in women with diabetes. Weight loss is a big challenge—nearly an obsession—with many women in this day and age. Our society is so hung up on being thin, and these women begin to feel that taking the right amount of insulin is causing them to gain weight, so they start cutting back, letting their blood sugars run high to stay thin."

The Weight Watchers Generation

The baby boomer generation is the first generation to be raised by mothers who were highly weight conscious, Chalmers believes. "Baby boomers have been called the children of the Weight Watchers generation," says Chalmers. "As a result, we have more of a dieter's mentality.

"When I asked the group at the seminar 'How many people have ever been on a diet?' every hand went up. 'Five diets?' Still every hand went up. About half the people in the seminar had been on 10 diets or more. I had a woman in my office recently who had spent over $10,000 on diets in the past seven years, and she's now the heaviest she's ever been in her life."

"People attending the seminar were comfortable enough in the hour-long session to admit in front of others that they manipulate their insulin dosages to lose weight." But as Chalmers explained to them, it's not their insulin alone which is causing them to gain weight or preventing them from losing weight. And while taking less than the correct amount of insulin will lead to rapid weight loss, the weight lost will be mostly water and muscle being broken down, and not all fat. "And losing weight that quickly is unhealthy—not to mention the fact that keeping your blood sugars high makes you increasingly prone to long-term diabetes complications," she says.

High Sugars Equal Weight Loss

But how do so many women come to believe that insulin is a root cause of their weight loss battle?

"When you don't take the right amount of insulin and your blood sugars run high, you can become dehydrated—which makes you think you've lost weight, but you've only lost water," Chalmers says. "Then, when you start taking your insulin in the appropriate amounts again, you start over-retaining fluids initially to make up for your dehydration, which makes you think you've rapidly gained a lot of weight. You associate it with taking insulin, but really what is happening is taking your insulin properly is just enabling your body to better use food and maintain a proper water balance."

"Or, maybe you are using less insulin and as a result your blood sugars will run high. High blood sugars can make you feel more hungry because not all the food you are eating is able to get into the cells as energy to nourish the cells. Then, when you've lost the weight you wanted to lose, you start taking the right amount of insulin again—and continue to eat the same amount of food. Only this time, because your body has enough insulin to process the food you're eating, you gain weight. Before, you were getting away with eating more food because your body couldn't use it properly But once your blood sugars are in a more normal range, you're just using the food properly—and you gain weight."

Others who are using intensive insulin therapy may find they are gaining weight simply because they are over-treating low blood sugar reactions with too many calories, she says.

Some of the women on intensive therapy noted that the results of a clinical trial showed that people on intensive therapy are prone to modest weight gain. "So they ask me, "How do you expect me to lose weight when I'm on intensive insulin therapy? Doesn't insulin prompt you to cause your body to store weight as fat?' But that isn't what's happening at all. It's these other metabolic processes that are causing the weight loss, and the weight gain."

Weight Gain Principles—Women Are Different

Women are more prone to weight gain—whether they have diabetes or not—for a variety of biological and lifestyle reasons. For example, women store fat more easily than men because female hormones tend to promote the formation of fat. Before puberty, boys and girls have about the same amount of body fat. Then after puberty (by around age 20), girls have 22 percent body fat, and active boys only have about 10 percent.

"In a nutshell, male hormones keep muscle mass high and fat levels low. Female hormones do just the opposite," says Chalmers.

The specific way men and women gain weight is different too. Women deposit fat from the bottom up—they gain weight in the thighs and buttocks first, then the stomach, and then finally on the upper body and arms. Men gain weight first in the stomach. Whatever fat is gained first is the last to be shed—which is why it is so hard for women to lose weight on their thighs and rear end, and why weight loss seems to happen first in the face, neck, and upper body.

Why Skipping Meals Promotes Weight Gain

There are a host of lifestyle reasons that lead to weight gain, too. Skipping meals actually causes your body to gain weight over the long haul, because when you skip meals, your body slows down its metabolism and becomes very efficient at conserving calories (instead of burning calories). Your body does this to protect you, because your body doesn't know when you'll feed it again—it stores more calories as fat so you'll have reserves on hand for the next time you skip a meal.

So if you eat little or nothing during the day and only eat at night, you're promoting higher weight—even if you aren't eating more total calories than you might have eaten if you ate three square meals a day—because your body is going to conserve more of those calories as fat.

The same thing happens to those who go on super low calorie diets. "If you are on too low a calorie amount, your metabolism is going to slow down and your body will adapt to being starved. So, super low calorie diets do not work long-term," Chalmers says.

The key to weight loss is not fooling with your insulin, or skipping meals or following the fad low-calorie diet of the week, explains Chalmers.

The Weight Loss Key—Keep Metabolism Up

The best way to lose weight is by keeping your metabolism sped up by spreading calories over the day, exercising regularly, and not skipping meals or following a diet too low in calories. If you are on a 1500 calorie a day diet, be sure you spread those calories over three meals and one to two snacks throughout the day. By doing that, fewer of the calories will be stored as fat than if you ate all the calories at one time. This will help keep your metabolism steady.

Chalmers also encourages people to move beyond the diet mentality and to learn more about the "set-point theory." "If you ask most people, they'll tell you that no matter how many diets they go on, their weight tends to go back to a certain weight—their 'set-point'—within a few weeks or months. Our set point tends to rise with age."

You Can Help Reset or Lower Your Set Point

You can help reset or lower your set point by:

- drastically reducing the fat in your diet
- exercising regularly

"I tell people to focus on the quality, not just the quantity of food they eat when they are trying to lose weight or reset their set point," says Chalmers. "If you can change the quality, you most likely will lower the set point. So once you lower the set point you can eat a normal low-fat meal and maintain the set point weight."

You have to be patient, she points out. "We've got to help people— especially women—get off this diet merry-go-round. Stop looking for the perfect diet. There isn't one. Why are there so many diets out there? Because none of them work. If one did, everyone would use it."

"There are people—many of us—who define food as good or bad. Their whole day revolves around food. They take their failure to lose weight as a personal failure. They lose a lot of their self-esteem, when the real truth is that diets just don't work unless they are individualized and relevant to one's lifestyle and food preferences."

"People with diabetes may let their sugars run high to lose weight," Chalmers says. "Imagine. You're risking your long-term health to lose weight."

For those whose problem isn't just weight, but an obsession with food, thinness, and losing weight, there are also people and programs who can help. The test will help you determine whether you may be too concerned about food and your weight and need some additional help because you have an eating disorder.

Certain antidepressant medications have been known to help patients with eating disorders begin to put food and their weight in perspective.

"Don't let food, and the desire to be thin, run your life," notes Chalmers. "We have to stop feeling guilty and punishing ourselves around food."

Why women are prone to weight gain as fat:

- Female hormones tend to encourage storage of calories as fat
- Less muscle than men
- Always dieting (which is the best way to gain weight)

505

- Women frequently have two jobs (work and home) and often can't exercise as much

A Self-Diagnosis Checklist for Food Addiction

For many, food addiction is a self-diagnosable disease. See how many of these questions you answer with "Yes."

- Do you frequently lose weight only to regain it?
- Have you been on five or more weight-loss diets in the past five years?
- Do you think you have a problem with food?
- Do you eat large amounts of food in a short space of time?
- Do you have trouble controlling the amount you eat?
- Do you seem to constantly crave food?
- Do you eat until you feel uncomfortably full?
- Does your eating always seem to interfere with your diabetes control?
- Has your weight ever affected any part of your life?
- Do you weigh yourself every day? More than once a day?
- Do you often eat more than you planned to eat?
- Do you worry about your weight or body size or weight?
- Do you prefer to eat alone?
- Do you avoid mirrors?

How many of these methods of weight loss have you tried?

- Diuretics/laxatives
- Self-induced vomiting
- Fasting/starvation
- Amphetamines or over-the-counter diet pills
- Compulsive exercise
- Insulin manipulation
- Liquid diets (supervised or unsupervised)
- Hypnosis
- Special foods and drinks from individual weight loss programs

If your answers to these questions concern you, you may need additional help. Discuss your answers to this quiz with your physician or your registered dietitian.

Chapter 52

Women and Respiratory Disease

Almost 22 percent of all American adult women (22.2 million) are smokers. Although fewer women smoke than men, the percentage difference between the two has continued to decrease year to year. The lung cancer incidence rate in women for 1999 was 50.1 per 100,000. In 1987, lung cancer surpassed breast cancer as the leading cause of cancer deaths among women in the United States. Smoking is directly responsible for 87 percent of all lung cancer cases in America each year.

- Current female smokers aged 35 or older are 12 times more likely than nonsmoking females to die prematurely from lung cancer. In 2002, an estimated 65,700 women will die of lung cancer.

- Current female smokers aged 35 or older are 10.5 times more likely than nonsmoking females to die from emphysema or chronic bronchitis.

- Cigarette smoking during pregnancy can cause serious health problems for an unborn child. Cigarette smoking not only passes nicotine on to the fetus; it also prevents as much as 25

"Women and Smoking," reprinted with permission. © 2003 American Lung Association. For more information on how you can support the fight against lung disease, the third leading cause of death in the U.S., please contact The American Lung Association at 1-800-LUNG-USA (1-800-586-4872) or visit the website at www.lungusa.org.

percent of oxygen from reaching the placenta. Smoking during pregnancy accounts for up to 14 percent of preterm deliveries and about 10 percent of all infant deaths. Maternal smoking has also been linked to asthma among infants and young children.

- Mothers who smoke and breast-feed their babies pass nicotine to their children through breast milk. Additionally, infants are more likely to develop colds, bronchitis, and other respiratory diseases if secondhand smoke is present in the home or day care center.

- The sales and advertising drive for women's cigarettes in the late 1960's and early 1970's coincided with sharp increases in the number of girls aged 12-17 who began smoking. From 1967 to 1973, when sales of women's cigarettes skyrocketed, smoking rates more than doubled among 12-year-old girls.

- Teenage girls often start to smoke to avoid weight gain. They also seek to identify themselves as independent and glamorous, which reflect images projected by tobacco ads.

- Social images can convince teens that being slightly overweight is worse than smoking. Cigarette advertising portrays cigarettes as causing slimness and implies that cigarette smoking suppresses appetite.

- In 2001, 27.7 percent of high school girls were current smokers, meaning they smoked at least once in the 30 days preceding the survey. In addition, 12.9 percent were frequent smokers, indicating that they smoked on 20 or more of the 30 days before the survey was taken.

- Since the 1920's, the tobacco industry has targeted women with images ranging from liberation, glamour, slimness, and feminism.

- Women join smoking cessation groups more often than men for social support, but they are somewhat less successful than men in quitting smoking.

- Women who quit smoking relapse for different reasons than men. Stress, weight control, and negative emotions, lead to relapse among women.

- Research in the past 20 years has consistently shown that cigarette smoking causes skin wrinkling that could make smokers appear less attractive and prematurely old.

For more information call the American Lung Association at (800) LUNG-USA (800-586-4872).

Additional American Lung Association Resources

Call your local American Lung Association at 1-800-LUNG-USA (1-800-586-4872) to find out more about how to stop smoking for good. The Lung Association is offering a new way to stop smoking through its Freedom From Smoking® online smoking cessation clinic.

The program is based on the Lung Association's Freedom From Smoking® program, which has already helped thousands of smokers quit smoking for good. The Freedom From Smoking® online smoking cessation clinic can be accessed day or night, seven days a week, on any schedule a smoker chooses.

Visit www.ffsonline.org and stop smoking today!

Chapter 53

Women and Asthma

Asthma is a chronic inflammatory disorder of the airways producing episodes of wheezing, chest tightness, shortness of breath, and coughing. Episodes are triggered by allergens, tobacco smoke and other irritants, exercise, and infections of the respiratory tract. The number of asthma sufferers increased by 75 percent between 1980 and 1993 to 1994 and, by 1996, it was the third most common chronic condition in the U.S. With effective management, however, persons with asthma can enjoy normal activities.

While 7.2 percent of U.S. adults had asthma in 2000, women had higher rates than men, 9.1 percent compared to 5.1 percent respectively. This higher prevalence appeared to be concentrated among middle-aged adults. In 1999, more than twice as many women as men aged 45-64 had asthma, though the rates were more comparable among men and women in younger and older age groups. In addition to higher prevalence, women were more likely than men to use health care for asthma, including hospitalizations and emergency room visits, and they were also more likely to die from asthma. Higher prevalence, morbidity, and mortality among women may be associated with hormones, obesity, or other characteristics, although it is unclear whether this variation is due to a real difference in prevalence, reporting, or other factors.

Excerpted from "*Women's Health USA 2002*," U.S. Department of Health and Human Services, Health Resources and Services Administration, Maternal and Child Health Bureau, Rockville, Maryland: U.S. Department of Health and Human Services, 2002.

511

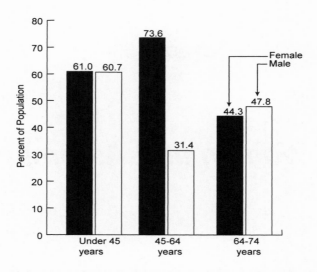

Figure 53.1. *Persons diagnosed with asthma, by age and sex, 1999. Source: (II.20): National Health Interview Survey.*

Chapter 54

Women and Stroke

Cerebrovascular accidents (CVAs), also known as strokes, are potentially fatal events in which oxygen-rich blood flow to the brain is restricted, often because of an obstructing blood clot. They strike an estimated 600,000 Americans each year, making them the leading cause of disability in the United States and the third leading cause of death. Although strokes occur with equal frequency in both men and women, women are more likely to have a stroke at a younger age (40s or 50s) and to die from stroke. Female victims account for more than 60 percent of the annual deaths due to stroke, making strokes the second leading cause of death among American women.

Fortunately, stroke is one of the most preventable neurological disorders. Many strokes can be prevented by controlling weight, blood pressure, cholesterol levels, and other risk factors. One of the best ways for women to prevent a stroke is to learn about these risk factors and to make healthy lifestyle changes accordingly. To survive a stroke, women are also encouraged to learn how they can recognize the symptoms of a stroke and what to do if they are having a stroke.

How dangerous are strokes for women?

Stroke is a very real threat to women's lives and well-being. Of those who survive a stroke, many face permanent losses of movement, speech, clear thinking, and other abilities. In the United States, there are over 4,500,000 stroke survivors, over half of them female, and many of them seriously disabled by their strokes. Strokes also tend to affect women at a much younger age than men, often striking women in their 40s or 50s. Among elderly women, it is a leading cause of both mental and physical disability.

In addition to the risk of disability, women also face the risk of death from a stroke. Though men and women are affected about equally by the 600,000 new or recurrent strokes that strike each year, women comprise more than half of those who die from them. In addition, 25 percent of women who have suffered a stroke will die within a year, and about 50 percent of female stroke survivors will die within eight years. That means that stroke claims dramatically more female lives than breast cancer does. For every American woman who dies of breast cancer, two more die of stroke. Many health care professionals are advocating that the same urgency associated with the prevention, recognition, and treatment of breast cancer be applied to the prevention, recognition, and treatment of stroke in women.

What are the risk factors for stroke in women?

Both men and women share many of the same risk factors for stroke, including the following:

- Advanced age
- High blood pressure (hypertension)
- Atrial fibrillation (associated with 15 percent of strokes)
- Carotid artery dissection (a tear in the inner lining of the carotid artery, creating a space between the inner and outer layers that could cause a stroke if blood leaked into it)
- Smoking habit (increases stroke risk up to three fold)
- High cholesterol levels and low levels of HDL ("good") cholesterol
- Diabetes
- History of irregular heart rhythms (arrhythmias) or other forms of heart disease
- Previous history of stroke or transient ischemic attack (TIA)

- Family history of stroke
- Excessive use of alcohol.
- Drug abuse (e.g., cocaine)
- Lack of exercise
- Obesity (more than 20 percent over one's ideal weight)
- Prior heart attack (according to the American Heart Association, 11 percent of women will have a stroke within six years after a heart attack)

Research has identified a number of additional risk factors that may play a role in the development of strokes in women. They include the following:

- Loss of estrogen. After menopause, women's lower estrogen levels can gradually increase their risk of stroke over time, unless they choose to take hormone replacement therapy or other options. Some evidence suggests that the abrupt loss of natural estrogen (as occurs in surgical removal of ovaries and uterus) can produce a more sharply increased risk for stroke.

- Birth control pills. While today's low-dose oral contraceptives carry a much lower risk than the earlier birth control pills, they still carry an increased risk of stroke for women who use them than for nonusers. The risk is more pronounced among smokers and women over the age of 40.

- Antiphospholipid syndrome. Some women who have had frequent miscarriages suffer from a condition called antiphospholipid syndrome, which causes an increased risk of stroke.

What can a woman do if she has symptoms of a stroke?

In general, men and women experience the same symptoms of stroke. The biggest challenge is recognizing them as soon as possible, avoiding the popular misconception that strokes are rare in women—even in their 40s or 50s.

A stroke is a true medical emergency and the following steps are strongly advised by health care professionals:

- Do not take aspirin unless directed by your physician. Although chewing adult-strength aspirin can be helpful for people who are having a heart attack, people who are having a hemorrhagic stroke can greatly worsen the situation by taking aspirin. However, only one out of every five strokes are hemorrhagic and patients who are at risk for the most common type of stroke (ischemic stroke) may be directed to take aspirin or other antiplatelet medicine by their physicians.

- Call 911 immediately. Studies have shown that stroke patients who arrived at a hospital by ambulance were seen by a physician 55 percent faster than those who arrived by private car. Women are encouraged to do everything they can to be seen as soon as possible. Recent studies have suggested that, in comparison with men having a stroke, women having a stroke take longer to get to a hospital and wait longer in the emergency room to see a physician.

- Note the time when the symptoms began and keep track of any symptoms as they appear or worsen.

How can strokes in women be prevented?

Women should be aware of the factors that may increase their risk of stroke, including high blood pressure (hypertension), smoking (increases stroke risk up to three fold), lack of exercise, and obesity.

For most women, the number one prevention against stroke is to reduce, control, or eliminate as many risk factors as possible. Specific prevention strategies include the following:

- Getting regular exercise. Regular physical activity can help middle-aged and elderly women reduce their risk of dying from stroke by 50 percent, according to a recent study published in the journal *Stroke: Journal of the American Heart Association*. The study found that the risk of dying from stroke declined as physical activity increased across all age groups strengthening the evidence that physical activity should be an important part of any strategy to prevent stroke in women at any age.

- Not smoking. Smoking is particularly dangerous for women, especially if they are also taking birth control pills.

- Eating a heart-healthy diet. People who eat at least five servings of fruit and vegetables every day are less likely to suffer from ischemic stroke (the most common form) than those who eat less than three servings a day. Eating foods rich in B-vitamins, antioxidants, fiber, and other heart-healthy substances is also important. Eating foods rich in omega 3 fatty acids, such as fish, helps increase levels of HDL ("good") cholesterol and may help reduce the risk of stroke. A study published in the *Journal of the American Medical Association* (January 2001) found that women who ate fish more than five or more times a week had a 52 percent lower risk of stroke than women who ate fish less than once a month. In the September 2000 issue of the same journal, researchers reported that women who eat large quantities of whole-grain foods have a decreased risk of ischemic stroke. Compared to women who ate little or no whole-grain foods, women who consumed these substances frequently had a 30 to 40 percent lower risk of stroke.

- Avoiding excessive alcohol use. Moderate alcohol use for women is typically defined as no more than one drink per day. One drink means 12 ounces of beer, 5 ounces of wine, or 1.5 ounces of liquor.

Women with multiple risk factors should speak with their physicians about being screened for carotid artery disease or other forms of peripheral arterial disease. The first level of screening is a simple physical examination in which the carotid artery is examined with a stethoscope. If the physician hears an abnormal sound (a carotid bruit), there is a higher chance of finding atherosclerosis or carotid artery disease—conditions that increase the risk of stroke.

If a carotid bruit is found, or if the physician finds other signs and symptoms that merit investigation, a carotid ultrasound may be recommended. A carotid ultrasound (or Duplex scan) is a painless strategy for assessing the presence of plaque in the carotid artery. It uses high-frequency sound waves to create an image of the arteries, including any blockage or narrowing that may be present.

Even in patients with a diagnosis of carotid artery disease, there are methods to reduce the risk of stroke. For instance, if the carotid artery is found to be more than 80 or 90 percent blocked, a physician may recommend a procedure called carotid endarterectomy. Carotid endarterectomy is a procedure in which plaque is stripped away from the carotid artery, increasing the space through which blood can flow through the arteries to the brain. As a result of the procedure, the patient has a lowered risk of the most common type of stroke (ischemic stroke).

About HeartCenterOnline

HeartCenterOnline is a cardiovascular specialized health care website providing tools to help patients and their families better understand the complex nature of heart-related conditions, treatments, and preventive care. The website includes a library of physician-edited patient education information, interactive health-tracking tools, and an online cardiovascular community for patients, their families and other site visitors.

HeartCenterOnline
1 South Ocean Boulevard
Suite 201
Boca Raton, FL 33432
Fax: (561) 620-9799
Website: http://www.heartcenteronline.com

Chapter 55

Osteoporosis

Chapter Contents

Section 55.1

Osteoporosis Overview

"Osteoporosis Overview" excerpted from the publication by the National
Institutes of Health, Osteoporosis and Related Bone Diseases National
Resource Center, October 2000. Available online at http://www.osteo.org;
accessed June 2003. "What about Falls?" excerpted from "Osteoporosis: The
Bone Thief," National Institute on Aging, August 2002. Available online
at http://www.nia.nih.gov; accessed June 2003.

Osteoporosis, or porous bone, is a disease characterized by low bone
mass and structural deterioration of bone tissue, leading to bone fra-
gility and an increased susceptibility to fractures of the hip, spine, and
wrist. Men as well as women suffer from osteoporosis, a disease that
can be prevented and treated.

Risk Factors

Certain factors are linked to the development of osteoporosis or
contribute to an individual's likelihood of developing the disease.
These are called risk factors. Many people with osteoporosis have several of these risk factors, but others who develop osteoporosis have
no identified risk factors. There are some risk factors that you cannot change, and others that you can.

Risk Factors You Cannot Change

- Gender—Your chances of developing osteoporosis are greater if
  you are a woman. Women have less bone tissue and lose bone more
  rapidly than men because of the changes involved in menopause.

- Age—the older you are, the greater your risk of osteoporosis.
  Your bones become less dense and weaker as you age.

- Body size—Small, thin-boned women are at greater risk.

- Ethnicity—Caucasian and Asian women are at highest risk.
  African-American and Latino women have a lower but significant risk.

- Family history—Susceptibility to fracture may be, in part, hereditary. People whose parents have a history of fractures also seem to have reduced bone mass and may be at risk for fractures.

Risk Factors You Can Change

- Sex hormones: abnormal absence of menstrual periods (amenorrhea), low estrogen level (menopause), and low testosterone level in men

- Anorexia

- A lifetime diet low in calcium and vitamin D

- Use of certain medications, such as glucocorticoids or some anticonvulsants

- An inactive lifestyle or extended bed rest

- Cigarette smoking

- Excessive use of alcohol

Prevention

To reach optimal peak bone mass and continue building new bone tissue as you get older, there are several factors you should consider.

Calcium. An inadequate supply of calcium over the lifetime is thought to play a significant role in contributing to the development of osteoporosis. Many published studies show that low calcium intakes appear to be associated with low bone mass, rapid bone loss, and high fracture rates. National nutrition surveys have shown that many people consume less than half the amount of calcium recommended to build and maintain healthy bones. Good sources of calcium include low fat dairy products, such as milk, yogurt, cheese and ice cream; dark green, leafy vegetables, such as broccoli, collard greens, bok choy and spinach; sardines and salmon with bones; tofu; almonds; and foods fortified with calcium, such as orange juice, cereals, and breads. Depending upon how much calcium you get each day from food, you may need to take a calcium supplement.

Calcium needs change during one's lifetime. The body's demand for calcium is greater during childhood and adolescence, when the skeleton is growing rapidly, and during pregnancy and breastfeeding. Postmenopausal women and older men also need to consume more calcium. This may be caused by inadequate amounts of vitamin D, which is necessary for intestinal absorption of calcium. Also, as you age, your body becomes less efficient at absorbing calcium and other nutrients. Older adults also are more likely to have chronic medical problems and to use medications that may impair calcium absorption.

Vitamin D. Vitamin D plays an important role in calcium absorption and in bone health. It is synthesized in the skin through exposure to sunlight. While many people are able to obtain enough vitamin D naturally, studies show that vitamin D production decreases in the elderly, in people who are housebound, and during the winter. These individuals may require vitamin D supplementation to ensure a daily intake of between 400 to 800 IU of vitamin D. Massive doses are not recommended.

Exercise. Like muscle, bone is living tissue that responds to exercise by becoming stronger. The best exercise for your bones is weight-bearing exercise, which forces you to work against gravity. These exercises include walking, hiking, jogging, stair-climbing, weight training, tennis, and dancing.

Smoking. Smoking is bad for your bones as well as for your heart and lungs. Women who smoke have lower levels of estrogen compared to nonsmokers and frequently go through menopause earlier. Postmenopausal women who smoke may require higher doses of hormone replacement therapy and may have more side effects. Smokers also may absorb less calcium from their diets.

Alcohol. Regular consumption of 2 to 3 ounces a day of alcohol may be damaging to the skeleton, even in young women and men. Those who drink heavily are more prone to bone loss and fractures, both because of poor nutrition as well as increased risk of falling.

Medications that cause bone loss. The long-term use of glucocorticoids (medications prescribed for a wide range of diseases, including arthritis, asthma, Crohn's disease, lupus, and other diseases of the lungs, kidneys, and liver) can lead to a loss of bone density and fractures. Other forms of drug therapy that can cause bone loss include long-term treatment with certain antiseizure drugs, such as phenytoin (Dilantin®) and barbiturates; gonadotropin releasing hormone (GnRH) analogs used to treat endometriosis; excessive use of aluminum-containing antacids; certain cancer treatments; and excessive

522

thyroid hormone. It is important to discuss the use of these drugs with your physician, and not to stop or alter your medication dose on your own.

Symptoms

Osteoporosis is often called the silent disease because bone loss occurs without symptoms. People may not know that they have osteoporosis until their bones become so weak that a sudden strain, bump, or fall causes a hip fracture or a vertebra to collapse. Collapsed vertebra may initially be felt or seen in the form of severe back pain, loss of height, or spinal deformities such as kyphosis, or severely stooped posture.

Detection

Following a comprehensive medical assessment, your doctor may recommend that you have your bone mass measured. Bone mineral density (BMD) tests measure bone density in the spine, wrist, and/or hip (the most common sites of fractures due to osteoporosis), while others measure bone in the heel or hand. These tests are painless, noninvasive, and safe. Bone density tests can:

- Detect low bone density before a fracture occurs

- Confirm a diagnosis of osteoporosis if you have already fractured

- Predict your chances of fracturing in the future

- Determine your rate of bone loss and/or monitor the effects of treatment if the test is conducted at intervals of a year or more

Treatment

A comprehensive osteoporosis treatment program includes a focus on proper nutrition, exercise, and safety issues to prevent falls that may result in fractures. In addition, your physician may prescribe a medication to slow or stop bone loss, increase bone density, and reduce fracture risk.

What about Falls?

When bones are weakened by osteoporosis, a simple fall can cause a fracture or break. This can result in a trip to the hospital, surgery, and possibly a long-lasting disabling condition in the case of a hip fracture. It is important to prevent falls. Some things you can do include:

- Make sure you can see and hear well. Use your glasses or a hearing aid if needed.

- Ask your doctor if any of the drugs you are taking can make you dizzy or unsteady on your feet.

- Use a cane or walker if your walking is unsteady.

- Wear rubber-soled and low-heeled shoes.

- Make sure all the rugs and carpeting in your house are firmly attached to the floor, or remove them.

- Keep your rooms well lit and the floor free of clutter.

- Use nightlights.

Section 55.2

Calcium Intake

Excerpted from the publication by the U.S. Department of Health and Human Services, National Women's Health Information Center (NWHIC), April 2001. Available online at http://www.4woman.gov; accessed June 2003.

What is the optimal calcium intake for women in different stages of their life?

Calcium is necessary for strong and healthy bones throughout life. A lack of calcium in the diet can lead to osteoporosis, or a condition of fragile, weakened bones that can break easily. Diet, hormones, drugs, age and genetic factors all influence the amount of calcium required for optimal skeletal health. Recommendations vary slightly. Tables 55.1 and 55.2 show the recommendations for different age groups based upon the most recent recommendations from the National Academy

Table 55.1. Recommended Daily Intake of Calcium for Women

Ages	Milligrams Per Day of Calcium
9-18	1300
19-50	1000
51 and older	1200

Note: The National Institutes of Health Consensus Conference and The National Osteoporosis Foundation support a higher calcium intake of 1,500 milligrams per day for postmenopausal women not taking estrogen and adults 65 years or older.

Table 55.2. Recommended Daily Intake of Calcium for Women Who Are Pregnant or Lactating

Ages	Milligrams Per Day of Calcium
Up to 18 years old	1300
19-50	1000

Table 55.3. Calcium Content of Some Common Foods

Source	Serving Size	Approximate Calcium (mg)
Fat free/non-fat milk; Lowfat, 2% milk; Whole milk; Chocolate milk, lowfat	8 oz.	300
Yogurt, plain, lowfat	8 oz.	415
Cheese, cheddar	1 oz.	204
Broccoli, cooked, fresh	1 cup	136
Ice cream, soft serve	1/2 cup	118
Bread, white or whole wheat	1 slice	20
Orange, medium	1	52
Macaroni and cheese	1/2 cup	180
Calcium-fortified orange juice	8 oz.	300
Pizza, cheese	1 slice	220

Note: Calcium content varies depending on ingredients. Source: National Institute of Child Health and Human Development, Milk Matters Campaign Fact Sheet.

of Sciences (1997) on optimal daily calcium intake. Table 55.3 lists the calcium content of common dairy products and some other foods high in calcium.

The guidelines are based on calcium received through diet and through calcium supplements. Calcium intake up to 2,000 mg/day appears to be safe in most individuals. Adequate vitamin D is essential for optimal calcium absorption, however most people receive enough Vitamin D through sunlight. If vitamin D supplements are necessary, no more than 800 International Units (IU) mg/day is recommended.

Part Eight

Physical Concerns of Special Significance for Women

Chapter 56

Migraine Pain

What You Should Know about Headache

During the past year, nearly 90% of men and 95% of women have had at least one headache. Most people with a headache use nonprescription pain relievers to treat their symptoms.

Store shelves hold a remarkable array of pain relievers, so you need more facts than ever to select one that best meets your needs. In light of the growing trend towards self-care, you have more responsibility than ever in safeguarding your and your family's health and well-being.

There are two main types of headache: primary and secondary.

- Primary headaches include tension-type, migraine, and cluster headaches and are not caused by other underlying medical conditions. More than 90% of headaches are primary.

- Secondary headaches result from other medical conditions, such as infection or increased pressure in the skull due to a tumor. These account for fewer than 10% of all headaches.

How Headaches Differ

Tension-Type Headaches

Tension type headaches are the most common, affecting upwards of 75% of all headache sufferers.

- As many as 90% of adults have had tension-type headache.
- Tension-type headaches are typically a steady ache rather than a throbbing one and affect both sides of the head.
- Some people get tension-type (and migraine) headaches in response to stressful events or a hectic day.
- Tension-type headaches may also be chronic, occurring frequently or even every day.
- Psychologic factors have been overemphasized as causes of headaches.

Migraine Headaches

Migraine headaches are less common than tension-type headaches. Nevertheless, migraines afflict 25 to 30 million people in the United States alone.

- As many as 6% of all men and up to 18% of all women (about 12% of the population as a whole) experience a migraine headache at some time.
- Roughly three out of four migraine sufferers are female.
- Among the most distinguishing features is the potential disability accompanying the headache pain of a migraine.
- Migraines are felt on one side of the head by about 60% of migraine sufferers, and the pain is typically throbbing in nature.
- Nausea, with or without vomiting, as well as sensitivity to light and sound often accompany migraines.
- An aura—a group of telltale neurologic symptoms—sometimes occurs before the head pain begins. Typically, an aura involves a disturbance in vision that may consist of brightly colored or blinking lights in a pattern that moves across the field of vision.
- About one in five migraine sufferers experiences an aura.
- Usually, migraine attacks are occasional, or sometimes as often as once or twice a week, but not daily.

Cluster Headaches

Cluster headaches are relatively rare, affecting about 1% of the population. They are distinct from migraine and tension-type headaches.

- Most cluster headache sufferers are male—about 85%.

- Cluster headaches come in groups or clusters lasting weeks or month.

- The pain is extremely severe but the attack is brief, lasting no more than an hour or two.

- The pain centers around one eye, and this eye may be inflamed and watery. There may also be nasal congestion on the affected side of the face.

- These "alarm clock" headaches may strike in the middle of the night, and often occur at about the same time each day during the course of a cluster.

- A history of heavy smoking and drinking is common, and alcohol often triggers attacks.

Rebound Headache

Rebound headache may occur among people with tension-type headaches as well as in those with migraines.

- It appears to be the result of taking prescription or nonprescription pain relievers daily or almost every day, contrary to directions on the package label.

- If prescription or nonprescription pain relievers are overused, headache may "rebound" as the last dose wears off, leading one to take more and more pills. This is a good reason to call your doctor!

Headache Triggers

No discussion of headache is complete without mention of headache triggers.

- Stress may be a trigger, but certain foods, odors, menstrual periods, and changes in weather are among many factors that may also trigger headache.

- Emotional factors such as depression, anxiety, frustration, letdown, and even pleasant excitement may be associated with developing a headache.

- Keeping a headache diary will help you determine whether factors such as food, change in weather, and/or mood have any relationship to your headache pattern.

Characteristics Associated with Primary Headaches Help Differentiate Tension-Type Headaches from Migraine

Table 56.1 shows the symptoms commonly seen in two types of headache. Compare your symptoms with those listed and determine what type of headache you may have by noting whether your symptoms are most like those in column A or B. Some people have both of these types of headache. If your headaches are very severe or if you think they are some other type, do not delay in seeking professional medical attention.

When to Call Your Doctor

Although very few headaches are signs of serious underlying medical conditions, call your doctor at once if any of the items below apply to you.

Table 56.1. Differentiating Tension-Type Headaches from Migraine

Symptom	A Tension	B Migraine
Intensity and Quality of Pain		
Mild-to-moderate	X	X
Moderate-to-severe	X	X
Intense, pounding, throbbing and/or debilitating		X
Distracting but not debilitating	X	
Steady ache	X	
Location of Pain		
One side of head		X
Both sides of head	X	X
Associated Symptoms		
Nausea/vomiting		X
Sensitivity to light and/or sounds		X
Aura before onset of headache such as visual symptoms		X

Note: Rebound headache may have features of tension and/or migraine headache.

Call your doctor if:

- You have three or more headaches per week.
- You must take a pain reliever every day or almost daily.
- You need more than recommended doses of over-the-counter medications to relieve headache symptoms.
- You have a stiff neck and/or fever in addition to a headache.
- Your headache is accompanied by shortness of breath, fever, and/or unexpected symptoms that affect your eyes, ears, nose, or throat.
- You are dizzy, unsteady, or have slurred speech, weakness, or changes in sensation (numbness and/or tingling) in addition to your headache.
- You experience confusion or drowsiness with your headache.
- Your headaches begin and persist after head injury.
- Your headache is triggered by exertion, coughing, bending, or sexual activity.
- Your headache keeps getting worse and won't go away.
- Your headaches have changed in character.
- Persistent or severe vomiting accompanies headache.
- You have your "first and/or worse" headache.
- Your headaches began after you reached the age of 50 and, finally, keep in mind that even if you have had headaches for many years, it's still possible to develop a new and possibly more serious type of headache.

Do You Need Migraine Prevention?

Migraine patients do not want to suffer from an attack, so prevention is important, even if they suffer from only one attack a year. Those who suffer from frequent attacks will need more aggressive prevention strategies that sometimes include medication. This decision is made by discussing treatment and management options with your physician. Additionally, nonpharmacological prevention may help if you have:

1. poor tolerance for specific pharmacological treatments,

2. medical contraindications for specific acute pharmacological treatments,

533

3. insufficient or no response to pharmacological treatment,

4. history of long-term, frequent, or excessive use of pain medications (analgesics) or acute medications that make headaches worse (or lead to decreased responsiveness to other pharmacotherapies), or

5. high stress levels or difficulty coping with stress.

Goals of Preventive Therapy

Migraine prevention is intended to reduce the suffering and disability associated with attacks. Unfortunately, preventive treatment strategies rarely eliminate migraine, but they can reduce the frequency and severity of attacks. Ideally, migraine sufferers should learn how to gain a sense of control over their attacks. This will lead to a better sense of well being and improved quality of life. The ultimate goals of migraine preventive therapy are to:

1. reduce frequency, severity, and duration of attacks,

2. improve responsiveness to treatment of acute attacks, and

3. reduce level of disability.

These goals can be achieved through a combination of education, lifestyle changes, and therapies (pharmacological [drug] and nonpharmacological [nondrug]). Specifically:

*   Learning about your specific migraine "triggers" may help you reduce the frequency of attacks.

*   Using a headache diary will help identify items that are associated with triggering migraine that you may have not been aware of such as menstruation, red wine, and caffeine, among others. The information collected in a headache diary also will allow your physician to review the severity, frequency, disability, and triggers associated with your attacks. A complete understanding of these details will help you and your doctor design a successful treatment plan.

Avoiding Triggers

"Triggers" are specific factors that may increase your risk of having a migraine attack. The migraine sufferer has inherited a sensitive nervous system that under certain circumstances, can lead to migraine.

Triggers do not "cause" migraine. Instead, they are thought to activate processes that cause migraine in people who are prone to the condition. A certain trigger will not induce a migraine in every person; and, in a single migraine sufferer, a trigger may not cause a migraine every time. By keeping a headache diary, you will be able to identify some triggers for your particular headaches.

Once you have identified triggers, it will be easier for you to avoid them and reduce your chances of having a migraine attack.

Common Triggers

The science linking triggers to migraine is not yet clearly established. Nonetheless, patients commonly report that they have migraine triggers.

Lifestyle Changes

Migraine is not a predictable disorder for all people. Simple things like changes to a normal routine can lead to a severely disabling migraine attack. Understanding how lifestyle impacts the severity and frequency of attacks can be a large part of successful migraine prevention.

Table 56.2. Common Migraine Triggers (continued on next page)

Categories	Triggers	Examples
Dietary	Skipping meals/fasting	MSG (monosodium glutamate)
	Food items	Chocolate
		Processed meats (containing nitrates)
		Aged cheese
		Alcohol/red wine
		Too much caffeine
	Medications	Nitroglycerine
Chronobiology	Change in sleep patterns	Napping
		Oversleeping
		Too little sleep
Environmental	Weather changes	Extreme heat or cold
	Bright lights	Office lighting
	Odors/pollution	Smog, perfumes, chemicals
		Flashing lights or screens

It is an unrealistic to expect anyone to completely change a certain life style. However, certain things are relatively easy to do. For example:

- Maintain regular sleep patterns. Go to sleep and wake up at the same time each day.

- Exercise regularly. For example, aerobic exercise for at least 30 minutes three times a week will help reduce frequency or severity of migraine.

- Eat regular meals, do not skip meals, and eat a good, healthy breakfast.

- Reduce stress. Limit stress by avoiding conflicts and resolving disputes calmly. Some people find it helpful to take a daily "stress break."

- Avoiding known triggers (see Table 56.2)

Establishing daily routines that help reduce migraine attacks is important for long-term migraine prevention. For example:

Table 56.2. Common Migraine Triggers (continued from previous page)

Hormonal	Estrogen level changes (rapid fluctuations in estrogen levels)	Menstruation Hormone replacement therapies Birth control pills Around the time of menopause
Stress	Work Home Family	Unrealistic timelines Financial issues Job changes Moving Childbirth Marriage Death/loss
Stress Letdown	Discontinuation of work	Weekends Vacations Ending a project or stressful task (such as a presentation)
Physical	Injuries Over-exertion	Marathon running Exercising when out of shape Exercising in heat

- Schedule a relaxation period that includes relaxation strategies. Take slow, deep breaths; focus the mind on a relaxing image or scene; or try soft relaxing lighting and sounds.

- Exercise on a regular basis, even if your daily routine changes (such as when traveling, when you have houseguests, or when your workload increases).

- Maintain the medication treatment plan designed by you and your physician. Early intervention may help prevent the migraine from progressing into a severe, disabling attack.

Nonpharmacological Strategies

You can do certain things that do not involve medications, and some of these have been discussed in the previous sections (Avoiding Triggers and Lifestyle Changes). Others involve techniques employed by trained practitioners. Many different kinds of "nonpharmacological techniques" are available, including behavioral and physical treatments.

Behavioral treatments:

- biofeedback therapy
- relaxation training
- cognitive-behavioral training (also known as stress-management training)
- hypnosis

Physical treatments:

- acupuncture
- massage
- cervical manipulation

Behavioral Treatments

Biofeedback therapy: Biofeedback is a technique where people learn to gain control of their body's internal functions. Specifically, biofeedback involves learning to sense changes in the body's activity, and using relaxation and other techniques to control the body's responses.

Biofeedback requires specific training sessions with a trained biofeedback therapist. This training usually takes one to two months of weekly 30-45 minute sessions, although many books and audiotapes are available to teach these techniques at home.

Biofeedback is monitored by measuring skin temperature and muscle tension. Changes in skin temperature and muscle tension indicate the level of activation of the patient's nervous system. Learning to control body functions, such as body temperature, is achieved by first learning to relax the skeletal muscles (muscles that support the bones). This relaxation is achieved through relaxation, visualization, and breathing techniques. Most important, though, is the daily practice of these techniques. The practice sessions can be only a few seconds or minutes long, but they need to be done frequently. A conscious effort is required in the first few weeks of training, but gradually, self-monitoring and very brief relaxation techniques become a subconscious habit.

Biofeedback allows many headache sufferers to lower tension throughout the body, which results in fewer headaches. Children adapt especially well to biofeedback training. They can often learn to prevent a headache in four to five sessions, and also they can learn to stop the headache once it begins.

Biofeedback therapy may be coupled with relaxation therapy. Relaxation therapy teaches a variety of relaxation strategies for reducing tension and stress throughout the body.

Cognitive-behavioral training (also known as stress-management training): This technique often is done with the help of a psychologist, psychiatrist, or other therapist. This training focuses on teaching migraine sufferers coping skills and other "cognitive" (thinking) strategies for managing stressful parts of their life.

Hypnosis: Hypnosis is now being studied in clinical trials for treatment of a variety of conditions including pain management. Little has been done so far about its use in preventing migraine.

Physical Treatments

Acupuncture: The ancient method of acupuncture recently received a boost in popularity because of the consensus statement released by a panel convened by the National Institutes of Health. This statement strongly suggests that acupuncture is in fact a legitimate therapy proven to be effective for some conditions, and acupuncture deserves additional studies for other conditions. The panel concluded that nausea and acute dental pain clearly respond to acupuncture. Many painful conditions, including headaches, may respond to acupuncture, but additional studies are needed.

Acupuncture treatment is done using very thin disposable needles, which cause very little discomfort or pain. For patients with chronic headaches, treatment involves 10 or more weekly 20-minutes sessions. Electric simulation of the needles is frequently used instead of the traditional manual twirling of the needles. Issues of cost, convenience, and patient preference should be taken into account when deciding whether to try this mode of treatment. Some insurance plans may cover this form of therapy.

Massage: Many migraine sufferers have tight, stiff, tender muscles in the back of the head, neck, and shoulders. If you feel these muscles, they often have tight bands or knots that are tender to pressure. Pressure on these points in the muscle may cause pain in the head, which is similar to the pain of a migraine. These points are often called trigger points. Massaging these trigger points can reduce the pain and tightness in the muscles and can decrease head pain and migraine in some sufferers.

Massage therapy is a healthy maneuver to reduce stress and tension. Its value in treating migraine, however, is not fully determined. Massage initially can be done once to twice a week for 4 to 6 weeks. Stretching and strengthening exercises should be continued even after therapy sessions have ended. Massage techniques can be taught to a spouse or significant other.

The likelihood of behavioral techniques working as preventive treatment for migraine depends upon appropriate training and discipline for the person using the technique. Headache sufferers must be willing to try these techniques and must be committed to maintaining the training programs designed by technicians and other professionals in order for them to be successful.

Preventive Medications

Preventive medications are taken daily to prevent the onset of migraine. They are not intended for use during a migraine attack.

Many different preventive medications are available, and the choice of medication depends on many factors such as co-existing conditions including high blood pressure, diabetes, or pregnancy (among others). Therefore, choosing medications for preventive therapy can be a complex process.

Before starting to take medications, several basic principles need to be considered:

1. The choice of a preventive medication needs to be tailored to meet each person's individual needs.

2. Co-existing medical conditions, drug side effects, other medications being taken, and individual patient needs will help determine which medication a physician chooses.

When deciding on preventive therapies, it is important to review with your doctor several important management principles:

- Low doses are used at first and gradually increased to higher doses as needed. Therefore, you may need to increase medication dose until the desired response is achieved.

- It may take 2 to 3 months before you notice a decrease in the frequency or severity of attacks.

- Treatment may be required for 6 to 12 months or longer.

- All medications have potential side effects so any unusual symptoms should be reported to your physician. It is important to discuss potential side effects, since some medications may be better tolerated than others.

- Side effects can often be limited by using low doses, increasing the dose slowly, or allowing time to adjust to the medication. If you are not tolerating the medication and if you start to have side effects, contact your doctor to discuss changes to the treatment plan.

- You should not suddenly stop taking preventive medications because of the risk of rebound headache or other side effects. Preventive medications need to be gradually tapered off after a period of sustained benefit.

Assessing Disability from Migraine

Disability caused by migraine can come from the pain of the attack itself or from non-headache symptoms associated with the attack, such as nausea or sensitivity to light and sound. Whether pain, nausea, or vomiting is the primary disabling feature, migraine prevents people from continuing with their daily routines. The goal of migraine prevention is to eliminate disability through pain management and treatment of associated symptoms. Disability created by migraine attacks can lead to:

- Time lost from school
- Time lost from work
- Time lost from household activities
- Reduced productivity and work performance

- Time lost from social activities and family activities
- Unemployment
- Strain in relationships with spouse or children

The fear of future migraine attacks can be just as disabling as the actual attack. For some people the fear of having another attack keeps

Table 56.3. Commonly Used Preventive Medications for Migraine

Type of medication	Medication class	Generic name	Side effects
Blood pressure medications	Beta-Blockers	Propranolol Timolol Metoprolol	Fatigue Depression Nausea Insomnia Dizziness
	Calcium channel blockers	Verapamil Diltiazem Nimodipine	Weight gain Constipation Dizziness Low blood pressure
Antidepressants	Tricyclic antidepressants	Amitriptyline Nortriptyline Imipramine	Dry mouth Sedation Decreased libido (sex drive) Low blood pressure
	Selective Serotonin Reuptake Inhibitors (SSRIs)	Fluoxetine Paroxetine Sertraline	Weight gain or loss Decreased libido
Anticonvulsants		Divalproex sodium Gabapentin Topiramate	Weight gain or loss Sedation Skin rash
Serotonin antagonists		Methysergide Methylergonovine	Blood vessel spasm Abdominal scarring (very rare)
Unconventional treatments	Magnesium salts	Magnesium oxide, magnesium, diglycinate, magnesium chloride slow release	Diarrhea
	Vitamins	Riboflavin	Urine discoloration
	Feverfew		Urine discoloration

them from taking part in activities such as vacations, parties, or having visitors.

Migraine also affects the sufferer's spouse, children, family, and friends. Coworkers are affected by a colleague's migraine because work plans may suddenly change, meetings may be canceled, work may not be done, responsibilities may be shifted, or the quality of work may be reduced.

The ultimate impact of a migraine disability may be underestimated and, in general, this information is poorly communicated between headache sufferers and their physicians. Measuring the total impact of migraine on your life will help you understand the severity of your illness and it will affect your physician's assessment of your need for treatment.

Several disability tools are available to assess the impact of migraine on your life. One such instrument is the MIDAS Questionnaire (Migraine Disability Assessment) which measures days missed or days with lower capacity to function due to migraine. Your physician can use this information to decide on need and choice of medications or other treatment strategies. Other disability assessment tools include IMPACT, PACE, and HDI. Importantly, prevention of migraine should be aimed at reducing disability and limiting disruption of your daily routine.

Monitoring Headaches

To fully understand the impact of migraine, it is important to keep track of your migraine attacks. Filling out a headache diary gives you and your physician an accurate picture of the frequency, severity, and disability of your attacks. It also provides a way to identify patterns, such as the association with the menstrual cycle.

Why use a headache diary?

- Triggers: migraine triggers may become more apparent as you monitor your migraines using a daily diary form.

- Track progress: diary forms also are an excellent way to track success, or failure, of treatment. For example, you may be thinking that your headaches are not getting better, but long-term improvement may only be detected by comparing regular reports of severity, frequency, duration, and disability from attacks.

Diary forms are easily available at this website location: http://www.achenet.org/your/diary1.php

Talk to Your Doctor

Three simple steps to taking better care of you and your migraine:

1. Keep monthly headache calendars.

2. Fill out a disability questionnaire.

3. Make an appointment to specifically talk with your doctor about your headaches. Many patients do not discuss migraine with their doctors and may suffer unnecessarily. Plan on discussing migraine as the main reason for the visit. You should not try and "squeeze" in a quick discussion about your headaches when your doctor has not scheduled enough time for a thorough headache evaluation. Designing a specific treatment plan that meets your individual needs will take additional time.

When going to the doctor's office remember to take with you:

- a list of all prescription medications you use.

- a list of all over-the-counter medications you use.

- a list of all dietary supplements you take, including vitamins, herbal therapies, and other nontraditional remedies.

- your completed headache diary.

- your completed MIDAS Questionnaire or other disability assessment tool, if you have one.

Remember

1. Be honest about the number of medications you use and how often you take them. This will help your physician determine how to properly treat your migraines, especially regarding your need for preventive therapies. Medication overuse is a common consequence of out-of-control migraine, not drug addiction.

2. Agree to a treatment plan that is appropriate to your specific needs. This includes assessing migraine severity and disability. Take into account your lifestyle, health, and any other issues that may affect the medications you take. For example, type of delivery (oral, nasal, liquid, tablet, suppository, injection); frequency of dosing (once, twice, three times or four

times a day); other existing health conditions (high blood pressure, depression, fatigue), and other health concerns (such as weight gain, drowsiness, desire to get pregnant).

3. Be sure that you understand your treatment plan when you leave the office. Taking medications incorrectly will decrease their effectiveness and could lead to additional side effects. Be sure the plan is written out. If it is not clear, ask to have it explained again or call back and ask to have it clarified. Changes in the treatment plan **must** be discussed with your doctor. Make sure you have a follow-up appointment when you leave the office, and be sure and keep the appointment, even if your headaches are doing better. Bring your completed diary to your follow-up visit. Treatment plans often require modifications and adjustments so do not give up if one particular plan is not working.

Remember, migraine can be effectively managed and treated. Patients do not need to "live with their migraine." A large number of medications and non-pharmacological treatment strategies are effective for treatment of migraine. Consult with you physician regularly to make sure you are getting the best possible care.

Chapter 57

Thyroid Disease

The thyroid is a gland that controls key functions of your body. Disease of the thyroid gland can affect nearly every organ in your body and harm your health. Thyroid disease is eight times more likely to occur in women than in men. In most cases, treatment of thyroid disease is safe and simple.

This chapter will tell you more about symptoms of thyroid disease, causes, and treatment. Once thyroid disease is diagnosed, it usually can be treated with success.

The Thyroid Gland

The thyroid gland is located at the base of your neck in front of your trachea (or windpipe). It has two sides and is shaped like a butterfly.

The thyroid gland makes, stores, and releases two hormones—T4 (thyroxine) and T3 (triiodothyronine). Thyroid hormones control the rate at which every part of your body works. This is called your metabolism. Your metabolism controls whether you feel hot or cold or tired or rested. When your thyroid gland is working the way it should, your metabolism stays at a steady pace—not too fast or too slow.

The thyroid gland is controlled by the pituitary gland (a gland in your brain). The pituitary gland makes thyroid-stimulating hormone (TSH). TSH tells the thyroid gland to make more hormone if needed.

American College of Obstetricians and Gynecologists. *Thyroid Disease.* (Patient Education Pamphlet No. AP128). Washington, DC. © ACOG 2002.

If there is not enough thyroid hormone in the bloodstream, the body's metabolism slows down. This is called hypothyroidism (underactive). If there is too much thyroid hormone, your metabolism speeds up. This is called hyperthyroidism (overactive). Certain disorders can cause the thyroid gland to make too much or too little hormone.

Diagnosing Thyroid Disease

Thyroid disease is diagnosed by your symptoms, an exam, and tests. Symptoms of thyroid disease can be much like symptoms of other health problems.

Your doctor will examine your neck while you swallow. The thyroid gland moves when you swallow. This makes it easier to feel. Your doctor also may examine your skin and eyes and check your weight and temperature.

Your doctor will use tests to help find the exact cause of the problem. You may have a:

- Blood test
- Thyroid scan
- Ultrasound

During a thyroid scan, you must drink a small amount of radioactive iodine. A special camera then detects the areas of thyroid gland that absorb the radioactive iodine. These are the problem areas. This will not be done if you are pregnant.

Hypothyroidism

Hypothyroidism occurs when the thyroid gland is not working hard enough (it's underactive). It is not making enough of the thyroid hormones to maintain your normal body metabolism.

Causes

The most common cause of hypothyroidism is a disorder known as thyroiditis—an inflammation of the thyroid gland. This also is called Hashimoto's disease. It causes the immune system—your body's natural defense against disease—to mistake cells in the thyroid gland for harmful invaders. Your body sends out white blood cells to destroy them. The pituitary gland then releases TSH to tell the thyroid gland to make more thyroid hormone. This demand on the thyroid gland can cause it to enlarge. This enlargement is called a goiter.

Hypothyroidism also can result from a diet that does not have enough iodine. The diet of most Americans is thought to have enough iodine because of the use of iodized salt. Other food sources of iodine include:

- Spinach
- Shrimp
- Oysters
- Lobster

Taking too high a dosage of medication to treat hyperthyroidism can lead to hypothyroidism, too.

Symptoms

The symptoms of hypothyroidism are slow to develop. You may have the condition but not have any symptoms for months or years. Common symptoms of hypothyroidism are:

- Fatigue or weakness
- Weight gain
- Decreased appetite
- Change in menstrual periods
- Loss of sex drive
- Feeling cold when others don't
- Constipation
- Muscle aches
- Puffiness around the eyes
- Brittle nails
- Hair loss

If your lab tests show that the hormone levels are normal, some other condition may be causing your symptoms.

Treatment

In most cases, hypothyroidism is treated with medication that contains thyroid hormone. The dose of the medication is increased slowly until a normal level has been reached in the blood.

Most people with hypothyroidism have to take the hormone for the rest of their lives. The dose may need to be changed from time to time. The level of the hormone in the blood is checked regularly.

Hyperthyroidism

Hyperthyroidism results when the thyroid gland is making too much thyroid hormone (it's overactive). This causes your metabolism to speed up.

Causes

The most common cause of hyperthyroidism is a disorder known as Graves' disease. It most often affects women between the ages of 20 and 40 years. Women with Graves' disease make a substance that causes the thyroid gland to make too much thyroid hormone. A late sign of Graves' disease is often a wide-eyed stare or bulging eyes.

Hyperthyroidism also may result from medication. Taking too much of thyroid hormone when being treated for hypothyroidism can lead to symptoms of an overactive thyroid. Lumps in the thyroid called hot nodules are another cause. These lumps produce too much thyroid hormone.

Symptoms

The more common symptoms of hyperthyroidism are:

- Fatigue
- Weight loss
- Nervousness
- Rapid heartbeat
- Increased sweating
- Feeling hot when others don't
- Changes in menstrual periods
- More frequent bowel movements
- Tremors

Treatment

Treatment for hyperthyroidism will lower the amount of thyroid hormone and relieve your symptoms. Antithyroid medication can be used to reduce the amount of thyroid hormone your body is making.

Medications known as beta blockers control rapid heartbeat. If these medications don't help, your doctor may suggest treatment with radioactive iodine to destroy parts of the thyroid gland. In some cases, surgery may be needed to remove the thyroid gland.

Thyroid Nodules

A nodule is a lump in the thyroid gland. You may notice the lump on your own, or your doctor may detect the lump during a routine exam.

When a thyroid nodule is found, it will be checked to see if it is benign (not cancer) or malignant (cancer).

Your doctor also may use ultrasound to examine the nodule. Nodules may be further examined by a procedure known as fine needle aspiration or biopsy.

If no cancer cells are found, your doctor may prescribe a thyroid hormone to decrease the size of your nodule. Or, your doctor may suggest surgery to remove it. If cancer cells are found, further treatment will be needed. Thyroid cancer usually can be treated with success.

Finally

Women are more likely than men to have thyroid problems. If you have symptoms of thyroid disease, you should see your doctor and be tested. Once thyroid disease is diagnosed, it usually can be treated with success.

Glossary

Fine Needle Aspiration: A procedure in which a needle and syringe are used to withdraw a small amount of tissue. The tissue sample is then examined under a microscope to look for cancer cells.

Goiter: An enlarged thyroid gland that causes a lump on the neck.

Hyperthyroidism: A condition in which the thyroid gland makes too much thyroid hormone.

Hypothyroidism: A condition in which the thyroid gland makes too little thyroid hormone.

Thyroid-Stimulating Hormone (TSH): A hormone made by the pituitary gland that encourages the thyroid gland to make more thyroid hormone.

Ultrasound: A test in which sound waves are used to create pictures of the internal organs.

Chapter 58

Chronic Fatigue Syndrome

What is chronic fatigue syndrome (CFS)?

Having chronic fatigue syndrome, or CFS, means more than just getting tired. With the busy lives American women lead, we all get tired from time to time. But, the fatigue with CFS is extreme and overwhelming, and doesn't get better with bed rest. And, it is often made worse with physical or mental activity.

This illness seems to happen all of a sudden—one day you may notice that you are very tired and can't manage your normal activities. Your energy level is lower and you often get tired for no reason. You may also feel weak and have muscle pain, difficulty focusing, or insomnia (not being able to sleep). After you engage in physical activity or exert yourself, you may feel tired for more than 24 hours. The extreme fatigue may then come and go, giving you times when your energy level is normal. Sometimes, though, the extreme tiredness never stops, leaving you feeling exhausted and depleted all the time. You notice that you can't get done in a day what you normally would have been able to, before having this condition.

CFS is diagnosed only when other possible causes of the fatigue are ruled out, and the fatigue has lasted for at least 6 months. There are treatments to help a person cope with CFS, some of which include

Excerpted from the publication by the U.S. Department of Health and Human Services, National Women's Health Information Center (NWHIC), September 2002. Available online at http://www.4woman.gov; accessed July 2003.

medication. Sometimes CFS goes away on its own or a person can have long periods of time, even years, without symptoms.

What causes CFS?

No one knows for sure what causes CFS. For more than 100 years, doctors have reported seeing illnesses like CFS. Some causes of CFS offered over the years by health experts include anemia (low iron in the blood); hypoglycemia (low blood sugar); environmental allergies; and candidiasis (yeast infection) in the entire body.

Sometimes CFS develops on its own, for no reason. But, most persons with CFS say that it started after having a cold, bronchitis, hepatitis, or an intestinal virus. It can also follow a bout of infectious mononucleosis (mono), the kissing disease that drains the energy of many teenagers and young adults. Some persons with CFS say their illness began after a time of extreme stress, such as the loss of a loved one or undergoing major surgery.

It can be hard to figure out if a person has CFS. This is because many illnesses have extreme fatigue as a symptom and many treatments, such as chemotherapy, can cause extreme fatigue.

What are the signs of CFS?

CFS symptoms either stay with a person or come and go for more than 6 months. Initial symptoms can feel like you have the flu. Besides extreme fatigue and weakness, CFS symptoms include:

- Headaches of a new type, pattern, or intensity
- Tender lymph nodes
- Sore throat
- Muscle pain or aches
- Pain or aches in several joints without swelling or redness
- Not being able to concentrate, focus, or remember
- Feeling tired even if sleeping
- Feeling discomfort or out of sorts after physical exertion

How common is CFS? Who gets it?

The Centers for Disease Control and Prevention estimates as many as half a million Americans have a CFS-like condition. In the early 1980s it was first called the yuppie flu because mostly well-educated women with high incomes in their 30s and 40s sought help for CFS-like symptoms. It is now known that this illness affects people of all ages, racial/ethnic backgrounds, and economic situations. And, it isn't just an American illness—people all over the world are affected by CFS.

More women than men are diagnosed with CFS. But, it isn't known for sure that this illness affects women more than men. Women may be more likely than men to talk to their doctors about symptoms like exhaustion and pain.

How is CFS treated?

Right now, there is no treatment that works to cure CFS. The good news is there are things you can do to feel better, increase the level at which you can function, and improve your quality of life.

Talking with your health care provider about treatments for your symptoms, along with ways to manage your fatigue, is a good place to start. And building a good relationship with your provider is key to managing your illness over time. This will help you to talk more freely with your provider about your symptoms, which can improve the treatment of your illness. Keep in mind your provider may need to learn more about CFS to better help you. If you feel your provider doesn't know a lot about CFS or has doubts about whether it is a real illness, see another provider for a second opinion. Try a local university medical school or research center for help with finding providers with expertise in CFS.

Medications can work to relieve the symptoms of CFS. Nonsteroidal anti-inflammatory drugs, or ibuprofen (Advil, Motrin, Aleve), can help with body aches, headaches, and muscle and joint pain. Non-drowsy antihistamines can relieve allergy symptoms, such as runny nose and itchy eyes. While there is no proof these practices help, some people report symptom relief with massage, acupuncture, and chiropractic care. Physical activity and exercise can also help with symptom relief, but be sure to talk with your provider about developing an activity and exercise program that's best for you. For some people, physical activity and exercise can worsen symptoms.

Drugs used to treat depression, or antidepressants, are sometimes used to treat CFS. This is because studies have found that people with fibromyalgia, an illness similar to CFS, get relief from taking these drugs. Some experts believe these drugs improve the quality of sleep, helping decrease fatigue with CFS. Two types of antidepressants are most often prescribed by providers—low-dose tricyclic antidepressants or the newer selective serotonin reuptake inhibitors (SSRIs).

Chapter 59

Fibromyalgia

What is fibromyalgia (FM)?

Fibromyalgia (FM), is a disorder with symptoms of widespread muscle pain, fatigue (feeling tired and having low energy), and multiple tender points. A tender point is tenderness that occurs in certain areas of the body. Tender points are located in the neck, spine, shoulders, hips, and knees and are painful when pressure is applied to them. People with FM often have sleep problems and may have many other symptoms. FM is not thought to be an autoimmune disease at this time, but it shares symptoms with several autoimmune illnesses.

What are the symptoms of fibromyalgia?

The main symptoms of FM include:

- Muscle pain in many areas of the body
- Fatigue
- Tender points in specific areas of the body that are painful when pressure is applied to them

In addition to these symptoms, other common symptoms of FM include:

Excerpted from "Fibromyalgia," U.S. Department of Health and Human Services, National Women's Health Information Center (NWHIC), August 2002. Available online at http://www.4woman.gov; accessed August 2003.

- Sleep problems. People with FM often have poor quality sleep that is not refreshing.
- Depression or anxiety.
- Stiffness, especially in the morning.
- Problems with thinking and concentrating.
- Headaches, jaw pain, or abdominal pain.
- Digestive problems such as bloating and trouble swallowing.
- Bladder problems such as interstitial cystitis.
- Feelings of numbness or tingling in hands, feet, or other areas.

Other conditions sometimes found in FM patients include irritable bowel syndrome (IBS), restless legs syndrome (RLS), periodic limb movement disorder (PLMD), temporomandibular joint (TMJ) pain, and myofascial pain syndrome (MPS).

How common is fibromyalgia? Who is mainly affected by it?

The National Institute of Arthritis and Musculoskeletal and Skin Diseases (NIAMS) estimates that the number of adults in the United States with FM is about 3.7 million. Other organizations estimate that the number may be as high as 8 million. It mainly occurs in women of childbearing age, but children, the elderly, and men are sometimes diagnosed with FM.

What causes fibromyalgia?

Although the cause of FM is unknown, researchers have several theories about causes or triggers of the disorder. Some scientists believe that an injury or trauma may sometimes cause the syndrome. This injury may affect the central nervous system. FM may be linked to muscle changes that cause fatigue and decreased strength. Others believe that an infection caused by a virus or other agent may trigger FM in susceptible people.

Other possible factors in FM include psychological stress, hormonal changes, or other changes in body chemicals such as serotonin and Substance P. The hormones produced by the hypothalamus-pituitary-adrenal (HPA) axis may be important in FM. Sleep problems, so common in people with FM, may be a cause as well as a symptom of FM. Increased sensitivity to and perception of pain seems to be involved.

How is fibromyalgia diagnosed?

Fibromyalgia is hard to diagnose because many of the symptoms are like those of other disorders. There is no lab test for FM. The American College of Rheumatology (ACR) has developed criteria for FM. According to ACR criteria, a person is considered to have FM if he or she has widespread pain for at least 3 months, and tenderness in at least 11 of 18 specific tender point sites in the neck, spine, shoulders, hips, and knees.

There is some controversy about the criteria for diagnosing FM. Some experts believe that it is not necessary to have at least 11 tender points for diagnosis, or pain that affects all segments of the body at the same time.

How is fibromyalgia treated?

If you have FM, you may need to work with your doctor to find a treatment plan that helps you. FM patients may benefit from a combination of exercise, medicine, physical therapy, and relaxation. There are medicines that may help elevate mood, improve quality of sleep, reduce pain, and relax muscles.

Drug therapies used in fibromyalgia include:

- Drugs for pain. These include aspirin, ibuprofen, and other pain relievers.

- Antidepressants. These drugs can help relieve depression and may also help with sleep. Low doses of certain tricyclic antidepressants and the newer serotonin boosters (SSRIs) are often used.

- Drugs for anxiety (anxiolytics). These medicines can help with anxiety and with sleep.

- Muscle relaxants such as cyclobenzaprine.

Exercise, including low-impact aerobic exercise (such as walking and swimming) and strength training have been found to be helpful in FM patients. But it is important to pace yourself and not overdo it. Exercise may help you increase your flexibility and strength, help with pain and sleep, and make you feel better in general. Heat and massage may also give short-term relief from pain and stiffness.

Cognitive behavioral therapy (focuses on helping you develop ways to manage your illness) is another form of treatment that can be helpful. Stress reduction and a healthy lifestyle are also important.

Chapter 60

Lupus

What is systemic lupus erythematosus (SLE) or lupus?

SLE, usually referred to as lupus, is an autoimmune disease. Autoimmune diseases are illnesses in which the immune system becomes overactive and attacks healthy body tissue. This tendency for the immune system to become overactive seems to run in families. Other factors, such as exposure to infections or other environmental triggers, are also thought to be involved. Lupus affects many more women than men, and black women more than white women.

Lupus can affect the joints, skin, kidneys, heart, lungs, blood vessels, and brain, causing inflammation and damage. For most people, lupus is a mild disease affecting only a few organs. For others, it can be disabling and cause serious and even life-threatening problems. One in five people with the disease are disabled, most commonly from fatigue and joint and muscle pain. Fifteen to 20 percent of all cases of lupus result in death, often from kidney disease, infection, and cardiovascular disease.

Currently, there is no cure for lupus. However, with early diagnosis and treatment, symptoms can usually be managed. Most people with the disease can lead active, healthy lives.

Excerpted from the publication by the U.S. Department of Health and Human Services, National Women's Health Information Center (NWHIC), August 2002. Available online at http://www.4woman.gov; accessed July 2003.

Who has lupus?

Surveys have shown that lupus affects up to 2 million people in the United States. About 9 out of 10 people who have lupus are women. Lupus is three times more common in black women than in white women. It is also more common in women of Hispanic, Asian, and Native American descent. Researchers are trying to learn why these women are more likely to get lupus.

The disease often starts between the ages of 15 and 44. In some people, lupus becomes active after exposure to sunlight, infections, or certain medicines.

What are the different kinds of lupus?

There are several forms of lupus:

- Systemic lupus erythematosus (SLE) is the form of the disease that most people are referring to when they say lupus. SLE can affect many parts of the body including joints, skin, kidney, lungs, heart and brain. Its symptoms can range from mild to serious. Although SLE usually develops in people between the ages of 15 and 44 years, it can occur in childhood or later in life as well.

- Discoid lupus erythematosus (DLE) mainly affects the skin. It causes a red, raised rash on the face, scalp, or other parts of the body. The rash may become thick and scaly and may last for days or years. A small percentage of people with DLE later develop SLE.

- Drug-induced lupus is a rare reaction to some prescription medicines. It resembles SLE, but is less serious. Symptoms go away when the drug is stopped.

- Neonatal lupus can affect some newborn babies of women with SLE or certain other immune system disorders. Babies with neonatal lupus may have a serious heart defect. Other affected babies may have a skin rash, liver problems, or low blood counts. Neonatal lupus is very rare, and most infants of mothers with SLE are healthy.

How is lupus treated?

Because the signs of lupus often differ from one person to another, treatment varies. There is no known cure today for lupus. However, in many cases, symptoms of the disease can be relieved. The good news is that with the correct medicine and by taking care of themselves, most persons with lupus can hold jobs, have children, and lead full lives.

Once lupus has been diagnosed, the doctor will develop a treatment plan. The plan is based on the person's age, gender, health, symptoms, and lifestyle. Tailored to the person's needs, this plan may change over time. Treatment is used to prevent flares, to effectively treat them when they do occur, and to reduce complications.

Treatment may include:

- Aspirin or similar medicine to treat the painful, swollen joints and the fever
- Creams to treat the rash
- Stronger medicines for more serious problems, based on the person's individual symptoms and needs
- Physical and emotional rest
- Protection from direct sunlight
- A healthful diet and exercise
- Prompt treatment of infections
- Avoidance of known allergens and aggravating factors

Drugs used in treating lupus include:

- Nonsteroidal anti-inflammatory drugs (NSAIDs)
- Antimalarial drugs
- Corticosteroid hormones
- Immunosuppressive agents

New drug treatments are being tested, including hormonal treatments. Working closely with the doctor helps ensure that treatments for lupus are as successful as possible. Because some treatments may cause harmful side effects, it is important to promptly report any new symptoms to the doctor.

It is also important not to stop or change treatments without talking to the doctor first. With early diagnosis and the correct treatment and medication, most people with lupus can maintain an overall high quality of life.

Chapter 61

Carpal Tunnel Syndrome

What is carpal tunnel syndrome (CTS)?

Carpal tunnel syndrome occurs when tendons in the wrist become inflamed after being aggravated. Tendons can become aggravated when the carpals (a tunnel of bones) and the ligaments in the wrist narrow, pinching nerves that reach the fingers and the muscle at the base of the thumb. Repetitive flexing and extension of the wrist may cause a thickening of the protective sheaths that surround each of the tendons, which narrows the tunnel. Women are three times more likely to develop CTS than men, and the risk increases with age. People between the ages of 40 and 60 are more commonly affected.

What are the symptoms of CTS?

The first symptoms usually appear at night. Symptoms range from a burning, tingling numbness in the fingers (especially the thumb and the index and middle fingers) to difficulty in gripping or making a fist. Many patients with CTS are unable to differentiate hot from cold by touch, and they experience an apparent loss of strength in their fingers. They might appear clumsy because they have trouble performing simple tasks such as tying their shoes or picking up small objects.

Excerpted from the U.S. Department of Health and Human Services, National Women's Health Information Center (NWHIC), June 2001. Available online at http://www.4woman.gov; accessed August 2003.

In advanced cases, the thenar muscle at the base of the thumb atrophies, and strength is lost.

What causes CTS?

Although there are many reasons for developing this swelling of the tendon, it can result from repetitive and forceful movements of the wrist during work and leisure activities. Research by the National Institute for Occupational Safety and Health (NIOSH) indicates that job tasks involving highly repetitive manual acts, or necessitating wrist bending or other stressful wrist postures, are connected with incidents of CTS or related problems. Moreover, it is apparent that this hazard is not confined to a single industry or job but occurs in many occupations, especially those in the manufacturing sector. Jobs involving cutting, small parts assembly, finishing, sewing, and cleaning seem predominantly associated with the syndrome. The factor common in these jobs is the repetitive use of small hand tools. CTS can also be due to trauma from repetitive work such as that of supermarket checkers, checkers in other types of stores, assembly line workers, meat packers, typists, word-processors, accountants, and writers.

How is CTS treated?

CTS is treated by immobilizing the wrist in a splint. Then, either anti-inflammatory drugs or injections of cortisone are used to reduce swelling in the wrist. There is also a surgical procedure in which doctors can open the wrist and cut the ligament at the bottom of the wrist to relieve the pressure. However, only a small percentage of patients require surgery.

Is there a cure for CTS?

Most people with CTS recover completely and can avoid re-injury by changing the way they do repetitive movements, the frequency with which they do the movements, and the amount of time they rest between periods when they perform the movements. Approximately 1 percent of individuals with CTS develop permanent injury.

How can I prevent CTS?

You can help prevent CTS by taking the following precautions:

- Reduce your force and relax your grip. Studies show that most people use four to five times more force than necessary to perform most tasks involving the hands. If your work involves hitting keys, hit them softly. If you frequently write by hand, use a big pen with an oversized, soft grip adapter and free-flowing ink. This way, you will not have to grip the pen tightly or press hard on the paper.

- Take frequent breaks. Every 15 to 20 minutes, give your hands and wrists a break by gently stretching and bending them. Also alternate tasks when possible. For example, type for 15 minutes then do some phone work for 5 minutes. If you use equipment that vibrates or on which you exert a great amount of force, taking breaks is even more important.

- Watch your form. Avoid bending your wrist all the way up or down. A relaxed middle position is best. If you use a keyboard, keep it at elbow height or slightly lower.

- Improve your posture. The tendency to roll the shoulders forward shortens the neck and shoulder muscles, compressing nerves in the neck. This, in turn, can affect the wrist, fingers, and hand.

- Keep your hands warm. You're more likely to develop carpal tunnel syndrome if you work in a cold environment. If you can't control the temperature at work, put on fingerless gloves that keep your hands and wrists warm.

- Use ergonomically designed equipment. If you use a computer, try using a track ball instead of a mouse if you're on a computer all day, or position your keyboard at elbow height or lower so that it reduces stress and increases efficiency. Also try to use proper seating. The height of your seat and position of your backrest should be adjustable. The chair should be on wheels so you can move easily, and arm rests are also helpful.

On a large scale, the Centers for Disease Control and Prevention (CDC) recommends the redesign of tools or tool handles to enable the user's wrist to maintain a more natural position during work. Other recommendations have involved modifying the layouts of workstations. Other approaches include altering the existing method for performing the job task, providing more frequent rest breaks, and rotating workers across jobs.

Chapter 62

Urinary Tract Disorders

Chapter Contents

Section 62.1

Urinary Incontinence in Women

Excerpted from "Urinary Incontinence in Women," produced by the National Institutes of Health, National Institute of Diabetes and Digestive and Kidney Diseases, NIH Pub. No. 02-4132, April 2002. Available online at http://www.niddk.nih.gov; accessed July 2003.

Urinary incontinence is an inability to hold your urine until you get to a toilet. More than 13 million people in the United States—male and female, young and old—experience incontinence. It is often temporary, and it always results from an underlying medical condition.

Women experience incontinence twice as often as men. Pregnancy and childbirth, menopause, and the structure of the female urinary tract account for this difference. But both women and men can become incontinent from neurologic injury, birth defects, strokes, multiple sclerosis, and physical problems associated with aging.

Older women, more often than younger women, experience incontinence. But incontinence is not inevitable with age. Incontinence is treatable and often curable at all ages. If you experience incontinence, you may feel embarrassed. It may help you to remember that loss of bladder control can be treated. You will need to overcome your embarrassment and see a doctor to learn if you need treatment for an underlying medical condition.

Incontinence in women usually occurs because of problems with muscles that help to hold or release urine. The body stores urine—water and wastes removed by the kidneys—in the bladder, a balloon-like organ. The bladder connects to the urethra, the tube through which urine leaves the body.

During urination, muscles in the wall of the bladder contract, forcing urine out of the bladder and into the urethra. At the same time, sphincter muscles surrounding the urethra relax, letting urine pass out of the body. Incontinence will occur if your bladder muscles suddenly contract or muscles surrounding the urethra suddenly relax.

What Are the Types of Incontinence?

Stress Incontinence

If coughing, laughing, sneezing, or other movements that put pressure on the bladder cause you to leak urine, you may have stress incontinence. Physical changes resulting from pregnancy, childbirth, and menopause often cause stress incontinence. It is the most common form of incontinence in women and is treatable.

Pelvic floor muscles support your bladder. If these muscles weaken, your bladder can move downward, pushing slightly out of the bottom of the pelvis toward the vagina. This prevents muscles that ordinarily force the urethra shut from squeezing as tightly as they should. As a result, urine can leak into the urethra during moments of physical stress. Stress incontinence also occurs if the muscles that do the squeezing weaken.

Stress incontinence can worsen during the week before your menstrual period. At that time, lowered estrogen levels might lead to lower muscular pressure around the urethra, increasing chances of leakage. The incidence of stress incontinence increases following menopause.

Urge Incontinence

If you lose urine for no apparent reason while suddenly feeling the need or urge to urinate, you may have urge incontinence. The most common cause of urge incontinence is inappropriate bladder contractions.

Medical professionals describe such a bladder as unstable, spastic, or overactive. Your doctor might call your condition reflex incontinence if it results from overactive nerves controlling the bladder.

Urge incontinence can mean that your bladder empties during sleep, after drinking a small amount of water, or when you touch water or hear it running (as when washing dishes or hearing someone else taking a shower).

Involuntary actions of bladder muscles can occur because of damage to the nerves of the bladder, to the nervous system (spinal cord and brain), or to the muscles themselves. Multiple sclerosis, Parkinson's disease, Alzheimer's disease, stroke, and injury—including injury that occurs during surgery—all can harm bladder nerves or muscles.

Functional Incontinence

People with functional incontinence may have problems thinking, moving, or communicating that prevent them from reaching a toilet.

A person with Alzheimer's disease, for example, may not think well enough to plan a timely trip to a restroom. A person in a wheelchair may be blocked from getting to a toilet in time. Conditions such as these are often associated with age and account for some of the incontinence of elderly women in nursing homes.

Overflow Incontinence

If your bladder is always full so that it frequently leaks urine, you have overflow incontinence. Weak bladder muscles or a blocked urethra can cause this type of incontinence. Nerve damage from diabetes or other diseases can lead to weak bladder muscles; tumors and urinary stones can block the urethra. Overflow incontinence is rare in women.

Other Types of Incontinence

Stress and urge incontinence often occur together in women. Combinations of incontinence—and this combination in particular—are sometimes referred to as mixed incontinence.

Transient incontinence is a temporary version of incontinence. It can be triggered by medications, urinary tract infections, mental impairment, restricted mobility, and stool impaction (severe constipation), which can push against the urinary tract and obstruct outflow.

How Is Incontinence Evaluated?

The first step toward relief is to see a doctor who is well acquainted with incontinence to learn the type you have. A urologist specializes in the urinary tract, and some urologists further specialize in the female urinary tract. Gynecologists and obstetricians specialize in the female reproductive tract and childbirth. A urogynecologist focuses on urological problems in women. Family practitioners and internists see patients for all kinds of complaints. Any of these doctors may be able to help you.

To diagnose the problem, your doctor will first ask about symptoms and medical history. Your pattern of voiding and urine leakage may suggest the type of incontinence. Other obvious factors that can help define the problem include straining and discomfort, use of drugs, recent surgery, and illness. If your medical history does not define the problem, it will at least suggest which tests are needed.

Your doctor will physically examine you for signs of medical conditions causing incontinence, such as tumors that block the urinary tract, stool impaction, and poor reflexes or sensations, which may be evidence of a nerve-related cause.

Your doctor will measure your bladder capacity and residual urine for evidence of poorly functioning bladder muscles. To do this, you will drink plenty of fluids and urinate into a measuring pan, after which the doctor will measure any urine remaining in the bladder.

Your doctor may also recommend

- Stress test—You relax, then cough vigorously as the doctor watches for loss of urine.

- Urinalysis—Urine is tested for evidence of infection, urinary stones, or other contributing causes.

- Blood tests—Blood is taken, sent to a laboratory, and examined for substances related to causes of incontinence.

- Ultrasound—Sound waves are used to see the kidneys, ureters, bladder, and urethra.

- Cystoscopy—A thin tube with a tiny camera is inserted in the urethra and used to see the inside of the urethra and bladder.

- Urodynamics—Various techniques measure pressure in the bladder and the flow of urine.

Your doctor may ask you to keep a diary for a day or more, up to a week, to record when you void. This diary should note the times you urinate and the amounts of urine you produce. To measure your urine, you can use a special pan that fits over the toilet rim.

Section 62.2

Bladder Control for Women

Excerpted from "Bladder Control for Women," a booklet produced by the National Institutes of Health, National Institute of Diabetes and Digestive and Kidney Diseases, NIH Pub. No. 03-4195, May 2003. Available online at http://www.niddk.nih.gov; accessed July 2003.

Why Talk about Bladder Control?

Women of all ages have bladder control problems. Some younger women find they can't hold their urine after having a baby. Others have problems when they stop having periods. Many women over the age of 75 also have bladder control problems.

You may feel ashamed about bladder control problems. Remember that it's a medical problem and it's not your fault. Millions of women have the same problem.

Don't believe people who tell you that urine leakage is normal. It isn't. Most of the time it can be improved.

Your health care team can help you. Nearly everyone with a bladder control problem can be helped. Call your clinic and find out how.

What Does the Doctor Need to Know?

You will need to keep a record. Try to write down the times when you go to the bathroom. Write down when you have accidents, too. Do this for a day or more. This record is called a bladder control diary. Diaries help your doctor or nurse learn the cause of your problem.

Will the Doctor Do Tests?

You will probably have a physical exam. The exam can show the reasons for your bladder control problem. First, your health care team will look for a simple cause. It could be an infection in the urinary tract. This can be treated easily.

The reason for your problem may be harder to find. Then the doctor or nurse may want to do some tests:

- Check to see how well the bladder muscles are doing their jobs.

- Take samples of urine and blood for tests.

- Look for something blocking the urine flow—like a stone, a growth, or hard bowel movement or stool.

- Take pictures of your bladder, using special machines.

What Is the Treatment for Bladder Control Problems?

Your treatment will depend on the type of bladder control problem you have. Some treatments are simple. Others are more complicated.

Your health care team may suggest one of the following treatments:

Do-It-Yourself Treatments

- Pelvic muscle exercises. You can learn simple exercises that can strengthen the muscles near the urethra. These are called pelvic muscle exercises or Kegel exercises and take only a few minutes a day.

- Bladder training. You can train your bladder to hold urine better. Follow a timetable to store and release urine. You can also learn to decrease the urge to urinate.

- Weight loss. Sometimes extra weight causes bladder control problems. A good meal plan and exercise program can lead to weight loss.

- Food and drink. Some drinks and foods may make urine control harder. These include foods with caffeine (coffee, tea, cola, or chocolate) and alcohol. Your health care team can suggest how to change your diet for better bladder control.

Muscle Therapy

- Electrical stimulation. Certain devices stimulate the muscles around the urethra. This makes the muscles stronger and tighter.

- Biofeedback. This takes the guesswork out of pelvic muscle exercise. A therapist places a patch over the muscles. A wire connects the patch to a TV screen. You watch the screen to see if you are exercising the right muscles. The therapist will help you. Soon you learn to control these muscles without the patch or screen.

573

Medical Treatments

- Medicines. Certain drugs can tighten or strengthen urethral and pelvic floor muscles. Other medicines can calm overactive bladder muscles and nerves. A skin patch can be worn to treat symptoms of overactive bladder.

- Surgery. Some bladder control problems can be solved by surgery. Many different operations can improve bladder control. The operation depends on what is causing the problem. In most cases, the surgeon changes the position of the bladder and urethra. After the operation, the bladder control muscles work better.

Devices

- Pessary. Your doctor can place a special device called a pessary in the vagina. The device will hold up the bladder to prevent leakage.

- Urethral inserts. Your doctor may give you a small device that goes directly in the urethra. You can learn to insert the device yourself. It's like a little plug. You remove the device when it is time to go to the bathroom and then replace it until it's time to go again.

- Urine seals. This is a small foam pad you place over the urethra opening. There it seals itself against your body to keep urine from leaking. When you go to the bathroom, you remove the pad and throw it away.

Soon you will be able to buy new products to help control leaks. However, they do not cure the causes of bladder control problems.

Dryness Aids

- Pads or diapers. Pads or diapers help many people. But diapers do not cure bladder control problems. See a doctor or nurse, even if diapers are working for you.

- Bedside urinal. Some people use a bed pan or a bedside chair urinal or commode.

- Assistance. If you are disabled, health care workers can help you move more easily to a toilet. Your doctor or nurse may teach you to urinate on a schedule that prevents wetting.

- Renovations. Sometimes, you just need a carpenter to make changes to your house. Perhaps you need a hallway light. Or a downstairs bathroom. Another solution could be widening a bathroom door to fit a wheelchair.

Section 62.3

Exercising Your Pelvic Muscles

Excerpted from "Exercising Your Pelvic Muscles," produced by the National Institutes of Health, National Institute of Diabetes and Digestive and Kidney Diseases, NIH Pub. No. 02-4188, April 2002. Available online at http://www.niddk.nih.gov; accessed July 2003.

Why Exercise Pelvic Muscles?

Life's events can weaken pelvic muscles. Pregnancy, childbirth, and being overweight can do it. Luckily, when these muscles get weak, you can help make them strong again.

Pelvic floor muscles are just like other muscles. Exercise can make them stronger. Women with bladder control problems can regain control through pelvic muscle exercises, also called Kegel exercises.

Pelvic Fitness in Minutes a Day

Exercising your pelvic floor muscles for just 5 minutes, three times a day can make a big difference to your bladder control. Exercise strengthens muscles that hold the bladder and many other organs in place.

The part of your body including your hip bones is the pelvic area. At the bottom of the pelvis, several layers of muscle stretch between your legs. The muscles attach to the front, back, and sides of the pelvis bone.

Two pelvic muscles do most of the work. The biggest one stretches like a hammock. The other is shaped like a triangle. These muscles prevent leaking of urine and stool.

How Do You Exercise Your Pelvic Muscles?

Find the right muscles. This is very important. Your doctor, nurse, or physical therapist will help make sure you are doing the exercises the right way.

You should tighten the two major muscles that stretch across your pelvic floor. They are the hammock muscle and the triangle muscle. Here are three methods to check for the correct muscles.

- Try to stop the flow of urine when you are sitting on the toilet. If you can do it, you are using the right muscles.

- Imagine that you are trying to stop passing gas. Squeeze the muscles you would use. If you sense a pulling feeling, those are the right muscles for pelvic exercises.

- Lie down and put your finger inside your vagina. Squeeze as if you were trying to stop urine from coming out. If you feel tightness on your finger, you are squeezing the right pelvic muscle.

Don't squeeze other muscles at the same time. Be careful not to tighten your stomach, legs, or other muscles. Squeezing the wrong muscles can put more pressure on your bladder control muscles. Just squeeze the pelvic muscle. Don't hold your breath.

Repeat, but don't overdo it. At first, find a quiet spot to practice—your bathroom or bedroom—so you can concentrate. Lie on the floor. Pull in the pelvic muscles and hold for a count of 3. Then relax for a count of 3. Work up to 10 to 15 repeats each time you exercise.

Do your pelvic exercises at least three times a day. Every day, use three positions: lying down, sitting, and standing. You can exercise while lying on the floor, sitting at a desk, or standing in the kitchen. Using all three positions makes the muscles strongest.

Be patient. Don't give up. It's just 5 minutes, three times a day. You may not feel your bladder control improve until after 3 to 6 weeks. Still, most women do notice an improvement after a few weeks.

Exercise aids. You can also exercise by using special weights or biofeedback. Ask your health care team about these exercise aids.

Hold the Squeeze until after the Sneeze

You can protect your pelvic muscles from more damage by bracing yourself.

Think ahead, just before sneezing, lifting, or jumping. Sudden pressure from such actions can hurt those pelvic muscles. Squeeze your pelvic muscles tightly and hold on until after you sneeze, lift, or jump.

After you train yourself to tighten the pelvic muscles for these moments, you will have fewer accidents.

Section 62.4

Urinary Tract Infections

Excerpted from "Urinary Tract Infections," U.S. Department of Health and Human Services, National Women's Health Information Center (NWHIC), October 2002. The complete document is available online at http://www. 4woman.gov; accessed July 2003.

What is the urinary tract?

Your urinary tract includes the organs that collect and store urine and release it from your body. These organs include the kidneys, which remove liquid waste from the blood in the form of urine, keep a balance of salts and other substances in the blood, and produce a hormone that helps form red blood cells. It also includes the ureters or narrow tubes that carry urine from the kidneys to the bladder, the triangle-shaped chamber in the lower abdomen that stores urine; and the urethra, a tube that carries the urine as it leaves the body.

What are urinary tract infections (UTIs)?

A urinary tract infection (UTI) is an infection anywhere in the urinary tract. Normal urine is sterile. It contains fluids, salts, and waste products, but it is free of bacteria, viruses, and fungi. An infection occurs when microorganisms, usually bacteria from the digestive tract, cling to the urethra, or opening to the urinary tract, and begin to multiply.

What causes UTIs?

Most infections are caused by one type of bacteria, *Escherichia coli* (*E. coli*), which normally live in the colon. In most cases, bacteria first begin growing in the urethra and often move on to the bladder, causing a bladder infection or cystitis. If an infection is not treated quickly, bacteria could then travel up the ureters to infect the kidneys. This serious condition is called pyelonephritis.

Microorganisms called chlamydia and mycoplasma can also cause UTIs in both women and men. These infections usually occur in the urethra and reproductive system (the uterus, or womb, and the ovaries and fallopian tubes). Unlike *E. coli*, chlamydia and mycoplasma can be sexually transmitted, and both partners should be treated for the infection.

Some women have a long-lasting condition called interstitial cystitis, also known as painful bladder syndrome or frequency-urgency-dysuria syndrome. With this condition, the wall of the bladder becomes inflamed or irritated, which affects the amount of urine the bladder can hold. Interstitial cystitis can cause scarring, stiffening, and bleeding in the bladder. This complex condition is different from a UTI, and scientists do not know what causes it.

What are the symptoms of a UTI?

Not everyone with a UTI has symptoms, but most people get at least some signs. They can range from slightly irritating to very painful. Symptoms include a frequent urge to urinate, but only passing a small amount of urine and a burning sensation, pressure, or pain in the area of the bladder or when urinating. The urine itself may look milky or cloudy, even reddish if blood is present. It is not unusual to feel tired, shaky or washed out. Often, women feel an uncomfortable pressure above the pubic bone, and some men feel fullness in the rectum. A fever may mean the infection has reached the kidneys. Other symptoms of a kidney infection include pain in your back or your side below the ribs, nausea or vomiting, and chills. It is very important to see your health care provider at the first sign of pain, irritation, or blood when you urinate or if you have discomfort in or near your abdomen, back, or sides. An untreated UTI can lead to a kidney infection. An untreated or recurrent kidney infection can lead to scarring of the kidneys and permanent kidney damage.

How is a UTI diagnosed?

To find out whether you have a UTI, your health care provider will test a sample of urine for pus and bacteria. You will be asked to give a clean catch urine sample by washing the genital area and collecting a midstream sample of urine in a sterile container. (This method of collecting urine helps prevent bacteria around the genital area from getting into the sample and confusing the test results.) The urine sample is then sent to the laboratory to be examined for white and red blood cells and bacteria. Then the bacteria are allowed to multiply in a culture. After the bacteria grow, it is tested against different antibiotics to see which drug best destroys the bacteria. This last step is called a sensitivity test. Although your health care provider may begin treatment before the bacterial cultures are back from the lab, the cultures will confirm the diagnosis and may cause a change in the antibiotic your health care provider chooses for you.

If the UTI doesn't clear up with treatment, or if you have had several bladder infections, you may need a test called a cystoscopy. A flexible tube with a light and camera is inserted into the bladder to remove samples of urine and tissue. Your health care provider might order other tests that produce pictures, or images, of the urinary tract, such as the intravenous pyelogram (IVP). This text provides x-ray images of the bladder, kidneys, and ureters. Another imaging test you might need is an ultrasound exam, which gives pictures from the echo patterns of sound waves bounced back from internal organs.

One test allows women with frequent infections to test their first-morning urine sample by themselves. Dipsticks (a type of testing paper that looks like a stick, which you can dip into a sample of your urine) that change color when an infection is present are now available in drug stores without a prescription.

How is a UTI treated?

UTIs are treated with antibiotics (a medicine that kills bacteria), usually for seven to ten days. For some infections, however, you may only need a single dose of an antibiotic. The choice of antibiotic and length of treatment depend on your health history and the type of bacteria causing the infection. The antibiotic drugs most often used to treat UTIs are

- trimethoprim (Trimpex)
- trimethoprim/sulfamethoxazole or TMP/SMZ (Bactrim, Septra, Cotrim)
- amoxicillin (Amoxil, Trimox, Wymox)
- nitrofurantoin (Macrodantin, Furadantin)
- ampicillin

Other antibiotics are sometimes used as well, including ofloxacin (Floxin), norfloxacin (Noroxin), ciprofloxacin (Cipro), and trovafloxacin (Trovan). Some antibiotics are not safe to take during pregnancy. Talk with your health care provider about the risks and benefits of taking the different medications.

Getting proper treatment will prevent your urinary tract problems from getting worse and affecting other parts of your body. You can help prevent kidney infections by seeing your health care provider as soon as you have symptoms of a UTI. If you are in pain, ask your health care provider to prescribe a pain reliever since various drugs are available. A heating pad may also help.

What if I keep getting UTIs?

Most healthy women do not get repeat infections. However, women who have had three UTIs are likely to continue having them. Four out of five of these women get another UTI within 18 months of the last UTI. Many women have them even more often. If you have frequent infections (three or more a year), ask your health care provider about one of the following treatment options:

- Taking low doses of an antibiotic, such as TMP/SMZ or nitrofurantoin, daily for six months or longer. Research has shown this therapy to be effective without causing serious side effects.

- Taking a single dose of an antibiotic after sexual intercourse.

- Taking a short course (one or two days) of antibiotics when symptoms appear.

Are there steps I can take to prevent a UTI?

Drink plenty of water every day to help flush bacteria out of your system. Some health care providers suggest drinking cranberry juice or taking Vitamin C (ascorbic acid) supplements, which keep the number of bacteria in your system down. Cleanse the area around the rectum and vagina each day. Urinate when you feel the need (or about every two to three hours, and before and after sex). Wipe the genital area from front to back to prevent bacteria from entering the vagina or urethra. It also helps to take showers instead of baths; avoid irritating douches and feminine hygiene sprays; and wear panties with a cotton crotch, which absorbs moisture. Some women say drinking a lot of water after sexual activity helps to prevent new infections.

Section 62.5

Interstitial Cystitis

Excerpted from "Interstitial Cystitis," U.S. Department of Health and Human Services, National Women's Health Information Center (NWHIC), October 2002. Available online at http://www.4woman.gov; accessed July 2003.

What is interstitial cystitis?

Interstitial cystitis (IC) is a chronic bladder condition that can cause pain and other symptoms. People with IC have an inflamed or irritated bladder wall. This inflammation can lead to: scarring and stiffening of the bladder; less bladder capacity (the bladder is able to hold less urine); and pinpoint bleeding in the bladder lining. In rare cases, ulcers form in the bladder lining.

Of the more than 700,000 Americans estimated to have IC, about 90 percent are women. Severe cases of IC can be very disabling.

What are the causes of interstitial cystitis?

No one knows what causes interstitial cystitis. Because IC varies so much in symptoms and severity, most researchers believe that it may actually be several diseases. One theory being studied is that IC is an autoimmune response following a bladder infection. Another theory is that there are substances in urine which are irritating to people with IC. Other theories are also being studied. Interstitial cystitis is different from urinary tract infections, which are caused by bacteria and can be treated with antibiotics. Studies have shown that antibiotics are not useful for treating IC.

What are some symptoms and signs of interstitial cystitis?

The symptoms of IC vary from person to person and even in the same person. People with IC may experience mild discomfort, pressure, tenderness, or intense pain in the bladder and surrounding pelvic area. Symptoms may include an urgent need to urinate (urgency), frequent need to urinate (frequency), or a combination of these symptoms. Pain may change in intensity as the bladder fills with urine or as it empties. Women's symptoms often get worse during their periods. Pain during sex is common.

Some people find that their bladders cannot hold much urine, which increases the frequency of urination. Yet some people with severe frequency have bladders that can hold a normal amount of urine. People with severe cases of IC may urinate as many as 60 times during a 24-hour period.

How is interstitial cystitis diagnosed?

The first step in diagnosing IC is to rule out other conditions that may be causing the symptoms. Other possible causes of the symptoms found in IC include urinary tract or vaginal infections, bladder cancer, endometriosis, sexually transmitted diseases, and kidney stones. Various tests on the patient's urine, bladder, and urinary tract may be done.

The most important test to confirm IC is a cystoscopy done under anesthesia. This test uses an instrument called a cystoscope to see inside the bladder. A liquid or gas is used to stretch the bladder. Anesthesia is required because stretching the bladder can be very painful for a person with IC. This test can detect bladder wall inflammation, pinpoint bleeding or ulcers, a thick, stiff bladder wall, and maximum bladder capacity.

Diagnosis of IC is based on: the presence of urinary urgency, urinary frequency, or bladder/pelvic pain; bladder wall inflammation, including pinpoint bleeding or ulcers, found by cystoscopy; the absence of other diseases that could cause the symptoms.

Is there a cure for interstitial cystitis?

Scientists have not yet found a cure for interstitial cystitis, nor can they predict who will respond best to which treatment. Symptoms may go away for no reason or at the same time as a change in diet or treatment. Even when symptoms go away, however, they may return after days, weeks, months, or years. Scientists do not know why. Because the causes of IC are unknown, treatments are aimed at relieving symptoms.

How is interstitial cystitis treated?

Treatments for IC include:

- Oral medicines, including pentosan polysulfate sodium (Elmiron), which the Food and Drug Administration (FDA) approved for IC treatment in 1996. (Because Elmiron has not been tested in pregnant women, it is not recommended for use during pregnancy, except in severe cases.) Other oral medicines used include aspirin and ibuprofen, stronger painkillers, antidepressants, and antihistamines.

- Bladder instillation (a bladder wash or bath). During bladder instillation, the bladder is filled with a solution that is held for varying periods of time before being emptied. The only drug approved to date by the FDA for use in bladder instillation is dimethyl sulfoxide (DMSO). Other drugs for this use are being studied.

- Transcutaneous electrical nerve stimulation (TENS), which delivers mild electric pulses to the bladder area. Scientists do not know exactly how TENS works, but it helps relieve pain and urinary frequency in some people. Sacral nerve stimulation implants are being studied as another way to relieve IC symptoms.

- Self-help strategies such as bladder training, dietary changes, stress reduction, and low-impact exercise.

- Surgery, considered a treatment of last resort. Surgery does not necessarily improve symptoms.

How does diet affect interstitial cystitis?

There is no scientific evidence linking diet to IC, but some people believe that alcohol, tomatoes, spices, chocolate, caffeinated and citrus beverages, and high-acid foods may add to bladder irritation and inflammation. Others notice that their symptoms get worse after eating or drinking products containing artificial sweeteners. If you believe certain foods or drinks make your symptoms worse, try avoiding those products. You can reintroduce them one at a time to see which, if any, affect symptoms. It is important, however, to maintain a well-balanced and varied diet.

Chapter 63

Spider and Varicose Veins

What are spider and varicose veins?

Spider veins are formed by the dilation of a small group of blood vessels located close to the surface of the skin. Although they can appear anywhere on the body, spider veins are most commonly found on the face and legs. They usually pose no health hazard but may produce a dull aching in the legs after prolonged standing.

Varicose veins are abnormally swollen or enlarged blood vessels caused by a weakening in the vein's wall. They can be harmful to a patient's health because they may be associated with the development of one or more of the following conditions: phlebitis or inflamed tender vein; thrombosis or a clot in the vein; and venous stasis ulcers or open sores from inadequate tissue oxygen and fluid retention.

Who develops spider and varicose veins?

The exact cause of spider and varicose veins is unknown, although heredity, pregnancy, and hormonal influences are believed to be primary factors contributing to both conditions. More than 20 percent of women have some form of varicose conditions, and more women than men have varicose veins.

Reprinted with permission from the American Society for Dermatologic Surgery, www.asds-net.org. © 2002 American Society for Dermatologic Surgery.

What is sclerotherapy?

Sclerotherapy is considered the gold standard treatment for removing spider and some varicose leg veins. It is a very cost-effective procedure that seldom leaves a scar or produces adverse effects. It is typically performed on an outpatient basis by a dermatologic surgeon. A concentrated saline or specially developed chemical solution is injected with a very small needle into the spider or varicose vein. The solution causes the vein to close up or collapse and become scar tissue that is eventually absorbed by the body. The work of carrying the blood is shifted to other healthy blood vessels nearby.

Sclerotherapy generally requires multiple treatment sessions. One to three injections are usually required to effectively treat any vein. The same area should not be retreated for four to six weeks to allow for complete healing, although other areas may undergo treatment during this time.

Post-treatment therapy includes wearing bandages and support hose for two days to three weeks following treatment. Walking and moderate exercise may also help speed recovery. Although sclerotherapy works for existing spider veins, it does not prevent new ones from developing.

Are there side effects or complications?

Most patients report few, if any minor side effects, which usually disappear in time. Temporary reactions can include a slight swelling of the leg or foot, minor bruising, itching, redness, and moderate soreness.

What are other treatments for vein conditions?

Laser surgery. Laser therapy and intense pulsed light therapy may be effective for certain leg veins and facial blood vessels. The heat from the high-intensity laser beam selectively destroys the abnormal veins.

Electrodesiccation. The veins are sealed off with the application of electrical current. The treatment may leave scars.

Surgical ligation and stripping. Certain varicose veins may require an in-hospital procedure, usually performed by a vascular surgeon, that involves making an incision in the skin and either tying off or removing the damaged blood vessel.

Ambulatory phlebectomy. Removal of undesired veins through a series of tiny incisions along the path of an enlarged vein.

Combined approaches. Your dermatologic surgeon may utilize a combination of techniques and technologies to provide an optimal treatment program for your individual condition and lifestyle.

Chapter 64

Women's Podiatric Concerns

Active Women's Feet

As women move into the U.S. workforce in greater numbers, a lot of them are finding that their professional and white-collar employment brings job satisfaction, but that it's tempered by other realities. One is that the new responsibilities probably haven't replaced those of the woman's once-traditional role as homemaker and mother.

Those roles remain, and many women find themselves not only holding down a full-time salaried position, but still doing the marketing, the child-rearing, and the laundry. Women probably were on their feet a lot more than men before work outside the home beckoned, and their new situations certainly haven't alleviated that. Their feet are taking even more punishment, and the footwear that some feel obliged to wear in the work place may be playing a role.

All this adds up to a need for women to pay more attention to foot care, to avoid subjecting themselves to unnecessary foot problems, particularly those that might be caused by improper footwear and hosiery.

High Heels: Use and Abuse

The wearing of high-heeled shoes is a prime example of women inviting foot problems. Doctors of podiatric medicine see no value in

Reprinted with permission from "Your Podiatric Physician Talks about Women's Feet," a brochure produced by the American Podiatric Medical Association, www.apma.org. © 1997 APMA. Reprinted with permission. Reviewed by David A. Cooke, M.D. on June 30, 2003.

high heels (generally defined as pumps with heels of more than two inches). They believe them to be biomechanically and orthopedically unsound, citing medical, postural, and safety faults of such heels.

They know, for example, that high heels may contribute to knee and back problems, disabling injuries in falls, shortened calf muscles, and an awkward, unnatural gait. In time, high heels may cause enough changes in the feet to impair their proper function. Most women admit high heels make their feet hurt, but they tolerate the discomfort in order to look taller, stylish, and more professional. In a Gallup Poll, 37 percent of the women surveyed said they would continue to wear high heels, even though they did not think them comfortable.

Toward Greater Comfort

If women persist in wearing high heels, there are ways to relieve some of the abusive effects; they can limit the time they wear them, for example, alternating with good-quality oxford-type shoes or flats for part of the day. High heels that are too tight compound the abuse; it's good advice to buy shoes in the afternoon because feet tend to increase in size later in the day.

Women have other heel-size choices, fortunately. They don't have to endure pain at the expense of their foot health. The key is wearing the right shoe for the right activity—and that means varying heel height, determining what heel is most suitable.

For example, there are comfortable and attractive walking pumps (also called comfort or performance pumps) for women for work and social activities. The shoe manufacturers who have introduced them seek a marriage of fashion considerations and comfort, offering fashionable pumps with athletic shoe-derived construction, with reinforced heels and wider toe room. They are using space-age materials, like long-lasting memory cushioning that acts as a shock absorber. And the soles are more pliable.

Several companies have also designed footwear for certain athletic activities, including aerobics, specifically for women.

Perhaps the best shoe for women, from an orthopedic point of view, is a walking shoe with ties (not a slip-on), a Vibram type composition sole, and a relatively wider heel, no more than a half or three-quarters of an inch in height—even though such a shoe may not be widely acceptable in the workplace.

What about Stockings?

Women who always wear nylon pantyhose are also inviting foot problems. Nylon is occlusive—it doesn't breathe—and the heat that it generates and traps causes excessive perspiration. A warm, damp area is an ideal place for the encouragement of fungal infections such as athlete's foot. (Pantyhose aren't the only apparel that cause excessive perspiration; the dress boots and shoe boots many women don in cold weather shouldn't be worn all day in an office.) Nylon, which tends to be abrasive, is even more so when it's damp; in a tight shoe that's already irritating, it offers little protection against blisters. Support hose, because they're so much tighter, can be the worst culprits of all.

Inexpensive nylon pantyhose can also cause forefoot problems, because the stretch mechanism constricts normal expansion of the foot when walking, and may pull the toes backward when the pantyhose ride up. The cramping and pressure of the hose can contribute to ingrown toenails and hammertoes. A better quality nylon will provide a better fit, and the better the fit, the less likely it is that cramping will occur. Women's feet have grown larger because of improved health care and nutrition. The one-size-fits-all stocking no longer is the universal answer, if it ever was. Attention to proper fit is essential.

Pregnancy

Pregnant women need to observe good foot health to prevent pain and discomfort. Since the body undergoes changes and acquires a new weight-bearing stance, women should wear shoes with broad-based heels that provide support and absorb shock. Additional body weight also calls for more support, to prevent foot breakdown.

The expectant mother often experiences more than ordinary swelling of her feet and ankles, which can aggravate existing foot conditions and promote inflammation or irritation. Pregnancy also triggers the release of hormones that enhance laxity in ligaments, which can contribute to foot strain. If problems develop, she should see a podiatric physician.

Women over 65

Older women have more trouble with their feet than younger ones, for the simple reason that fat pads on the bottom of the feet tend to deteriorate in the aging process. They can alleviate some foot problems by wearing properly fitted, well-constructed shoes—shoes which provide cushioning and have a soft, flexible upper that will conform to the shape of their feet. They also need leather shoes that breathe and can reduce the possibility of skin irritation. Soles should be lightweight, with enough flexibility and shock-absorbing quality to provide solid footing and not be slippery. Low-heeled shoes provide greater stability, more protection for the feet, and greater comfort. Because older women often have circulatory problems, they have a special need to keep their feet warm in cold weather, to prevent frostbite or chilblains.

Women's Foot Afflictions

Whether the sources are congenital problems, foot abuse, high heels, poorly fitting shoes, or other maltreatment of the feet, women are subject to a number of afflictions involving the feet (most of which can also occur to men):

- **Achilles tendinitis:** inflammation of the Achilles tendon, the link between the calf muscle and heel bone. Those who wear high heels regularly can expect to acquire shortened tendons; switching to low heels for strenuous physical activity without appropriate warm-up exercises creates an ideal scenario for Achilles tendinitis.

- **Bunions:** misaligned big toe joints that become swollen and tender. Bunions tend to be familial, but the tendency can be aggravated by shoes that are too narrow in the forefoot and toe.

- **Hammertoe:** a condition in which the toe is contracted in a claw-like position. Although the condition usually stems from muscle imbalance, it is often aggravated by ill-fitting shoes, socks, or hosiery that cramp the toes.

- **Metatarsalgia:** general pain in the ball of the foot; often caused by wearing high heels.

- **Neuromas:** enlarged, benign growths of nerves, most commonly between the third and fourth toes. They may stem, in part, from ill-fitting shoes, resulting in pain, burning, tingling, or numbness between the toes and in the ball of the foot. Treatment includes orthotic devices and/or steroid injections, and sometimes surgery.

- **Plantar fasciitis:** inflammation of the long band of connective tissue running from the heel to the ball of the foot, a main cause of rear-foot pain. This condition is sometimes caused by shoes that cramp the feet, especially in the arch area.

- **Pump bump (Haglund's deformity):** a bone enlargement at the back of the heel bone, in the area where the Achilles tendon attaches to the bone. The deformity generally is the result of faulty biomechanics causing increased motion of the heel bone against the shoe counter.

Chapter 65

Cosmetics and Health

Chapter Contents

Section 65.1

Cosmetic Allergies

"Allergies: The Culprit Could Be Hiding In Your Cosmetic Bag,"
reprinted with permission from the American Academy of Dermatology.
All rights reserved. March 2000.

The average adult uses at least seven different skin care products each day, including fragrances, moisturizers, sunscreens, skin cleansers, hair care items, deodorants/antiperspirants, and cosmetics. So when a patient is suffering from a cosmetic allergy, the task of identifying the culprit is an investigative process for a dermatologist.

Dermatologist Anthony F. Fransway, MD, of Fort Myers, Fla., discussed the antigens commonly used in cosmetics that cause adverse reactions and the extensive testing necessary to identify the source of the problem.

Studies suggest that up to 10 percent of the population may have some adverse reaction to a cosmetic item over the course of his or her lifetime. These reactions are not gender-specific, but typically women are affected more than men since they tend to use more cosmetic items. Men see the most reactions from aftershave, cologne, and shampoos. Women react most commonly to moisturizers/sunscreens, makeup ingredients (specifically makeup bases and eye care products like mascara, eyeliners, and eye shadows), perfume, hair care products, and nail products.

Fragrance is the number-one cause of allergic cosmetic reactions. There are more than 5,000 basic fragrances, but this encompasses far more than cologne or perfume. Countless skin care products, soaps, shampoos, lipsticks, sunscreens, and lotions contain fragrance. Some people are sensitive to the fragrance chemical used in these various products. Other antigens in cosmetics may include preservative chemicals, which are needed to prevent skin care products from spoiling, antioxidants, sunscreen ingredients, and other inactive ingredients.

Fragrance-free products can be safely used by those with a fragrance allergy, but even products labeled unscented may contain a masking fragrance added to cover up the chemical smell. Unscented products are not necessarily fragrance-free. "There are very few truly preservative-free products," warned Dr. Fransway. "Most cosmetic items have an aqueous base or compartment in which bacterial and fungal overgrowth and spoilage may occur. Once a preservative allergy is identified through specific testing, cosmetics free of the offending agent may be identified and used safely."

The face, lips, eyes, ears, and neck are the most common locations for cosmetic allergy. Additionally, hands can be affected by moisturizers or nail products. Adverse reactions include irritant contact dermatitis, which produces burning, stinging, itching, and redness. The most common skin irritants are bath soaps, detergents, antiperspirants, astringents, eye makeup, moisturizers, permanent hair solutions, and shampoos.

Allergic contact dermatitis afflicts those who are allergic to a specific ingredient or ingredients in a product. Symptoms include redness, swelling, itching, and fluid-filled blisters. Reactions can occur whenever an individual is exposed to the ingredient, although symptoms may take several days to appear.

Irritant reactions to cosmetics typically occur within days of initial use, but a true allergic reaction can take anywhere from a week to 10 days. In some cases, an allergic reaction is years in the making, and the catalyst for reaction is the condition of the skin and the immune system.

The first step in managing allergic dermatitis is one month to six weeks of strict avoidance of the suspected products. This allows the immune response to settle down and become less active, and the skin to heal.

"A dermatologist is an expert in recognizing cosmetic allergies," said Dr. Fransway. "It is important to consult a dermatologist early if you experience a reaction to cosmetics. Reactions range from mild to severe.

In severe or continuously bothersome cases, medical intervention is necessary to find the source of the reaction. A meticulous exposural history is done, followed by patch testing."

Dermatologists recommend that people who experience allergic contact dermatitis adhere to the following program to avoid some of the most probable offending agents, with specific patch testing performed once the dermatitis is clear:

- For clothing care, double rinse all detergents and avoid all fabric softeners.

- Try to wear pure, untreated cotton in light colors. Avoid permanent press or cotton blends. Silk and polyester are acceptable.

- Wash all new clothing items five times before wearing.

- Use only fragrance-free soaps, body cleansers, shampoos, and conditioners.

- Avoid all perfumes, colognes, and aftershaves.

- Do not use any fingernail care products or hairspray.

Section 65.2

Hair-Care Irritants and Allergies

"Heading Off Hair-Care Disasters: Use Caution With Relaxers and Dyes," U.S. Food and Drug Administration, *FDA Consumer*, January-February 2001. By Michelle Meadows.

According to the Food and Drug Administration's Office of Cosmetics and Colors, hair straighteners and hair dyes are among its top consumer complaint areas. Complaints range from hair breakage to symptoms warranting an emergency room visit. Reporting such complaints is voluntary, and the reported problem is often due to incorrect use of a product rather than the product itself. FDA encourages consumers to understand the risks that come with using hair chemicals, and to take a proactive approach in ensuring their proper use. The agency doesn't have authority under the Federal Food, Drug, and Cosmetic Act to require premarket approval for cosmetics, but it can take action when safety issues surface.

Safer Straightening

FDA has received complaints about scalp irritation and hair breakage related to both lye and "no lye" relaxers. Some consumers falsely assume that compared to lye relaxers, no-lye relaxers take all the worry out of straightening.

"People may think because it says 'no lye' that it's not caustic," says FDA biologist Lark Lambert. But both types of relaxers contain ingredients that work by breaking chemical bonds of the hair, and both can burn the scalp if used incorrectly. Lye relaxers contain sodium hydroxide as the active ingredient. With no-lye relaxers, calcium hydroxide and guanidine carbonate are mixed to produce guanidine hydroxide.

Research has shown that this combination in no-lye relaxers results in less scalp irritation than lye relaxers, but the same safety rules apply for both. They should be used properly, left on no longer than the prescribed time, carefully washed out with neutralizing shampoo, and followed up with regular conditioning. For those who opt to straighten their own hair, it's wise to enlist help simply because not being able to see and reach the top and back of the head makes proper application of the chemical and thorough rinsing more of a challenge.

Some stylists recommend applying a layer of petroleum jelly on the scalp before applying a relaxer because it creates a protective barrier between the chemical and the skin. Scratching, brushing, and combing can make the scalp more susceptible to chemical damage and should be avoided right before using a relaxer. Parents should be especially cautious when applying chemicals to children's hair and should keep relaxers out of children's reach. There have been reports of small children ingesting straightening chemicals and suffering injuries that include burns to the face, tongue, and esophagus.

Hair Dye Reactions

As with hair relaxers, some consumers have reported hair loss, burning, redness, and irritation from hair dyes. Allergic reactions to dyes include itching, swelling of the face, and even difficulty breathing.

Coal tar hair dye ingredients are known to cause allergic reactions in some people, FDA's Lambert says. Synthetic organic chemicals, including hair dyes and other color additives, were originally manufactured from coal tar, but today manufacturers primarily use materials derived from petroleum. The use of the term "coal tar" continues because historically that language has been incorporated into the law and regulations.

The law does not require that coal tar hair dyes be approved by FDA, as is required for other uses of color additives. In addition, the law does not allow FDA to take action against coal tar hair dyes that are shown to be harmful, if the product is labeled with the prescribed caution statement indicating that the product may cause irritation in certain individuals, that a patch test for skin sensitivity should be done, and that the product must not be used for dyeing the eyelashes or eyebrows. The patch test involves putting a dab of hair dye behind the ear or inside the elbow, leaving it there for two days, and looking for itching, burning, redness, or other reactions.

"The problem is that people can become sensitized—that is, develop an allergy—to these ingredients," Lambert says. "They may do the patch test once, and then use the product for 10 years" before having an allergic reaction. "But you're supposed to do the patch test every time," he says, even in salons.

When using all hair chemicals, it's critical to keep them away from children to prevent ingestion and other accidents, and to follow product directions carefully. It sounds basic, but some people don't do it, says FDA's Halper. "If it says leave on hair for five minutes, seven minutes doesn't make it better," he says. "In fact, it could do damage."

Look out for Your Eyes

Whether applying hair chemicals at home or in a hair salon, consumers and beauticians should be careful to keep them away from the eyes. FDA has received reports of injuries from hair relaxers and hair dye accidentally getting into eyes. And while it may be tempting to match a new hair color to eyebrows and eyelashes, consumers should resist the urge. The use of permanent eyelash and eyebrow tinting and dyeing has been known to cause serious eye injuries and even blindness. There are no color additives approved by FDA for dyeing or tinting eyelashes and eyebrows.

The law does not require that coal tar hair dyes be approved by FDA, as is required for other uses of color additives. In addition, the law does not allow FDA to take action against coal tar hair dyes that are shown to be harmful, if the product is labeled with the following caution statement: "Caution—This product contains ingredients which may cause skin irritation on certain individuals and a preliminary test according to accompanying directions should first be made. This product must not be used for dyeing the eyelashes or eyebrows; to do so may cause blindness."

Michelle Meadows is a staff writer for *FDA Consumer*.

Part Nine

Women's
Emotional and Mental Health

Chapter 66

Depressive Disorders

Chapter Contents

Section 66.1

Depression: What Every Woman Should Know

National Institutes of Health, National Institute of Mental Health,
NIH Publication No. 00-4779. Published August 2000; updated February 2003.
Available online at http://www.nimh.nih.gov; accessed May 2003.

The Types of Depressive Illness

In major depression, sometimes referred to as unipolar or clinical depression, people have some or all of the symptoms listed below for at least 2 weeks but frequently for several months or longer. Episodes of the illness can occur once, twice, or several times in a lifetime.

In dysthymia, the same symptoms are present though milder and last at least 2 years. People with dysthymia are frequently lacking in zest and enthusiasm for life, living a joyless and fatigued existence that seems almost a natural outgrowth of their personalities. They also can experience major depressive episodes.

Manic-depression, or bipolar disorder, is not nearly as common as other forms of depressive illness and involves disruptive cycles of depressive symptoms that alternate with mania. During manic episodes, people may become overly active, talkative, euphoric, irritable, spend money irresponsibly, and get involved in sexual misadventures. In some people, a milder form of mania, called hypomania, alternates with depressive episodes. Unlike other mood disorders, women and men are equally vulnerable to bipolar disorder; however, women with bipolar disorder tend to have more episodes of depression and fewer episodes of mania or hypomania.

Symptoms of Depression and Mania

A thorough diagnostic evaluation is needed if three to five or more of the following symptoms persist for more than 2 weeks (1 week in the case of mania), or if they interfere with work or family life. An evaluation involves a complete physical checkup and information gathering on family health history. Not everyone with depression experiences each of these symptoms. The severity of the symptoms also varies from person to person.

Depression

- Persistent sad, anxious, or empty mood
- Loss of interest or pleasure in activities, including sex
- Restlessness, irritability, or excessive crying
- Feelings of guilt, worthlessness, helplessness, hopelessness, pessimism
- Sleeping too much or too little, early-morning awakening
- Appetite and/or weight loss or overeating and weight gain
- Decreased energy, fatigue, feeling slowed down
- Thoughts of death or suicide or suicide attempts
- Difficulty concentrating, remembering, or making decisions
- Persistent physical symptoms that do not respond to treatment, such as headaches, digestive disorders, and chronic pain

Mania

- Abnormally elevated mood
- Irritability
- Decreased need for sleep
- Grandiose notions
- Increased talking
- Racing thoughts
- Increased activity, including sexual activity
- Markedly increased energy
- Poor judgment that leads to risk-taking behavior
- Inappropriate social behavior

Causes of Depression

Genetic Factors

There is a risk for developing depression when there is a family history of the illness, indicating that a biological vulnerability may be inherited. The risk is somewhat higher for those with bipolar disorder. However, not everybody with a family history develops the illness. In addition, major depression can occur in people who have had no family members with the illness. This suggests that additional factors, possibly biochemistry, environmental stressors, and other psychosocial factors, are involved in the onset of depression.

Biochemical Factors

Evidence indicates that brain biochemistry is a significant factor in depressive disorders. It is known, for example, that individuals with major depressive illness typically have dysregulation of certain brain chemicals, called neurotransmitters. Additionally, sleep patterns, which are biochemically influenced, are typically different in people with depressive disorders. Depression can be induced or alleviated with certain medications, and some hormones have mood-altering properties. What is not yet known is whether the biochemical disturbances of depression are of genetic origin, or are secondary to stress, trauma, physical illness, or some other environmental condition.

Environmental and Other Stressors

Significant loss, a difficult relationship, financial problems, or a major change in life pattern have all been cited as contributors to depressive illness. Sometimes the onset of depression is associated with acute or chronic physical illness. In addition, some form of substance abuse disorder occurs in about one third of people with any type of depressive disorder.

Other Psychological and Social Factors

Persons with certain characteristics—pessimistic thinking, low self-esteem, a sense of having little control over life events, and a tendency to worry excessively—are more likely to develop depression. These attributes may heighten the effect of stressful events or interfere with taking action to cope with them or with getting well. Upbringing or sex role expectations may contribute to the development of these traits. It appears that negative thinking patterns typically develop in childhood or adolescence. Some experts have suggested that the traditional upbringing of girls might foster these traits and may be a factor in women's higher rate of depression.

Women Are at Greater Risk for Depression Than Men

Major depression and dysthymia affect twice as many women as men. This two-to-one ratio exists regardless of racial and ethnic background or economic status. The same ratio has been reported in ten other countries all over the world. Men and women have about the same rate of bipolar disorder (manic-depression), though its course in women typically has more depressive and fewer manic episodes. Also, a greater number of women have the rapid cycling form of bipolar disorder, which may be more resistant to standard treatments.

A variety of factors unique to women's lives are suspected to play a role in developing depression. Research is focused on understanding these, including: reproductive, hormonal, genetic or other biological factors; abuse and oppression; interpersonal factors; and certain psychological and personality characteristics. And yet, the specific causes of depression in women remain unclear; many women exposed to these factors do not develop depression. What is clear is that regardless of the contributing factors, depression is a highly treatable illness.

The Many Dimensions of Depression in Women

Investigators are focusing on the following areas in their study of depression in women:

The Issues of Adolescence

Before adolescence, there is little difference in the rate of depression in boys and girls. But between the ages of 11 and 13 there is a precipitous rise in depression rates for girls. By the age of 15, females are twice as likely to have experienced a major depressive episode as males. This comes at a time in adolescence when roles and expectations change dramatically. The stresses of adolescence include forming an identity, emerging sexuality, separating from parents, and making decisions for the first time, along with other physical, intellectual, and hormonal changes. These stresses are generally different for boys and girls, and may be associated more often with depression in females. Studies show that female high school students have significantly higher rates of depression, anxiety disorders, eating disorders, and adjustment disorders than male students, who have higher rates of disruptive behavior disorders.

Adulthood: Relationships and Work Roles

Stress in general can contribute to depression in persons biologically vulnerable to the illness. Some have theorized that higher incidence of depression in women is not due to greater vulnerability, but to the particular stresses that many women face. These stresses include major responsibilities at home and work, single parenthood, and caring for children and aging parents. How these factors may uniquely affect women is not yet fully understood.

For both women and men, rates of major depression are highest among the separated and divorced, and lowest among the married, while remaining always higher for women than for men. The quality of a marriage, however, may contribute significantly to depression. Lack of an intimate, confiding relationship, as well as overt marital disputes, have been shown to be related to depression in women. In fact, rates of depression were shown to be highest among unhappily married women.

Reproductive Events

Women's reproductive events include the menstrual cycle, pregnancy, the postpregnancy period, infertility, menopause, and sometimes, the decision not to have children. These events bring fluctuations in mood that for some women include depression. Researchers have confirmed that hormones have an effect on the brain chemistry that controls emotions and mood; a specific biological mechanism explaining hormonal involvement is not known, however.

Many women experience certain behavioral and physical changes associated with phases of their menstrual cycles. In some women, these changes are severe, occur regularly, and include depressed feelings, irritability, and other emotional and physical changes. Called premenstrual syndrome (PMS) or premenstrual dysphoric disorder (PMDD), the changes typically begin after ovulation and become gradually worse until menstruation starts. Scientists are exploring how the cyclical rise and fall of estrogen and other hormones may affect the brain chemistry that is associated with depressive illness.

Postpartum mood changes can range from transient blues immediately following childbirth to an episode of major depression to severe, incapacitating, psychotic depression. Studies suggest that women who experience major depression after childbirth very often have had prior depressive episodes even though they may not have been diagnosed and treated.

Pregnancy (if it is desired) seldom contributes to depression, and having an abortion does not appear to lead to a higher incidence of depression.

Women with infertility problems may be subject to extreme anxiety or sadness, though it is unclear if this contributes to a higher rate of depressive illness. In addition, motherhood may be a time of heightened risk for depression because of the stress and demands it imposes.

Menopause, in general, is not associated with an increased risk of depression. In fact, while once considered a unique disorder, research has shown that depressive illness at menopause is no different than at other ages. The women more vulnerable to change-of-life depression are those with a history of past depressive episodes.

Specific Cultural Considerations

As for depression in general, the prevalence rate of depression in African-American and Hispanic women remains about twice that of men. There is some indication, however, that major depression and dysthymia may be diagnosed less frequently in African American and slightly more frequently in Hispanic than in Caucasian women. Prevalence information for other racial and ethnic groups is not definitive.

Possible differences in symptom presentation may affect the way depression is recognized and diagnosed among minorities. For example, African Americans are more likely to report somatic symptoms, such as appetite change and body aches and pains. In addition, people from various cultural backgrounds may view depressive symptoms in different ways. Such factors should be considered when working with women from special populations.

Victimization

Studies show that women molested as children are more likely to have clinical depression at some time in their lives than those with no such history. In addition, several studies show a higher incidence of depression among women who have been raped as adolescents or adults. Since far more women than men were sexually abused as children, these findings are relevant. Women who experience other commonly occurring forms of abuse, such as physical abuse and sexual harassment on the job, also may experience higher rates of depression. Abuse may lead to depression by fostering low self-esteem, a sense of helplessness, self-blame, and social isolation. There may be biological and environmental risk factors for depression resulting from growing up in a dysfunctional family. At present, more research is needed to understand whether victimization is connected specifically to depression.

Poverty

Women and children represent seventy-five percent of the U.S. population considered poor. Low economic status brings with it many stresses, including isolation, uncertainty, frequent negative events, and poor access to helpful resources. Sadness and low morale are more common among persons with low incomes and those lacking social supports. But research has not yet established whether depressive illnesses are more prevalent among those facing environmental stressors such as these.

Depression in Later Adulthood

At one time, it was commonly thought that women were particularly vulnerable to depression when their children left home and they were confronted with empty nest syndrome and experienced a profound loss of purpose and identity. However, studies show no increase in depressive illness among women at this stage of life.

As with younger age groups, more elderly women than men suffer from depressive illness. Similarly, for all age groups, being unmarried (which includes widowhood) is also a risk factor for depression. Most important, depression should not be dismissed as a normal consequence of the physical, social, and economic problems of later life. In fact, studies show that most older people feel satisfied with their lives.

Depression Is a Treatable Illness

Even severe depression can be highly responsive to treatment. Indeed, believing one's condition is incurable is often part of the hopelessness that accompanies serious depression. Such individuals should be provided with the information about the effectiveness of modern treatments for depression in a way that acknowledges their likely skepticism about whether treatment will work for them. As with many illnesses, the earlier treatment begins, the more effective and the greater the likelihood of preventing serious recurrences. Of course, treatment will not eliminate life's inevitable stresses and ups and downs. But it can greatly enhance the ability to manage such challenges and lead to greater enjoyment of life.

The first step in treatment for depression should be a thorough examination to rule out any physical illnesses that may cause depressive symptoms. Since certain medications can cause the same symptoms as depression, the examining physician should be made aware of any medications being used. If a physical cause for the depression is not found, a psychological evaluation should be conducted by the physician or a referral made to a mental health professional.

Types of Treatment for Depression

The most commonly used treatments for depression are antidepressant medication, psychotherapy, or a combination of the two. Which of these is the right treatment for any one individual depends on the nature and severity of the depression and, to some extent, on individual preference.

In mild or moderate depression, one or both of these treatments may be useful, while in severe or incapacitating depression, medication is generally recommended as a first step in the treatment. In combined treatment, medication can relieve physical symptoms quickly, while psychotherapy allows the opportunity to learn more effective ways of handling problems.

Medications

There are several types of antidepressant medications used to treat depressive disorders. These include newer medications—chiefly the selective serotonin reuptake inhibitors (SSRIs)—and the tricyclics and monoamine oxidase inhibitors (MAOIs). The SSRIs-and other newer medications that affect neurotransmitters such as dopamine or norepinephrine generally have fewer side effects than tricyclics. Each acts on different chemical pathways of the human brain related to moods.

Antidepressant medications are not habit-forming. Although some individuals notice improvement in the first couple of weeks, usually antidepressant medications must be taken regularly for at least 4 weeks and, in some cases, as many as 8 weeks, before the full therapeutic effect occurs. To be effective and to prevent a relapse of the depression, medications must be taken for about 6 to 12 months, carefully following the doctor's instructions. Medications must be monitored to ensure the most effective dosage and to minimize side effects. For those who have had several bouts of depression, long-term treatment with medication is the most effective means of preventing recurring episodes.

The prescribing doctor will provide information about possible side effects and, in the case of MAOIs, dietary and medication restrictions. In addition, other prescribed and over-the-counter medications or dietary supplements being used should be reviewed because some can interact negatively with antidepressant medication. There may be restrictions during pregnancy.

For bipolar disorder, the treatment of choice for many years has been lithium, as it can be effective in smoothing out the mood swings common to this disorder. Its use must be carefully monitored, as the range between an effective dose and a toxic one can be relatively small. However, lithium may not be recommended if a person has pre-existing thyroid, kidney, or heart disorders or epilepsy. Fortunately, other medications have been found helpful in controlling mood swings. Among these are two mood-stabilizing anticonvulsants, carbamazepine (Tegretol®) and valproate (Depakote®). Both of these medications have gained wide acceptance in clinical practice, and valproate has been approved by the Food and Drug Administration for first-line treatment of acute mania. Studies conducted in Finland in patients with epilepsy indicate that valproate may increase testosterone levels in teenage girls and produce polycystic ovary syndrome in women who began taking the medication before age 20. Therefore, young female patients should be monitored carefully by a physician. Other anticonvulsants that are being used now include lamotrigine (Lamictal®) and gabapentin (Neurontin®); their role in the treatment hierarchy of bipolar disorder remains under study.

Most people who have bipolar disorder take more than one medication. Along with lithium and/or an anticonvulsant, they often take a medication for accompanying agitation, anxiety, insomnia, or depression. Some research indicates that an antidepressant, when taken without a mood stabilizing medication, can increase the risk of switching into mania or hypomania, or of developing rapid cycling, in people with bipolar disorder. Finding the best possible combination of these medications is of utmost importance to the patient and requires close monitoring by the physician.

Herbal Therapy

In the past few years, much interest has risen in the use of herbs in the treatment of both depression and anxiety. St. John's wort (*Hypericum perforatum*), an herb used extensively in the treatment of mild to moderate depression in Europe, has recently aroused interest in the United States. St. John's wort, an attractive bushy, low-growing plant covered with yellow flowers in summer, has been used for centuries in many folk and herbal remedies. Today in Germany, *Hypericum* is used in the treatment of depression more than any other antidepressant. However, the scientific studies that have been conducted on its use have been short-term and have used several different doses.

The Food and Drug Administration issued a Public Health Advisory on February 10, 2000. It stated that St. John's wort appears to affect an important metabolic pathway that is used by many drugs prescribed to treat conditions such as heart disease, depression, seizures, certain cancers, and rejection of transplants. Therefore, health care providers should alert their patients about these potential drug interactions. Any herbal supplement should be taken only after consultation with the doctor or other health care provider.

Psychotherapy

In mild to moderate cases of depression, psychotherapy is also a treatment option. Some short-term (10 to 20 week) therapies have been very effective in several types of depression. Talking therapies help patients gain insight into and resolve their problems through verbal give-and-take with the therapist. Behavioral therapies help patients learn new behaviors that lead to more satisfaction in life and unlearn counter-productive behaviors. Research has shown that two short-term psychotherapies, interpersonal and cognitive-behavioral, are helpful for some forms of depression. Interpersonal therapy works to change interpersonal relationships that cause or exacerbate depression. Cognitive-behavioral therapy helps change negative styles of thinking and behaving that may contribute to the depression.

Electroconvulsive Therapy

For individuals whose depression is severe or life threatening or for those who cannot take antidepressant medication, electroconvulsive therapy (ECT) is useful. This is particularly true for those with extreme suicide risk, severe agitation, psychotic thinking, severe weight loss or physical debilitation as a result of physical illness. Over the years, ECT has been much improved. A muscle relaxant is given before treatment, which is done under brief anesthesia. Electrodes are placed at precise locations on the head to deliver electrical impulses. The stimulation causes a brief (about 30 seconds) seizure within the brain. The person receiving ECT does not consciously experience the electrical stimulus. At least several sessions of ECT, usually given at the rate of three per week, are required for full therapeutic benefit.

Treating Recurrent Depression

Even when treatment is successful, depression may recur. Studies indicate that certain treatment strategies are very useful in this instance. Continuation of antidepressant medication at the same dose that successfully treated the acute episode can often prevent recurrence. Monthly interpersonal psychotherapy can lengthen the time between episodes in patients not taking medication.

The Path to Healing

Depressive illnesses make you feel exhausted, worthless, helpless, and hopeless. Such feelings make some people want to give up. It is important to realize that these negative feelings are part of the depression and will fade as treatment begins to take effect.

Along with professional treatment, there are other things you can do to help yourself get better. Some people find participating in support groups very helpful. It may also help to spend some time with other people and to participate in activities that make you feel better, such as mild exercise or yoga. Just don't expect too much from yourself right away. Feeling better takes time.

Section 66.2

Seasonal Affective Disorder

What Is Seasonal Affective Disorder?

Some people suffer from symptoms of depression during the winter months, with symptoms subsiding during the spring and summer months. This may be a sign of Seasonal Affective Disorder (SAD). SAD is a mood disorder associated with depression episodes and related to seasonal variations of light.

SAD was first noted before 1845, but was not officially named until the early 1980s. As sunlight has affected the seasonal activities of animals (i.e., reproductive cycles and hibernation), SAD may be an effect of this seasonal light variation in humans. As seasons change, there is a shift in our biological internal clocks or circadian rhythm, due partly to these changes in sunlight patterns. This can cause our biological clocks to be out of step with our daily schedules. The most difficult months for SAD sufferers are January and February, and younger persons and women are at higher risk.

Symptoms of SAD

Symptoms include:

- regularly occurring symptoms of depression (excessive eating and sleeping, weight gain) during the fall or winter months

- full remission from depression in the spring and summer months

- symptoms occurring in the past two years, with no nonseasonal depression episodes

- seasonal episodes substantially outnumber nonseasonal depression episodes

- a craving for sugary and/or starchy foods

Possible Cause of This Disorder

Melatonin, a sleep-related hormone secreted by the pineal gland in the brain, has been linked to SAD. This hormone, which may cause symptoms of depression, is produced at increased levels in the dark. Therefore, when the days are shorter and darker the production of this hormone increases.

Treatments

Phototherapy or bright light therapy has been shown to suppress the brain's secretion of melatonin. Although, there have been no research findings to definitely link this therapy with an antidepressant effect, many people respond to this treatment. The device most often used today is a bank of white fluorescent lights on a metal reflector and shield with a plastic screen. For mild symptoms, spending time outdoors during the day or arranging homes and workplaces to receive more sunlight may be helpful. One study found that an hour's walk in winter sunlight was as effective as two and a half hours under bright artificial light.

If phototherapy doesn't work, an antidepressant drug may prove effective in reducing or eliminating SAD symptoms, but there may be unwanted side effects to consider. Discuss your symptoms thoroughly with your family doctor and/or mental health professional.

Section 66.3

Premenstrual Dysphoric Disorder

Reprinted with permission from the American Psychiatric Association and Medem, Inc. © 2001 American Psychiatric Association and Medem, Inc.

What is premenstrual dysphoric disorder (PMDD)?

A woman who has PMDD experiences severe depression, irritability and/or mood swings, which interfere with relationships, social functioning, and work or school. The symptoms of PMDD start seven to 14 days before menstruation, and they resolve a few days after menstruation starts.

The term premenstrual dysphoric disorder is a medical term that makes sense when broken down into its individual parts. Disorder is a term used to describe a group of symptoms that impair health. The symptoms are described as premenstrual because they occur before menstruation. The word dysphoric is a Greek word, which literally means ill-being. Dysphoria is the opposite of a more common word, euphoria (or well-being).

How is PMDD different from premenstrual syndrome (PMS)?

Premenstrual syndrome (PMS) is a condition that affects some women before they menstruate each month. Physical symptoms—such as breast tenderness, cramps, abdominal bloating, headaches and cravings for starchy foods—are common. Mood symptoms include depression, anger, irritability, and anxiety. Other problems include social withdrawal and difficulty concentrating and thinking.

Many women have one or more of these symptoms before they menstruate, but the symptoms usually are mild and do not interfere with their ability to function. Making lifestyle changes—such as getting regular exercise, quitting smoking, drinking less caffeine and learning how to manage stress—may help relieve symptoms. For some women who have PMS, physicians may prescribe birth control pills or select a different birth control pill, which can relieve some symptoms. The physician also may prescribe diuretics, which help the body eliminate the excess water that causes bloating.

Although the mood symptoms associated with PMS sound similar to PMDD, they are different in one key respect: PMDD is much more severe. Premenstrual dysphoric disorder should be diagnosed only when mood symptoms seriously impact relationships and impair functioning at work or school. Depending on how broadly it is defined, between 20 percent and 50 percent of women live with PMS, but only 3 percent to 8 percent of women are estimated to have PMDD.

The term PMDD was added to the appendix of the *Diagnostic and Statistical Manual of Mental Disorders, Fourth Edition* in 1994. (The *DSM-IV* is the standard text of mental disorders published by the American Psychiatric Association). The psychiatrists who developed the *DSM-IV* added PMDD to the appendix to provide a common definition of the problem so scientists could study whether some women with premenstrual symptoms suffer so seriously that their symptoms should be considered a disease. Adding a condition to the appendix of the *DSM-IV* does not mean it is a disease. Only further study and scientific evidence can establish whether PMDD is a disease.

What are the symptoms of PMDD?

According to the research criteria in the *DSM-IV*, a woman may have PMDD if she has five or more of the following symptoms during the week before menstruating for most of her menstrual cycles in the last year. (It is important to note that a woman may have PMDD only if the symptoms are tied to the menstrual cycle. If they are not, then she may have another condition.)

- Depression (hopelessness; more than just feeling sad or blue)
- Anxiety (feeling keyed up or on edge)
- Severe mood swings (feeling suddenly sad or extremely sensitive to rejection)
- Anger or irritability

- Decreased interest in usual activities (work, school, friends, hobbies)

- Difficulty concentrating

- Decreased energy

- Appetite changes (overeating or cravings for certain foods)

- Sleep problems (insomnia, early morning waking, or oversleeping)

- Feeling overwhelmed or out of control

- Physical symptoms, such as bloating, breast tenderness or headaches

The symptoms of PMDD end with menopause, when menstruation stops and the levels of hormones in the body that regulate menstruation no longer rise and fall each month.

How is PMDD diagnosed?

According to the appendix of the *DSM-IV*, a physician can diagnose PMDD only if the woman has five or more of the symptoms described above for most menstrual cycles and if those symptoms seriously impair her relationships with others and her ability to be productive at work or school.

A psychiatrist or other physician also will need to consider and rule out other possible causes of the symptoms—such as thyroid problems or lupus—or another mental disorder, such as depression or an anxiety disorder. The symptoms of all these conditions may worsen before menstruation and so could be confused with PMDD.

To determine if a woman has PMDD, a psychiatrist or other physician will ask her to keep a mood and symptom journal every day for at least two months. It is easy in hindsight to think symptoms occurred around the time of menstruation. For this reason, keeping a journal over time is necessary to show with more certainty if the mood or functioning problems truly began one to two weeks before menstruation and improved within a few days of menstruation starting. Also, without the information provided in the journal, it could be difficult to identify another medical or mental health condition causing the symptoms.

Some physicians suggest keeping two separate records: a calendar marking the days of menstruation and a journal of mood and behavior throughout the entire month. Keeping these two records separate helps prevent incorrectly associating mood changes with the menstrual cycle.

How is PMDD treated?

The same lifestyle changes that sometimes help women with PMS may help relieve the symptoms of PMDD. In most cases, however, PMDD symptoms will persist despite such efforts.

Studies show some women with PMDD may benefit from treatment with antidepressants called selective serotonin reuptake inhibitors (SSRIs). These medications also are prescribed commonly for depression, but for women with PMDD they usually work more quickly and are prescribed in lower dosages to be taken for just part of each month.

The U.S. Food and Drug Administration has approved one SSRI, Sarafem™ (fluoxetine), for the treatment of PMDD. Sarafem is the same chemical compound as Prozac™, but the manufacturer renamed it for the treatment of PMDD. Recent studies have found that other SSRIs used to treat depression—such as sertraline, citalopram and paroxetine—also are effective for treating PMDD. Because different women will tolerate some medications better than others, a physician might prescribe one of these other SSRIs. It is a legal and common practice for physicians to prescribe medications off-label, which means that a medicine approved by the FDA to treat one illness can be prescribed to treat another illness.

With treatment, most women with PMDD will be able to lead more satisfying lives, without the cycles of severe distress and limited functioning caused by the disorder.

Section 66.4

Postpartum Depression

U.S. Department of Health and Human Services, National Women's
Health Information Center (NWHIC); July 2002. Available online at
http://www.4woman.gov; accessed July 2003.

Why do women get postpartum depression?

Having a baby can be one of the biggest and happiest events in a
woman's life. While life with a new baby can be thrilling and rewarding, it can also be hard and stressful at times. Many physical and
emotional changes can happen to a woman when she is pregnant and
after she gives birth.

These changes can leave new mothers feeling sad, anxious, afraid,
or confused. For many women, these feelings (called the baby blues)
go away quickly. But when these feelings do not go away or get worse,
a woman may have postpartum depression. This is a serious condition that requires quick treatment from a health care provider.

What is postpartum depression? Are the baby blues the same thing as postpartum depression?

Postpartum depression (PPD) is a condition that describes a range
of physical and emotional changes that many mothers can have after
having a baby. PPD can be treated with medication and counseling.
Talk with your health care provider right away if you think you have
PPD.

There are three types of PPD women can have after giving birth:

- The baby blues happen in many women in the days right after
  childbirth. A new mother can have sudden mood swings, such as
  feeling very happy and then feeling very sad. She may cry for no
  reason and can feel impatient, irritable, restless, anxious, lonely,
  and sad. The baby blues may last only a few hours or as long as
  1 to 2 weeks after delivery. The baby blues do not always require treatment from a health care provider. Often, joining a
  support group of new moms or talking with other moms helps.

- Postpartum depression (PPD) can happen a few days or even months after childbirth. PPD can happen after the birth of any child, not just the first child. A woman can have feelings similar to the baby blues—sadness, despair, anxiety, irritability—but she feels them much more strongly than she would with the baby blues. PPD often keeps a woman from doing the things she needs to do every day. When a woman's ability to function is affected, this is a sure sign that she needs to see her health care provider right away. If a woman does not get treatment for PPD, symptoms can get worse and last for as long as 1 year. While PPD is a serious condition, it can be treated with medication and counseling.

- Postpartum psychosis is a very serious mental illness that can affect new mothers. This illness can happen quickly, often within the first 3 months after childbirth. Women can lose touch with reality, often having auditory hallucinations (hearing things that aren't actually happening, like a person talking) and delusions (seeing things differently from what they are). Visual hallucinations (seeing things that aren't there) are less common. Other symptoms include insomnia (not being able to sleep), feeling agitated (unsettled) and angry, and strange feelings and behaviors. Women who have postpartum psychosis need treatment right away and almost always need medication. Sometimes women are put into the hospital because they are at risk for hurting themselves or someone else.

What are the signs of postpartum depression?

The signs of postpartum depression include:

- Feeling restless or irritable
- Feeling sad, depressed or crying a lot
- Having no energy
- Having headaches, chest pains, heart palpitations (the heart being fast and feeling like it is skipping beats), numbness, or hyperventilation (fast and shallow breathing)
- Not being able to sleep or being very tired, or both
- Not being able to eat and weight loss
- Overeating and weight gain

- Trouble focusing, remembering, or making decisions
- Being overly worried about the baby
- Not having any interest in the baby
- Feeling worthless and guilty
- Being afraid of hurting the baby or yourself
- No interest or pleasure in activities, including sex

A woman may feel anxious after childbirth but not have PPD. She may have what is called postpartum anxiety or panic disorder. Signs of this condition include strong anxiety and fear, rapid breathing, fast heart rate, hot or cold flashes, chest pain, and feeling shaky or dizzy. Talk with your health care provider right away if you have any of these signs. Medication and counseling can be used to treat postpartum anxiety.

Who is at risk for getting postpartum depression?

Postpartum depression (PPD) affects women of all ages, economic status, and racial/ethnic backgrounds. Any woman who is pregnant, had a baby within the past few months, miscarried, or recently weaned a child from breastfeeding can develop PPD. The number of children a woman has does not change her chances of getting PPD. New mothers and women with more than one child have equal chances of getting PPD. Research has shown that women who have had problems with depression are more at risk for PPD than women who have not had a history of depression.

How is postpartum depression treated?

It is important to know that postpartum depression (PPD) is treatable and that it will go away. The type of treatment will depend on how severe the PPD is. PPD can be treated with medication (antidepressants) and psychotherapy. Women with PPD are often advised to attend a support group to talk with other women who are going through the same thing. If a woman is breastfeeding, she needs to talk with her health care provider about taking antidepressants. Some of these drugs affect breast milk and should not be used.

Chapter 67

Anxiety Disorders

Chapter Contents

Section 67.1

Panic Disorder, Phobias, and Other Anxiety Disorders

Excerpted from "Anxiety Disorders," U.S. Department of Health and Human Services, National Women's Health Information Center (NWHIC), July 2002. Available online at http://www.4woman.gov; accessed July 2003.

What are anxiety disorders? Are they common?

Everybody knows what it's like to feel anxious—the butterflies in your stomach before a first date, the tension you feel when your boss is angry, the way your heart pounds if you're in danger. Anxiety isn't always a bad thing. It can help you cope with life's everyday stress. It makes you study harder for that exam, keeps you on your toes when you're making a speech, and helps you stay focused when looking for a job or asking for a raise.

But if you have an anxiety disorder, this normally helpful emotion can do just the opposite. It can keep you from coping and can disrupt your daily life. Anxiety disorders aren't just a case of nerves. They are serious illnesses that can grow worse when not treated. They are thought to be related to the biological makeup and life experiences of a person, and often run in families. Every year, more than 19 million American adults suffer from anxiety disorders. There are treatments for these disorders that can help people lead full and healthy lives. And, research is being done to find new ways to help people with anxiety disorders.

What are the different types of anxiety disorders and what are their symptoms?

There are five types of anxiety disorders, each with different symptoms. They include:

Generalized anxiety disorder (GAD)—constant and exaggerated (more than normal) worry and tension about everyday life events and decisions that lasts for at least six months. A person fears the worst, even though there may be little reason to expect so. Physical symptoms can also happen, such as fatigue, trembling, muscle tension, headache, or nausea.

Obsessive-compulsive disorder (OCD)—repeated, unwanted thoughts (obsessions) or ritual behaviors (compulsions) that a person feels they can't control or stop. A person can sometimes feel an urgent need to perform a ritual behavior, such as always washing hands three times because three is a good luck number and one isn't.

Panic disorder—feelings of extreme fear and dread that strike with no warning and for no reason. These feelings can happen over and over again. A person can have physical symptoms, such as chest pain, heart palpitations (heart beating fast or skipping beats), shortness of breath, dizziness, stomach problems, feeling disoriented or not real, and have a fear of dying.

Phobias—includes social phobia, an extreme fear of being embarrassed, judged, or made fun of in social or work situations and specific phobia, an extreme fear of an object or situation that poses little or no danger. People with phobias often avoid certain situations (like public speaking or parties) or objects (like elevators). Phobias can affect a person's career, relationships, and daily life activities.

Post-traumatic stress disorder (PTSD)—involves how a person reacts to a very frightening or stressful event, such as being tortured or put in a prison camp during a war, seeing another person being hurt or killed, or raped. With PTSD, a person can keep re-living the event with nightmares and flashbacks. They can feel numb, depressed, angry, irritable, and jumpy. Family members of victims can also develop PTSD.

How are anxiety disorders treated?

Anxiety disorders are among the most common of all the mental disorders. Many people misunderstand these disorders and think people should be able to overcome the symptoms by sheer willpower. But the symptoms can't be willed or wished away. There are treatments, developed through research, that work well for these disorders.

Anxiety disorders are treated in two ways—with medication and with certain types of psychotherapy (sometimes called talk therapy). Sometimes only one treatment is used or both treatments are combined.

621

If you have an anxiety disorder, talk with your doctor about what will work best for you. If you do choose psychotherapy, make sure the therapist is able to provide you with medication, if needed.

A number of drugs used for treating depression, called antidepressants, have been found to help with anxiety disorders as well. Monoamine oxidase inhibitors (MAOIs) are used, along with the newer selective serotonin reuptake inhibitors (SSRIs). Other medicines include anti-anxiety drugs called benzodiazepines and beta-blockers.

Treatment with psychotherapy includes cognitive-behavioral therapy (CBT) and behavioral therapy. In CBT, the goal is to change how a person thinks about, and then reacts to, a situation that makes them anxious or fearful. In behavioral therapy, the focus is on changing how a person reacts to a situation. CBT or behavioral therapy most often lasts for 12 weeks. It can be group or individual therapy. Some studies have shown that the benefits of CBT or behavioral therapy last longer than do those of medications for people with panic disorder, OCD, PTSD, and social phobia.

Keep in mind that it can be a challenge to find the right treatment for an anxiety disorder. But, if one treatment doesn't work, the odds are good that another one will. Your doctor and therapist will work together to help you find the best approach. New treatments are being developed through ongoing research. So don't give up hope. If you have recovered from an anxiety disorder and it comes back at a later date, don't think that you've failed. You can be treated again. And the skills you learned dealing with the disorder the first time can help you in coping with it again.

What should I do if I think I may have an anxiety disorder?

If you think you may have symptoms of anxiety, a visit to your doctor is the best place to start. Your doctor will perform a careful exam to figure out whether your symptoms are really due to an anxiety disorder, which disorder you have, and if there are any other problems present. Be aware that all anxiety disorders are not treated the same.

The next step your doctor may suggest is a visit with a mental health professional. This includes psychiatrists, psychologists, social workers, and counselors. It is best to look for a professional who has special training in cognitive-behavioral and/or behavioral therapy. Try to find someone who is open to the use of medications, should they be needed. And if they are not a medical doctor, be sure they work with one so medication can be prescribed. Keep in mind that when you start taking medicine, it may not start working right away. You need to give your body a few weeks to get used to the medicine. Then you and your doctor can decide if it's working.

It's very important that you feel comfortable with your treatment. If this is not the case, seek help elsewhere. If you've been taking medication, don't stop it all of a sudden. These drugs need to be tapered off slowly, under the care of your doctor. Talk with your doctor about how to stop the medication you're taking.

Section 67.2

Post-Traumatic Stress Disorder

Excerpted from "Escaping the Prison of a Past Trauma: New Treatment for Post-Traumatic Stress Disorder," U.S. Food and Drug Administration, *FDA Consumer*, May-June 2000. By Tamar Nordenberg.

In a given year, more than 10 million Americans (about 4 percent) will experience the life-disrupting symptoms of post-traumatic stress disorder (PTSD), which was first widely recognized during World War I and known as shell shock or battle fatigue.

Like combat horrors, other manmade tragedies such as criminal assaults or sexual attacks can provoke PTSD symptoms, as can a fire, earthquake, or other natural disaster. Accidents—car and airplane crashes, for example—are also common precipitators of PTSD.

By definition, the disorder can only develop in response to a traumatic event, says Edna Foa, Ph.D., director of the University of Pennsylvania's Center for the Treatment and Study of Anxiety. It can't arise from other seriously stressful occurrences that are less extreme—losing a job, say, or going through a divorce.

And, while not all life stressors are traumatic enough to lead to a PTSD diagnosis (but instead might cause generalized anxiety), not everyone who experiences a trauma will develop post-traumatic stress disorder, either.

As many as 70 percent of American adults have been through at least one major trauma, according to the *Expert Consensus Treatment*

Guidelines for Post-Traumatic Stress Disorder: A Guide For Patients and Families, a guide written by Foa and others based on a survey of 100 PTSD experts. But, Foa explains, "Most people who go through a traumatic event may be more frightened and act more cautiously than they used to, but don't develop the disorder. That is, they don't get symptoms that would disrupt their daily life in a significant way and render them dysfunctional on some level."

Experts divide symptoms that rise to the level of PTSD into these main types:

- **Re-experiencing the traumatic event.** Re-experiencing can refer to having intrusive memories of the ordeal, flashbacks when awake, recurring nightmares, and exaggerated emotional and physical responses to triggers that remind the person of the event. "Sometimes I've thought I was back in Vietnam. When you start dreaming, you can smell the flesh of your buddies burning," says veteran John Palmer Sr., who recalls being among 19 wounded survivors of a 1968 ambush by the North Vietnamese that killed the rest of his 59-strong battalion.

- **Avoidance.** After a trauma, people may lose interest in and avoid certain activities, places, and thoughts and feelings related to the trauma. July 4th is "really hard" for 51-year-old veteran Palmer because the loud noises remind him of wartime. And Palmer avoided seeing the critically acclaimed *Saving Private Ryan.* "I chose not to go," he explains, "even though some people thought it was pretty good . . . if there could be anything good about it. Watching movies about the war bothers me, and I start having nightmares."

- **Emotional detachment.** Foa's patients have told her, "I'm not the person I used to be. I don't trust people. I can't feel loving anymore." One of her patients, who had been injured in an explosion at his factory that killed many others, was "like a zombie emotionally," Foa says. The man's daughter complained, "He's not there for us. All he cares about is himself, and indulging in his own misery."

- **Increased arousal.** This symptom can show itself in difficulty sleeping, irritability or angry outbursts, difficulty concentrating, and unusually startled reactions in certain situations. Palmer says, "When I first came back [from Vietnam], people were afraid to be around me. I got in a lot of trouble, drinking and fighting, and I didn't really care."

People can have wide-ranging reactions to a certain stressor. Some people will have no long-lasting effects, while on the other end of the spectrum, people can have problems that last for months or years. The symptoms must last for at least a month, however, to be classified as post-traumatic stress disorder.

While symptoms usually begin immediately after a trauma or within the following few weeks, sometimes they can show up months or years later. Many of the World War II prisoners of war that Veterans Administration counselor James Boehnlein, M.D., talks with have had stable lives—were married long-term, raised children, and worked steadily—and developed delayed PTSD symptoms after they retired and when people their age began to die of natural causes. "Their losses brought back memories of their wartime sadness and loss," Boehnlein explains, "and they would start having nightmares of combat experience and being prisoners of war."

While Zoloft is the only drug approved by FDA to treat PTSD, doctors sometimes prescribe other drugs that they believe may improve a patient's condition. For PTSD, doctors sometimes prescribe drugs in the same class as Zoloft. These selective serotonin reuptake inhibitors, or SSRIs, include Paxil (paroxetine), Prozac (fluoxetine), Luvox (fluvoxamine), and Celexa (citalopram). Based on an individual patient's medical circumstances, a doctor may in some cases choose to prescribe other types of antidepressants or anti-anxiety medications.

Facing Fears

As an alternative to medication or coupled with it, some patients opt to rely on group or individual psychotherapy to manage their PTSD symptoms. Three types are considered especially effective, according to the expert consensus guidelines:

- **Exposure therapy.** To help patients confront the everyday reminders of their trauma, therapists sometimes use "exposure in the imagination" or "exposure in reality." In the first type, patients imagine the trauma and recount the memories in detail, over and over again, with a therapist they trust and at home between sessions. The goal of therapy: to give people an opportunity to reprocess what happened until the thoughts lose their distressful impact. Lyn Rezer, 35, re-examined a traumatic gang rape that had occurred when she was 12 years old and had haunted her for more than 20 years. Using this approach, Rezer says she conquered her feelings of worthlessness and despair. "I walked around for 23 years feeling extremely suicidal, wanting to flee, wanting to cry. I thought I was bad, I was filthy, I was nothing. I detached myself emotionally from a lot, and today I'm not detached. I feel everything, like a normal 35-year-old woman with normal impulses and instincts. I haven't had a suicidal thought since midway through treatment." With exposure in reality, therapists ask patients to gradually expose themselves to situations or places they had been avoiding because they are reminders of the trauma.

- **Cognitive behavioral therapy.** With CBT, therapists work on changing victims' irrational beliefs, such as self-blame for a rape, criminal assault, or accident.

- **Anxiety management.** This classification refers to techniques such as slow abdominal breathing to relax and avoid hyperventilation, and positive thinking and self-talk to replace negative thoughts.

Tamar Nordenberg is a staff writer for *FDA Consumer*.

Chapter 68

Eating Disorders

Chapter Contents

Section 68.1

Overview of Eating Disorders

Excerpted from "Eating Disorders," U.S. Department of Health and Human Services, National Women's Health Information Center (NWHIC), July 2002. Available online at http://www.4woman.gov; accessed July 2003.

What are eating disorders?

Eating disorders are real illnesses that can affect how we eat and how we feel about food. They can be treated to help people who have them have healthy and full lives. From time to time, we all change our eating habits. Sometimes we reduce the amount of food we eat or go on a diet to shed some pounds, or we eat more to gain weight. These can be healthy ways to control or reach our ideal body weight. But, people who have eating disorders have unhealthy ways, or patterns, of eating. They may eat too much and become overweight, or way too little and become very thin.

Sometimes a person can eat so little, or nothing at all, they actually begin to starve (called anorexia nervosa). A person can also eat an extreme amount of food all at once and then do things like vomit to rid the body of food (called bulimia nervosa). And, a person may not be able to control the need to overeat, often keeping it a secret (called binge eating disorder). People can also have wrong ideas, or misperceptions, of their body weight. People with eating disorders can feel certain they weigh too much, even though they may be well under the ideal body weight for a person their size.

Eating disorders affect people of all ages, race, and income levels. But, these disorders affect women much more than they do men. Women make up more than 90 percent of people with these disorders. Without treatment, an eating disorder can take over a person's life and cause serious illness and death. These disorders can increase risk for osteoporosis (thinning of the bones) and heart problems. People who have eating disorders can also have depression and anxiety, and may turn to alcohol and drugs for relief.

Who is at risk for eating disorders?

In the United States and other Western countries, women are more at risk for eating disorders than are men. These disorders affect 8 to 10 times more women than men. In the U.S., it was thought that eating disorders affected mostly white women. But, recent research has shown that black women are affected as well. One study found that black women were more likely than white women to have repeated episodes of binge eating disorder. This may put black women more at risk for obesity (being overweight).

Women may be more at risk for eating disorders because of a need to have the ideal figure often shown in the media (TV, magazines, movies). The "thin is best" view can affect girls and young women in particular. They often go on strict diets to look like the girls and women they see in the media. Pressure from friends to be thin and to diet can also happen. For women, body image, or how you feel about how you look, can affect feelings about body weight. Not liking how much you weigh, feeling fat, and wanting to be thin can make you worry more about how you look than other things, such as your own ideas or what you want to do in your life. Sometimes, young women who are at a normal weight, or even underweight, may feel that they are too fat. A woman may also feel that how she looks or how much she weighs makes up a major part of her self-esteem. While young women may be most at risk for eating disorders, these disorders are affecting older women in growing numbers.

What are the most common types of eating disorders? What effects do they have on a person's health?

The three most common types of eating disorders are:

• Anorexia nervosa

• Bulimia nervosa

• Binge eating disorder (BED)

There are two other types of eating disorders. Eating disorder not otherwise specified (EDNOS) is the name for disorders of eating that don't fit into one of the three disorders described above. With EDNOS, a person has some form of abnormal eating but not all the symptoms needed to be diagnosed with an eating disorder. For instance, a person with EDNOS may purge themselves after eating, but do so with less frequency or intensity than someone who has bulimia.

More common than eating disorders is a condition called disordered eating. This is when a person diets, binges, or purges, but doesn't do so often or severely enough to be diagnosed with an eating disorder. A person may change how they eat after a stressful event or an illness, before an important speech or work event, or before a sports competition. Disordered eating can lead to weight loss or weight gain, but rarely requires treatment. But, if the disordered eating becomes long lasting, causes upset and stress, changes the way a person feels about themselves or how they look, or starts to get in the way of daily activities, they need to get help right away. Don't wait to see if the problem goes away by itself, talk with a health care provider about where to go for help.

What are the treatments for eating disorders?

Eating disorders can be treated and a person can return to a healthy weight. Success in treating eating disorders is greatest when they are found early and treated right away. The longer abnormal ways of eating go on, the harder it is to overcome the disorder. Plus, more damage is done to the body over time, which can result in serious health problems.

There is no one, or best, way to treat these complex disorders. Most people with eating disorders are treated by a team of health care providers and receive medical care, psychotherapy (sometimes called talk therapy), and nutritional counseling. Professionals who provide psychotherapy can be therapists, psychologists, psychiatrists, social workers, or counselors. Types of psychotherapy include cognitive-behavioral therapy (changes how a person thinks about, and then reacts to, a situation that makes them anxious or fearful) family therapy, and group therapy. In some cases, a person may need to go into the hospital or into an inpatient or residential program. Medication is also sometimes used to treat the disorder and prevent relapse (or keep it from coming back). Certain antidepressants, called selective serotonin reuptake inhibitors or SSRIs, have been shown to help maintain weight and reduce anxiety for people with anorexia and bulimia. Training to build self-esteem can also be helpful.

Talk with your health care provider about treatment options. Also, look under mental health services in your local phone book or call the National Association of Anorexia Nervosa and Associated Disorders, (847) 831-3438, for referrals to service providers, treatment centers, and special programs.

Section 68.2

Anorexia Nervosa

Excerpted from "Anorexia Nervosa," U.S. Department of Health and Human Services, National Women's Health Information Center (NWHIC), October 2000. Available online at http://www.4women.gov; accessed June 2003.

What is anorexia nervosa?

People who intentionally starve themselves or severely restrict their food intake suffer from an eating disorder called anorexia nervosa. The disorder, which usually begins in young people around the time of puberty, involves extreme weight loss—at least 15 percent below a young woman's normal body weight. Those experiencing anorexia nervosa also have an intense fear of becoming fat, even though they are underweight. Many people with the disorder look emaciated but are convinced that they are overweight. Sometimes they must be hospitalized to prevent starvation, yet they often continue to deny the condition. Food and weight become obsessions. For some, the compulsiveness shows up in strange eating rituals or the refusal to eat in front of others. It is not uncommon for people with anorexia to collect recipes and prepare lavish gourmet feasts for family and friends, but not partake in the meals themselves. They may adhere to strict exercise routines to keep off weight. Ninety percent of all anorexics are women.

What problems are associated with anorexia?

There are many side effects of anorexia nervosa. Girls with anorexia usually stop having menstrual periods; this is a condition called amenorrhea. Anorexia may lead to dry skin and thinning hair. Anorexics may have a growth of fine hair all over their body as a natural defense mechanism against extreme weight loss. People suffering from anorexia may feel cold and are easily susceptible to illness. Mood swings are typical.

The National Institute of Mental Health estimates that one in ten anorexic cases ends in death from starvation, suicide, or medical complications like heart attacks or kidney failure. Physical problems also include anemia, heart palpitations, bone loss, tooth decay, as well as inflammation of the esophagus.

What is the treatment for anorexia?

Anorexia is a mental problem manifested in a physical form. Treatment for any eating disorder should include both a mental health professional as well as a primary health care physician. Essential components of successful treatments are ongoing medical care, regular therapy, nutritional counseling, and possibly medication. Eating disorders can be treated with antidepressants, however, this is less effective for anorexia nervosa. Physicians help monitor bone density loss and hear heart rhythm disturbances. Psychologists help identify the important issues and replace destructive thoughts and behaviors with more positive ones. Support groups also play a role in treating anorexia. Often groups of patients will meet weekly to discuss their fears and help each other recover. Most cases of anorexia can be treated successfully, but not instantly. For many patients, treatments may need to be long-term.

What are some of the warning signs of anorexia?

Possible warning signs include:

- Deliberate self-starvation with weight loss
- Intense fear of gaining weight
- Refusal to eat
- Denial of hunger
- Constant exercising
- Greater amounts of hair on the body or the face
- Sensitivity to cold
- Absent or irregular periods
- Loss of scalp hair
- A self-perception of being fat when the person is already too thin

Section 68.3

Bulimia Nervosa

Excerpted from "Bulimia Nervosa," U.S. Department of Health and Human Services, National Women's Health Information Center (NWHIC), June 2001. Available online at http://www.4women.gov; accessed June 2003.

What is bulimia nervosa?

Bulimia nervosa, often simply called bulimia, is an eating disorder. People with bulimia consume large amounts of food and then rid their bodies of the excess calories by purging (self-induced vomiting or misuse of laxatives or diuretics) or by nonpurging (excessive exercise and fasting) behaviors. Some bulimics use a combination of purging and nonpurging behaviors. The cycle of overeating and purging can quickly become an addictive behavior. Often, the individual will feel a loss of control during over eating and the purging/nonpurging behavior becomes a way of regaining control.

Who suffers from bulimia nervosa?

As with anorexia, bulimia typically begins during adolescence. The condition occurs most often in women, but is also found in men. Many people who suffer from bulimia binge and purge in secret. They may maintain normal or above normal body weight. Others may experience significant weight fluctuations. Bulimia can occur in those with anorexia nervosa or it can occur as a separate condition. The chances for recovery increase the earlier bulimia nervosa is detected.

What are some of the warning signs of bulimia?

The binge-purge cycle may be accompanied by self-deprecating thoughts, depression, and an awareness that the eating is abnormal and out of control. Bulimia may be present when a person frequently shows some of the following warning sings:

- Evidence of binge eating, including disappearance of large amounts of food in short periods of time or the existence of wrappers and containers indicating the consumption of large amounts of food.

- Evidence of purging behaviors, including frequent trips to the bathroom after meals, signs and/or smells of vomiting, presence of wrappers or packages of laxatives or diuretics.

- Excessive, rigid exercise regimen; the need to burn off calories taken in despite weather, fatigue, illness, or injury.

- Unusual swelling of the cheeks or jaw area.

- Calluses on the back of the hands and knuckles from self-induced vomiting.

- Discoloration or staining of the teeth.

- Creation of complex lifestyle schedules or rituals to make time for binge-and-purge sessions.

- Withdrawal from usual friends and activities.

In general, behaviors and attitudes indicating that weight loss, dieting, and control of food are becoming primary concerns.

What are the medical consequences of bulimia?

Bulimia can be extremely harmful to the body. The type of purging behavior used can have varied effects on different body systems. Most complications of bulimia result from electrolyte (salt in the blood) imbalance or trauma from repeated purging behaviors. Self-induced vomiting can erode tooth enamel, increase dental cavities, and create a sensitivity of the teeth to hot or cold food. Swelling and soreness in the salivary glands (cheek area) can occur. Also, repeat vomiting can result in irritation and tears in the lining of the throat, esophagus, and stomach (ulcers). The misuse of laxatives and diuretics results in the loss of sodium and potassium that can damage the heart muscle, increasing the risk for irregular heartbeats, heart failure, and death. Also, misuse of laxatives can result in chronic irregular bowel movements and constipation.

How is bulimia treated?

The treatment of bulimia should address both physical and psychological needs of the person. The ultimate outcome of treatment is to restore physical health and normal eating patterns. Many times treatment is undertaken by a team of medical, nutritional, and mental health professionals to evaluate the severity and meaning of the symptoms and to both prescribe and provide care. It is essential that team members communicate regularly about the patient and clarify their roles in treatment on an ongoing basis, to the patient and the family, as well as to each other.

Section 68.4

Binge Eating Disorder

Excerpted from "Binge Eating Disorder," U.S. Department of Health and Human Services, National Women's Health Information Center (NWHIC), October 2000. Available online at http://www.4women.gov; accessed June 2003.

What is binge eating disorder?

Binge eating disorder is an illness that resembles bulimia nervosa. Like bulimics, binge eaters have episodes of uncontrolled eating or bingeing. However, binge eating disorder differs from bulimia because its sufferers do not purge their bodies of excess food.

Individuals with binge eating disorders feel that they lose control of themselves when eating. They eat large quantities of food and do not stop until they are uncomfortably full. Usually, they have more difficulty losing weight and keeping it off than do people with other serious weight problems. Most people with the disorder are obese and have a history of weight fluctuations.

Who suffers from binge eating disorders?

Although it has only recently been recognized as a distinct condition, binge eating disorder is probably the most common eating disorder. Most people with binge eating disorder are obese (more than 20 percent above a healthy body weight), but normal-weight people also can be affected. Binge eating disorder probably affects 2 percent of all adults, or about 1 million to 2 million Americans. Among adolescent and young adult women of America, as much as 4 percent suffer from binge eating disorder. Recent research shows about 30 percent of people participating in medically supervised eating disorder programs suffer from binge eating.

Binge eating disorder is more common in women, with three women affected for every two men. The disorder affects blacks as often as whites; its frequency in other ethnic groups is not yet known. Obese people with binge eating disorder often became overweight at a younger age than those without the disorder. They also may have more frequent episodes of losing and regaining weight (yo-yo dieting).

How is binge eating treated?

Several studies have found that people with binge eating disorder may find it harder than other people to stay in weight loss treatment. Binge eaters also may be more likely to regain weight quickly. For these reasons, people with the disorder may require treatment that focuses on their binge eating before they try to lose weight. Even those who are not overweight are frequently distressed by their binge eating, and may benefit from treatment.

Several methods are being used to treat binge eating disorder. Like all eating disorders, binge eating should be treated on both a physical and psychological level. Physicians and nutritionists can help monitor weight gain or loss. Therapy can help modify behavior and attitude.

Cognitive behavioral therapy teaches patients techniques to monitor and change their eating habits as well as to change the way they respond to difficult situations. Interpersonal psychotherapy helps people examine their relationships with friends and family and to make changes in problem areas. Treatment with medications such as antidepressants may be helpful for some individuals. Self-help groups also may be a source of support.

Researchers are still trying to determine which method or combination of methods is the most effective in controlling binge eating disorder. The type of treatment that is best for an individual is a matter for discussion between the patient and her health care provider.

Chapter 69

Types of Violence That Affect Women

Chapter Contents

Section 69.1

Violence against Women

Excerpted from "Violence against Women," U.S. Department of Health and Human Services, National Women's Health Information Center (NWHIC), September 2001. The full document is available online at http://www. 4women.gov; accessed August 2003.

What are the types of violence against women?

Violence against women can take several forms including domestic violence, intimate partner violence, sexual assault and abuse, rape, incest, dating violence, and elder abuse. Violence includes both actual and threatened violent acts—physical, psychological, or sexual— against women. Battered is a term used to describe women involved and usually living with physically and/or psychologically abusive spouses or partners. Dating violence includes the use of date rape drugs such as Rohypnol, a drug that sedates and immobilizes a person, as well as impairs memory of a violent event. Elder abuse from individuals caring or living with an older person has increased dramatically since the 1980s, and is mostly committed by a family member.

Are some women more at risk for physical assault than others?

Violence against women does not discriminate. It affects women of all racial backgrounds, ages, and economic situations. But, research shows that some women may be more at risk for violence than others. It is estimated that between almost 10% to a little more than 20% of women in America have experienced intimate partner violence during pregnancy. Women in families with incomes under $10,000 are more likely than women with larger incomes to be victims of violence by an intimate partner. Women 19 to 29 years of age are more likely to be victims of violence by an intimate partner. Also, women living with HIV can be at increased risk for intimate partner violence. Research has shown that HIV positive women report emotional, physical, or sexual abuse at some time after their diagnosis.

What is intimate partner violence (or domestic violence)?

Intimate partner violence is the most frequent type of violence committed against women. Intimate partner violence—sometimes called domestic violence—is defined as abuse that is committed by a current or past spouse, boyfriend, or girlfriend. The types of abuse include actual or threatened physical and/or sexual assault, emotional abuse, or verbal abuse. These crimes occur in both heterosexual and same-sex relationships. Intimate partner abuse can have an extremely negative effect not just on the victim, but on other family members as well, particularly children.

Intimate partner violence is not confined to any one socioeconomic, racial/ethnic, religious, or age group. It is the leading cause of injury to women in the United States, where they are more likely to be assaulted, injured, raped, or killed by a male partner than by any other type of assailant. Accurate information on the extent of domestic violence is difficult to obtain because of extensive underreporting. However, it is estimated that as many as four million instances of domestic abuse against women occur annually in the U.S. About one fourth of all hospital emergency room visits by women result from domestic assaults.

What are the signs of intimate partner violence (or domestic violence)?

Intimate partner violence, or domestic violence, involves elements of control and the abuse of power by the person committing the violence. By using intimidation, coercion and threats, and emotional or economic abuse, these abusers exert their control over their victims. In many cases, victims are too frightened to ask for help or to report the acts of violence committed against them or their children.

A number of reasons could be given for an abuser's behavior, including economic hardship, growing up in a violent or abusive household, or abusing drugs or alcohol or both. There is no justification, however, for violent behavior. It is a very common problem and should be taken very seriously.

Here are some questions to ask yourself:

- Have you ever been physically hurt, such as being kicked, pushed or punched, by your partner or ex-partner?

- Has your partner ever used the threat of hurting you to get you to do something?

- Has your partner tried to keep you from seeing your family, going to school, or doing other things that are important to you?

- Do you feel like you are being controlled or isolated by your partner?

- Have you ever been forced by your partner to have sex when you did not want to?

- Has your partner ever insisted on having unsafe (not using protection for sexually transmitted infections or HIV) sex?

- Is your partner very jealous and always questioning whether you are faithful?

- Does your partner regularly blame you for things that you could not control or insult you?

- Are you ever afraid of your partner or of going home? Does he/she make you feel unsafe?

Other signs of intimate partner violence, or domestic violence, that observers might see in a relative or friend include:

- Being prone to accidents.

- Injuries that could not be caused by accident, or do not match the story of what happened to cause them.

- Injuries on many different areas of the body, especially areas that are less likely to get hurt, such as the face, throat, neck, chest, abdomen, or genitals.

- Many injuries that happened at different times.

- Bruises, burns, or wounds that are shaped like objects such as teeth, hands, belts, a cigarette tip, or look like the injured person has a glove or sock on (from having a hand or foot placed in boiling water).

- Seeking medical help a lot.

- Waiting to or not seeking medical help for serious injuries.

- Depression.

- Use of alcohol or drugs.

- Suicide attempts.

A "yes" answer to any of these questions means that your relative or friend may be in an abusive relationship and should get help immediately.

It is important to understand that an abusive partner chooses to be violent and it is not the victim's fault, no matter what the abuser might say. Also remember that abuse usually becomes worse over time. There are many places you or your friend can go to receive information or help. To find help near you, call the National Domestic Violence Hotline (800) 799-SAFE, the National Resource Center on Domestic Violence (800) 537-2238, or local telephone information for domestic violence programs and shelters in your area.

Section 69.2

Female Genital Cutting

Excerpted from "Female Genital Cutting: Frequently Asked Questions," U.S. Department of Health and Human Services, National Women's Health Information Center (NWHIC), August 2001. Available online at http://www.4woman.gov; accessed July 2003.

The following information is sensitive in nature and suited for mature readers only. Furthermore, this material should not be regarded as medical or legal advice.

What is female genital cutting (FGC)?

Female genital cutting (FGC) is the collective name given to traditional practices that involve the partial or total cutting away of the female external genitalia or other injury to the female genitals, whether for cultural or other non-therapeutic reasons. Historically, it has been also called female genital mutilation or female circumcision.

When is FGC carried out?

The age at which FGC is performed on women and girls varies. It may be performed during infancy, childhood, marriage, or during a first pregnancy. FGC is typically performed on young girls who are between 4 and 12 years old, however, by a medically untrained person—often an older woman—from the local culture or community.

Increasingly FGC is also performed by trained health personnel, including physicians, nurses and midwives.

Where is FGC practiced?

FGC is practiced predominantly in 28 countries in Africa. Eighteen African countries have prevalence rates of 50 percent or higher, but these estimates vary from country to country and within various ethnic groups. FGC also occurs in some Middle Eastern countries—Egypt, the Republic of Yemen, Oman, Saudi Arabia and Israel—and is found in some Muslim groups in Indonesia, Malaysia, Pakistan and India. Some immigrants practice various forms of FGC in other parts of the world, including Australia, Canada, New Zealand, the United States and in European nations.

Section 69.3

Sexual Assault

U.S. Department of Health and Human Services, National Women's Health Information Center (NWHIC), April 2001. Available online at http://www.4woman.gov; accessed July 2003.

What is sexual assault?

Sexual assault is any type of sexual activity that you do not want or agree to. It ranges from inappropriate touching to penetration or intercourse. It also can be verbal, visual, audio, or any other form which forces a person to participate in unwanted sexual contact or attention.

Sexual assault includes rape and attempted rape, child molestation, voyeurism, exhibitionism, incest, and sexual harassment. It can happen in different situations, such as: date rape, domestic or intimate partner violence; or by a stranger. All forms of sexual assault are crimes.

Sexual assault is an act of power and control and is not related to sexual urge. The offender, who often is an intimate partner, acquaintance, or family member, can plan the assault ahead of time. Nearly

6 out or 10 rape or sexual assault incidents are reported by victims to have occurred in their own home or at the home of a friend, relative, or neighbor (U.S. Department of Justice). No matter who attacks you, sexual assault is a crime.

Sometimes, the offender is able to take advantage of the victim because the victim is under the influence of alcohol or drugs. Rohypnol and GHB (gamma hydroxybutyrate) are commonly referred to as the date rape drugs since they have been given to victims without their knowledge, they make the victim unable to resist assault, and also cause an amnesia-like affect so the victim is uncertain about what happened. Even if you were drinking alcohol or taking drugs at the time of the attack, sexual assault is a crime.

Unfortunately, rape or sexual assault is the violent crime least often reported to law enforcement. Only 16% of rapes are ever reported to the police. In a survey of victims who did not report rape or attempted rape to the police, victims gave the following reasons for not making a report: 43% thought nothing could be done; 27% thought it was a private matter; 12% were afraid of police response; and 12% thought it was not important enough. Remember, sexual assault is against the law. You have the right to report this crime to the police, and to be treated fairly.

Who are the victims of sexual assault?

According to the U.S. Department of Justice, an estimated 91% of the victims of rape and sexual assault are female and 9% are male. (Nearly 99% of the reported offenders are male.) The National Victim Center reports that 683,000 women are raped per year, and 13.3% of college women say they had been forced to have sex in a dating situation. The National Violence Against Women Survey found of the women who reported being raped, 54% were under the age of 18 at the time of the first rape and 83% were under the age of 25. However, sexual assault affects women, children, and men of all ages, racial, cultural and economic backgrounds.

How can I help prevent being sexually assaulted?

In general, be alert to your surroundings. Walk with confidence and trust your instincts. If you feel uncomfortable in your surroundings, leave. When out with friends at social events, never leave with someone you've just met. Don't take drugs or alcohol, which might cloud your judgment. (Be wary of isolated spots, like underground garages, offices after business hours, and apartment laundry rooms. Avoid walking alone, especially at night. Never hitchhike or pick up a hitch-hiker. If possible, stay in areas where there are other people, and park your car in well-lighted areas. Always lock your car and have your key ready to use before you reach the car. If you think you are being followed, run towards a lighted house, restaurants, stores or other public places. If possible, always carry a cellular phone.

If your car breaks down, turn on your flashers, lock the doors, stay in your car, and call for help on the cellular phone. If you don't have a phone, put on the flashers, lift your hood, use flares if possible, get back in the car, and lock the doors. If someone stops to help you, roll the window down enough so he or she can hear you, and ask them to call the police or a tow service.

At home, never open your door to strangers. Always check the identification of salespersons or service people before opening the door. It also is a good idea to have another adult at home with you when service people come, if you can arrange it. Make sure all windows and doors are locked. Have a peephole in the door and well-lighted entrances. Know a neighbor you can call or rely on if something happens.

If you are in an abusive relationship, create a safety plan so you know what you would do in the event of an attempted attack. A safety plan includes: knowing possible escape routes to get away from the attacker (windows, stairwells, basement exits); knowing a safe place to go (a friend or family member you can trust); having a survival kit of money, keys, clothes, and important personal information like bank account numbers, phone numbers, and legal documents; knowing the number for a domestic violence hotline; avoiding arguments with the abuser in areas where there are potential weapons; having a personal savings account, separate from the abuser; and reviewing the plan monthly.

How do I handle a sexual assaulter?

The National Crime Prevention Council (NCPC) explains that there are no hard and fast, right or wrong answers to handle an attacker. It depends on your emotional state and physical state, the situation, and the attacker's personality. Surviving is the goal, but NCPC recommends the following:

- Try to escape. Scream. Be rude. Make noise to discourage your attacker from following.

- Talk, stall for time, and assess your options.

- If the attacker has a weapon, you may have no choice but to submit. Do whatever it takes to survive.

- If you decide to fight back, you must be quick, determined, and effective. Target the eyes or groin.

What do I do if I am sexually assaulted?

- Get away from the attacker to a safe place as fast as you can.

- Call a friend or family member you trust. You also can call a crisis center or a hotline to talk with a counselor. One national hotline is the National Domestic Violence Hotline 1-800-799-SAFE or 1-800-787-3224 (TDD). Do not feel ashamed or guilty. These feelings, as well as being afraid and shocked, are normal. It is important to get counseling from a trusted professional.

- Do not wash, comb, or clean any part of your body, or change clothes if possible. Do not touch or change anything at the scene of the assault; it is a crime scene. Then, go to your nearest hospital emergency room as soon as possible.

- You need to be examined, treated for any injuries, and screened for possible sexually transmitted diseases or pregnancy. The doctor will collect evidence that the attacker may have left behind, like clothing fibers, hairs, saliva, or semen. A standard rape kit is usually used to help collect these things. You, or the hospital staff can call the police from the emergency room to file a report.

Where else can I go for help?

If you are sexually assaulted, it is not your fault. Don't be afraid to ask for help or support. Help is available. You can call: National Domestic Violence Hotline 1-800-799-SAFE or 1-800-787-3224 (TDD).

Section 69.4

Dating Violence

"Dating Violence Fact Sheet," Centers for Disease Control and Prevention, National Center for Injury Prevention and Control, January 27, 2000. Available online at http://www.cdc.gov; accessed May 2003.

Dating violence may be defined as the perpetration or threat of an act of violence by at least one member of an unmarried couple on the other member within the context of dating or courtship. This violence encompasses any form of sexual assault, physical violence, and verbal or emotional abuse.

Violent behavior that takes place in a context of dating or courtship is not a rare event. Estimates vary because studies and surveys use different methods and definitions of the problem.

- A review of dating violence research found that prevalence rates of nonsexual, courtship violence range from 9% to 65%, depending on whether threats and emotional or verbal aggression were included in the definition.

- Summarizing many studies, the average prevalence rate for nonsexual dating violence is 22% among male and female high school students and 32% among college students. Females are somewhat more likely than males to report being victims of violence.

- In a national study of college students, 27.5% of the women surveyed said that they had suffered rape or attempted rape at least once since age 14. Only 5% of those experiences were reported to the police. The term hidden rape has emerged because this survey and many other studies found that sexual assaults are seldom reported to the police.

- Over half of a representative sample of more than 1,000 female students at a large urban university had experienced some form of unwanted sex. Twelve percent of these acts were perpetrated by casual dates and 43% by steady dating partners.

- Studies of college students and high school students suggest that both males and females inflict and receive dating violence in equal proportion, but the motivation for violence by women is more often for defensive purposes. Other studies have found that women and girls were victims of dating violence twice as often as men and boys, and that females suffer significantly more injuries than males.

- A recent National Crime Victimization survey found that women were 6 times more likely than men to experience violence at the hands of an intimate partner. Intimate partners include current or former spouses, boyfriends, girlfriends, dating partners, regardless of whether they are cohabiting or not.

- Nearly half of the 500,000 rapes and sexual assaults reported to the police by women of all ages were committed by friends or acquaintances. From 80% to 95% of the rapes that occur on college campuses are committed by someone known to the victim.

Section 69.5

Date Rape Drug (Rohypnol)

Excerpted from "Date Rape Drug (Rohypnol)," U.S. Department of Health and Human Services, National Women's Health Information Center (NWHIC); December 2000. Available online at http://www.4woman.gov; accessed August 2003.

What is the date rape drug?

The date rape drug is the common name for Rohypnol, generically called flunitrazepam. Rohypnol is manufactured by Hoffman-La Roche and prescribed as a sleeping pill in countries outside of the United States. It is used as a short-term treatment for insomnia, as a sedative hypnotic and a pre-anesthetic. It has physiological effects similar to Valium (diazepam), but is approximately ten times more potent. It is used also as an illicit drug, often in combination with other drugs, such as heroin, cocaine, and alcohol. Common names for Rohypnol include the following: rophies, roofies, R2, roofenol, Roche, roachies, la rocha, rope, rib, circles, Mexican valium, roach-2, roopies, and ropies. A similar drug is known as clonazepam (Klonopin in the U.S. and Rivotril in Mexico.)

What does Rohypnol look like?

Rohypnol tablets are white, scored on one side, with the word "ROCHE" and an encircled one or two (depending on the dosage) on the other. They are sold in pre-sealed bubble packs of one or two mg doses. Rohypnol can often be dissolved in a drink and may be undetectable.

What happens when you take Rohypnol?

Rohypnol intoxication is generally associated with impaired judgment and impaired motor skills and can make a victim unable to resist a sexual attack. The combination of alcohol and Rohypnol is also particularly hazardous because together, their effects on memory and judgment are greater than the effects resulting from either taken alone. Effects begin within thirty minutes, peak within two hours, and can persist for up to eight hours. It is commonly reported that persons who become intoxicated on a combination of alcohol and flunitrazepam have blackouts lasting eight to twenty-four hours following ingestion. Disinhibition (losing your social inhibitions) is another widely reported effect of Rohypnol, when taken alone or in combination with alcohol.

Adverse effects of Rohypnol use include, decreased blood pressure, memory impairment, drowsiness, visual disturbances, dizziness, confusion, gastrointestinal disturbances and urinary retention.

How can I avoid becoming a victim?

Here are a few suggestions for staying aware and alert:

- Be wary about accepting drinks from anyone you don't know well or long enough to trust. If you are accepting a drink, make sure it's from an unopened container and that you open it yourself.

- Don't put your drink down and leave it unattended, even to go to the restroom.

- Notify other females you know about the effects of this dangerous drug.

If you think that you have been a victim, notify the authorities immediately.

Section 69.6

Recovering from Rape

Excerpted from "Recovering from Rape," Health and Human Services, National Women's Health Information Center (NWHIC), May 2000. By Clare G. Holzman, Ph.D. Available online at http://www.4woman.gov; accessed July 2003.

Whether and Where to Get Medical Attention

Rape survivors often have physical injuries, including internal injuries, they may not be aware of. Treatment can also prevent pregnancy and sexually transmitted diseases. The medical exam also collects evidence that may help convict the rapist; the sooner the exam is done, the better the chances are that important evidence will be preserved. These services are available in hospital emergency rooms. Many hospitals treat rape survivors without advance payment, even if they have no insurance.

Whether to Report the Rape to the Police

Many rape survivors want to see the rapist punished, and protect others from being victimized. They want society to make a clear statement that rape is a crime that will not be tolerated. Playing a part in the rapist's arrest and conviction can make a woman feel more powerful and less like a helpless victim.

At a more practical level, a woman must report the rape to be eligible for Crime Victims' Compensation benefits. Crime Victims' Compensation can pay for medical expenses, other financial losses resulting from the rape, and even long-term psychotherapy. Information about how to apply can be obtained from the state Crime Victims Board, the police, or a rape crisis counseling program. On the other hand, a woman may choose not to report the rape. She or someone she knows may have been treated badly by the police in the past. The rapist may have threatened to harm her or her family if she reports the crime. Furthermore, pressing charges can be a long, painful process. Every woman must decide for herself, based on her own circumstances, whether it makes sense to go through it.

How to Make Space for Healing

Sometimes it can feel like recovering from rape is a full-time job all by itself. The survivor may be overwhelmed by confusing emotions—fear, grief, guilt, shame, rage. She may be unable to sleep at night and unable to stay awake during the day. She may have trouble thinking clearly, concentrating, and making decisions. Some women have no choice but to put their emotions aside and go on coping with the demands of their daily reality. Some find that they feel better if they carry on with their normal routine as much as possible.

Where to Seek Support

The best family members and friends to turn to are those who will stay calm and who will not blame, criticize, or try to take over. It's good to have more than one person to turn to; some people are duds at dealing with intense emotions, but terrific about practical things like baby sitting or providing transportation to a medical appointment.

A hot line counselor or an in-person rape crisis counselor can be a supportive listener when family and friends are unavailable or are too emotionally involved to be helpful. She can provide information about the recovery process and about available resources. She can be an advocate if the survivor runs into bureaucratic roadblocks in obtaining services.

After the initial crisis, a support group can help to break down isolation, secrecy, and shame. Because members of the group are at different stages of healing, she can gain perspective on how far she has come and see evidence that further progress is possible.

If the recovery process has stalled, psychotherapy may be the next step. A rape can bring up old anxieties and conflicts about issues like trust, control, sexuality, self-worth, etc. Sometimes it triggers feelings and memories related to earlier traumas, such as child sexual abuse. If depression or anxiety is severe and shows no signs of improving, medication may be useful.

Recovery from rape doesn't mean that it's as if the rape never happened. Most women find that in some ways they have changed permanently. Recovery does mean that, more and more of the time, the survivor is not thinking about the rape. Her emotions are no longer dominated by it. She is able to envision a future for herself, to set goals and work to achieve them. Her life moves forward.

Chapter 70

Drug and Alcohol Abuse among Women

Chapter Contents

Section 70.1

Alcohol Abuse and Treatment

U.S. Department of Health and Human Services, National Women's
Health Information Center (NWHIC), October 2000. Available online at
http://www.4woman.gov; accessed July 2003.

Opinions vary on the definition of alcohol abuse. Abuse can be regular usage that is turning into a dependency. Abuse can also be binge
drinking; consuming a large quantity of alcohol in a very short amount
of time, but not necessarily every day. Some believe that more than
one drink a day for most women is too much. A standard drink is generally considered to be 12 ounces of beer, 5 ounces of wine, or 1.5
ounces of 80-proof distilled spirits. It is generally believed that on any
given day, a woman should have no more than 2 drinks, and that a
woman should not drink every day.

However, defining abuse is difficult because the pattern of drinking is an important determinant of alcohol-related consequences. So,
while data is often collected in terms of the "average number of drinks
per week," one drink taken each day may have different consequences
than seven drinks taken on a Saturday night.

What is alcoholism?

Alcoholism, also known as alcohol dependence, is a disease. Alcoholism is a chronic, often progressive disease with symptoms that
include a strong need to drink despite negative consequences, such
as serious job, relationships, or health problems. Like many other diseases, it has a generally predictable course, has recognized symptoms,
and is influenced by both genetic and environmental factors that are
being increasingly well defined. The four known symptoms are:

- Craving: A strong need, or compulsion, to drink.

- Impaired control: The inability to limit one's drinking.

- Physical dependence: Withdrawal symptoms (nausea, sweating,
  shakiness, anxiety) when alcohol is stopped after a period of
  heavy drinking.

- Tolerance: The need for increasing amounts of alcohol in order to feel its effects.

Does a person have to be alcoholic to experience problems from alcohol abuse?

No. An alcoholic is dependent upon alcohol. This dependence grows as the disease progresses. A person who abuses alcohol may not be dependent upon it but still drinks excessively. Even if you are not an alcoholic, abusing alcohol has negative results. This includes failure to meet major work, school, or family responsibilities; alcohol-related legal trouble; automobile crashes due to drinking; as well as a variety of medical problems. Under some circumstances, problems can result from even moderate drinking—for example, when driving, during pregnancy, or when taking certain medicines.

Does alcohol affect women differently than men?

Yes. Increasing evidence suggests that the detrimental effects of chromic alcohol abuse are more severe for women than men. Women develop alcoholic liver diseases, particularly alcoholic cirrhosis and hepatitis, after a comparatively shorter period of heavy drinking and at a lower level of daily drinking than men. Proportionately, more alcoholic women die of cirrhosis than do alcoholic men. Women also become more intoxicated than do men, after drinking the same amount of alcohol. This is due to differences in body weight and hormone releases. Alcohol dependence and related medical problems, such as brain and liver damage, progress more rapidly in women.

Does heavy drinking affect your menstrual period?

Yes. Menstrual disorders (e.g., painful menstruation, heavy flow, premenstrual discomfort, and irregular or absent cycles) have been associated with chronic heavy drinking. These disorders can have adverse effects on fertility. Further, continued drinking may lead to early menopause.

What effect does drinking during pregnancy have on the baby?

Fetal Alcohol Syndrome (FAS) describes the pattern of abnormalities observed in children born to alcoholic mothers. These abnormalities include low birth weight, behavioral dysfunction, brain malformation, physical deformities, and mental retardation. Prenatal alcohol exposure is one of the leading known causes of mental retardation in the Western world. Moderate drinkers can also pass on milder forms of these serious health risks to their children. These are termed fetal alcohol effects (FAE) and can have serious implications in the development of the child.

The Centers for Disease Control in the Department of Health and Human Service found that the rate of frequent drinking among pregnant women increased fourfold between 1991 and 1995.

How is alcoholism treated?

Alcoholism is a disease and has no cure, but can be managed with medical treatment and social support groups. This means that even if an alcoholic has been sober for a long time and has regained health, he or she may relapse, and must continue to avoid all alcoholic beverages. The most common and most effective way to combat alcohol abuse is through a systematic support group, with advice and support from a health care professional.

What do I do if I think I may be drinking too much?

If you think you may have a drinking problem, talk to your doctor, a close friend, or a family member you trust. It is important to recognize the problem and get help. You can also contact the Center for Substance Abuse Treatment at (800) 662-HELP. This Center has specific information about treatment programs. Alcoholics Anonymous runs local support meetings and local phone numbers are in the phone book. It takes courage to admit you don't have control over alcohol; asking for help is an important first step.

Section 70.2

Drug Abuse and Treatment

U.S. Department of Health and Human Services, National Women's
Health Information Center (NWHIC), October 2000. Available online at
http://www.4woman.gov; accessed July 2003.

What are the consequences of drug abuse for women?

Research indicates that women can become addicted quickly to
certain drugs, such as crack cocaine, even after casual or experimen-
tal use. Therefore, by the time a woman enters treatment, she may
be severely addicted, making treatment more difficult. This is also true
when a woman becomes dependent on prescription painkillers.

What happens during treatment?

Treatment should include an evaluation of other serious health
problems associated with drug abuse. For women, some of these problems are: poor nutrition and below-average weight; low self-esteem;
depression; physical abuse; if pregnant, preterm labor or early delivery; and serious medical and infectious diseases (e.g., increased blood
pressure and heart rate, STDs, HIV/AIDS).

Why do some women refuse to seek treatment?

Many drug-using women do not seek treatment because they are
afraid, they worry they won't be able to keep or care for their children, they fear reprisal from their spouses or boyfriends, and they fear
punishment from authorities in the community. Many women report
that their drug-using male sex partners initiated them into drug abuse
and then sabotaged their efforts to quit using drugs.

Is there a connection between drug abuse and HIV/AIDS?

Yes. AIDS is now the fourth leading cause of death among women
of childbearing age in the United States. It is the leading cause of
death for African-American women between the ages of 25 and 44.

Because HIV/AIDS often is transmitted through shared needles or syringes, women who inject drugs or share drug paraphernalia are at an increased risk of getting the deadly disease. In addition, under the influence of illicit drugs and alcohol, a woman's judgment can become impaired. As a result, women may engage in unprotected sex, which also increases their risk for contracting or transmitting HIV/AIDS. Among the 1.5 million injecting drug users, 14% are known to be infected with HIV.

What treatment is available for women?

Research shows that women receive the most benefit from drug treatment programs that provide comprehensive services for meeting their basic needs, including access to: food, clothing, and shelter; transportation; job counseling and training; legal assistance; literacy training and educational opportunities; parenting training; family therapy; medical care; child care; social services; social support; psychological assessment and mental health care; assertiveness training; and family planning services.

Traditional male-oriented drug treatment programs may not be appropriate for women because those programs may not provide these services. Research also indicates that for women in particular, treatment is more successful when they stay in regular touch with their treatment provider. When a woman lapses during the treatment and recovery process; it is important that they get the support of the community and encouragement of those closest to them. After completing a drug treatment program, women also need services to assist them in sustaining their recovery and in rejoining the community.

Where can I call if I have questions related to drug abuse?

A toll-free hotline is available to provide free, confidential answers to women seeking help for themselves or for someone they care about, or to provide referral to a local drug treatment program. The National Drug Information, Treatment, and Referral Line is reached through 1-800-662-HELP (1-800-66-AYUDA for Spanish-speaking callers.) The hotline operates Monday through Friday from 9 a.m. to 3 a.m. and Saturday and Sunday from 12 noon to 3 a.m.

Chapter 71

Women and Stress

Chapter Contents

Section 71.1

Coping with Stress

Excerpted from "Stress," U.S. Department of Health and Human Services, National Women's Health Information Center (NWHIC), September 2001. Available online at http://www.4woman.gov; accessed July 2003.

What are some of the most common causes of stress?

Stress can arise for a variety of reasons. Stress can be brought about by a traumatic accident, death, or emergency situation. Stress can also be a side effect of a serious illness or disease. There is also stress associated with daily life, the workplace, and family responsibilities.

What are some early signs of stress?

Stress can take on many different forms, and can contribute to symptoms of illness. Common symptoms include headache, sleep disorders, difficulty concentrating, short temper, upset stomach, job dissatisfaction, low morale, depression, and anxiety.

Is there any way to relieve your stress?

There are many stress management programs that can teach you about the nature and sources of stress, the effects of stress on health, and personal skills to reduce the effects of stress. Examples of stress reducing skills include time management and physical exercise.

For more serious stress related disorders, like PTSD, research has demonstrated the effectiveness of cognitive-behavioral therapy, group therapy, and exposure therapy, in which the patient repeatedly relives the frightening experience under controlled conditions to help him or her work through the trauma. Studies have also shown that medications help ease associated symptoms of depression and anxiety and help promote sleep.

Section 71.2

Caregiver Stress

Excerpted from "Caregiver Stress," U.S. Department of Health and Human Services, National Women's Health Information Center (NWHIC), August 2002. Available online at http://www.4woman.gov; accessed June 2003.

What is caregiving?

Caregiving means caring for others, whether friends or relatives, who have health problems or disabilities and need help. Caregivers provide many kinds of help to care receivers, from grocery shopping to helping with daily tasks such as bathing, dressing, and eating. Most people who need help from caregivers are elderly.

What is caregiver stress?

Caregiver stress is a daily fact of life for many caregivers. Caregiving often takes a great deal of time, effort, and work. Many caregivers struggle to balance caregiving with other responsibilities including full-time jobs and caring for children. Constant stress can lead to burnout and health problems for the caregiver. Caregivers may feel guilty, frustrated, and angry from time to time.

Caregivers often need help caring for an elderly or disabled care receiver. Sometimes other family members or friends and neighbors are able to help, but many caregivers do most or all of the caregiving for a loved one alone. Research has shown that caregivers often are at increased risk for depression and illness. This is especially true if they do not receive enough support from family, friends, and the community.

Caring for a person with Alzheimer's disease (AD) or other kinds of dementia at home can be overwhelming. The caregiver must cope with declining abilities and difficult behaviors. Basic activities of daily living often become hard to manage for both the care receiver and the caregiver. As the disease worsens, the care receiver usually needs 24-hour care.

What can caregivers do to prevent stress and burnout?

Caregivers can call upon others for support and assistance. Other family members, friends, and neighbors may be able to help in different ways. It may not be easy to ask for help, and you may need to make very specific requests. But getting help from others will benefit you and the person you are caring for.

Respite care can be a good way to get a break (respite) from constant caregiving. If other caregivers aren't available to fill in for the main caregiver, respite care services may be available in the community.

As a caregiver, you can take steps to take care of your own health:

• Eat a healthy diet rich in fruits, vegetables, and whole grains and low in saturated fat. Ask your health care provider about taking a multivitamin as well.

• Try to get enough sleep and rest.

• Find time for some exercise most days of the week. Regular exercise can help reduce stress and improve your health in many ways.

• See your health care provider for a checkup. Talk to your provider about symptoms of depression or illness that you may be having. Get counseling if needed.

• Stay in touch with friends. Social activities can help keep you feeling connected and help with stress. Faith-based groups can offer support and help to caregivers.

• Find a support group for other caregivers in your situation (such as caring for a person with dementia). Many support groups are available online through the Internet.

Part Ten

Additional
Help and Information

Chapter 72

Glossary of Terms
Related to Women's Health

Amenorrhea: Absence or abnormal cessation of the menses.

Anorexia nervosa: A mental disorder manifested by extreme fear of becoming obese and an aversion to food, usually occurring in young women and often resulting in life-threatening weight loss, accompanied by a disturbance in body image, hyperactivity, and amenorrhea.

Areola: A circular pigmented area surrounding the nipple.

Bacterial vaginosis: Infection of the human vagina that may be caused by anaerobic bacteria, especially by *Mobiluncus* species or by *Gardnerella vaginalis*. Characterized by excessive, sometimes malodorous, discharge.

Bulimia nervosa: A chronic morbid disorder involving repeated and secretive episodic bouts of eating characterized by uncontrolled rapid ingestion of large quantities of food over a short period of time (binge eating), followed by self-induced vomiting, use of laxatives or diuretics, fasting, or vigorous exercise in order to prevent weight gain; often accompanied by feelings of guilt, depression, or self-disgust.

Cervix: The lower part of the uterus extending from the isthmus of the uterus into the vagina.

Contraception: Prevention of conception or impregnation.

Definitions in this chapter were taken from *Stedman's Medical Dictionary, 27th Edition.* © 2000, Lippincott Williams & Wilkins. All rights reserved.

Domestic violence: Intentionally inflicted injury perpetrated by and on family member(s); varieties include spouse abuse, child abuse, and sexual abuse, including incest. Various kinds of abuse, such as sexual abuse, also happen outside the family unit.

Dysmenorrhea: Difficult and painful menstruation.

Dyspareunia: Occurrence of pain during sexual intercourse.

Endometriosis: Ectopic occurrence of endometrial tissue, frequently forming cysts containing altered blood.

Estrogen: Estrogens are formed by the ovary, placenta, testes, and possibly the adrenal cortex, as well as by certain plants; they stimulate secondary sexual characteristics, and exert systemic effects, such as growth and maturation of long bones, and are used therapeutically in any disorder attributable to estrogen deficiency or amenable to estrogen therapy, such as menstrual disorders and menopausal problems. They control the course of the menstrual cycle.

Fallopian tube: One of the tubes leading on either side from the upper or outer extremity of the ovary. It provides the path by which the ovum travels from ovary to uterus where, if it is fertilized in the tube, it will implant as a zygote.

Fetus: In humans, the product of conception from the end of the eighth week to the moment of birth.

Fibromyalgia: A syndrome of chronic pain of musculoskeletal origin but uncertain cause. The American College of Rheumatology has established diagnostic criteria that include pain on both sides of the body, both above and below the waist, as well as in an axial distribution (cervical, thoracic, or lumbar spine or anterior chest); additionally there must be point tenderness in at least 11 of 18 specified sites.

Gynecologist: A physician specializing in gynecology, the medical specialty concerned with diseases of the female genital tract, as well as endocrinology and reproductive physiology of the female.

Hormone replacement therapy (HRT): Administration of sex hormones to women after menopause or oophorectomy.

Hysterectomy: Removal of the uterus; unless otherwise specified, usually denotes complete removal of the uterus.

Interstitial cystitis: A chronic inflammatory condition of unknown etiology involving the epithelium and muscularis of the bladder, resulting in reduced bladder capacity, pain relieved by voiding, and severe bladder irritative symptoms

Laparoscopy: Examination of the contents of the abdominopelvic cavity with a laparoscope passed through the abdominal wall.

Lumpectomy: Removal of either a benign or malignant lesion from the breast with preservation of essential anatomy of the breast.

Lupus erythematosus: An illness that may be chronic (characterized by skin lesions alone), subacute (characterized by recurring superficial nonscarring skin lesions that are more disseminated and present more acute features both clinically and histologically than those seen in the chronic discoid phase), or systemic or disseminated (in which antinuclear antibodies are present and in which there is almost always involvement of vital structures).

Mammary gland: The potential and active milk-secreting gland that lies within the breast.

Mammogram: The record produced by mammography, which is radiologic examination of the female breast with equipment and techniques designed to screen for cancer.

Mastalgia: Pain in the breast.

Mastectomy: Excision of the breast.

Menopause: Permanent cessation of the menses; termination of the menstrual life.

Menstruation: Cyclic endometrial shedding and discharge of a bloody fluid from the uterus during the menstrual cycle.

Morning after pill: An oral drug that, when taken by a woman within 2–3 days after intercourse, reduces the probability that she will become pregnant.

Obstetrician: A physician specializing in the medical care of women during pregnancy and childbirth.

Oophorectomy: Excision of one or both ovaries.

Osteoporosis: Reduction in the quantity of bone or atrophy of skeletal tissue; an age-related disorder characterized by decreased bone mass and increased susceptibility to fractures.

Ovary: One of the paired female reproductive glands containing the ova or germ cells.

Ovulation: Release of an ovum from the ovarian follicle.

Ovum: The female sex cell. When fertilized by a sperm, an ovum is capable of developing into a new individual of the same species.

Pap Test: Microscopic examination of cells exfoliated or scraped from a mucosal surface after staining with Papanicolaou stain; used especially for detection of cancer of the uterine cervix.

Perimenopause: The 3–5-year period prior to menopause during which estrogen levels begin to drop.

Placenta: Organ of metabolic interchange between fetus and mother.

Polycystic ovary syndrome (PCOS): A condition commonly characterized by hirsutism [excessive body hair], obesity, menstrual abnormalities, infertility, and enlarged ovaries; thought to reflect excessive androgen secretion of ovarian origin.

Postmenopausal: Relating to the period following menopause.

Premenstrual dysphoric disorder (PMDD): A pervasive pattern occurring during the last week of the luteal phase in most menstrual cycles for at least a year and remitting within a few days of the onset of the follicular phase, with some combination of depressed mood, mood lability, marked anxiety, or irritability; various specific physical symptoms; and significant functional impairment; the symptoms are comparable in severity to those seen in a major depressive episode, distinguishing this disorder from the far more common premenstrual syndrome.

Premenstrual syndrome (PMS): In women of reproductive age, a constellation of emotional, behavioral, and physical symptoms that occur in the luteal (premenstrual) phase of the menstrual cycle and subside with the onset of menstruation; characterized by swelling and weight gain due to fluid retention, breast tenderness, irritability, mood swings, anxiety, depression, drowsiness, fatigue, difficulty concentrating, and changes in appetite and libido.

Progesterone: Used to correct abnormalities of the menstrual cycle and as a contraceptive and to control habitual abortion.

Toxic shock syndrome: Infection with toxin-producing staphylococci, occurring most often in the vagina of menstruating women using superabsorbent tampons but also prevalent in many soft tissue infections and characterized by high fever, vomiting, diarrhea, a scarlatiniform rash followed by desquamation, and decreasing blood pressure and shock, which can result in death

Uterus: The hollow muscular organ in which the impregnated ovum is developed into a child.

Vagina: The genital canal in the female, extending from the uterus to the vulva.

Vaginitis: Inflammation of the vagina.

Varicose veins: Permanent dilation and tortuosity [full of turns and twists] of veins, most commonly seen in the legs; there is a predisposition to varicose veins among persons in occupations requiring long periods of standing, and in pregnant women.

Vulva: The external genitalia of the female, comprised of the mons pubis, the labia majora and minora, the clitoris, the vestibule of the vagina and its glands, and the opening of the urethra and of the vagina.

Vulvodynia: Chronic vulvar discomfort with complaints of burning and superficial irritation.

Chapter 73

Organizations That Provide Information and Assistance for Victims of Domestic Violence or Sexual Assault

American Bar Association Commission on Domestic Violence
740 15th Street NW, 9th Floor
Washington, DC, 20005-1022
Toll-Free: (800) 799-SAFE
TTY: (800) 787-3224
Website: http://www.abanet.org/domviol/home.html
E-mail: cdv@staff.abanet.org

American Institute on Domestic Violence
2116 Rover Drive
Lake Havasu City, AZ 86403
Phone: (928) 453-9015
Fax: (775) 522-9120
Website: http://www.aidv-usa.com
E-mail: info@aidv-usa.com

American Women's Self-Defense Association
713 North Wellwood Avenue
Lindenhurst, NY 11757
Toll-Free: (888) STOP-RAPE
Website: http://www.awsda.org
E-mail: awsda@nvbb.net

Corporate Alliance to End Partner Violence
2416 East Washington Street
Suite E
Bloomington, IL 61704
Phone: (309) 664-0667
Fax: (309) 664-0747
Website: http://www.caepv.org
E-mail: caepv@caepv.org

Resources in this chapter were compiled from many sources deemed accurate; all contact information was verified and updated in July 2003.

End Violence Against Women
111 Market Place
Suite 310
Baltimore, MD 21202
Phone: (410) 659-6300
Fax: (410) 659-6266
Website: http://www.endvaw.org
E-mail: ertran@jhuccp.org

Family Violence and Sexual Assault Institute
6160 Cornerstone Court East
San Diego, CA 92121
Phone: (858) 623-2777
Fax: (858) 646-0761
Website: http://www.fvsai.org
E-mail: fvsai@alliant.edu

Family Violence Prevention Fund
383 Rhode Island Street
Suite 304
San Francisco, CA 94103-5133
Phone: (415) 252-8900
TTY: (800) 595-4889
Fax: (415) 595-4889
Website: http://endabuse.org
E-mail: info@endabuse.org

National Coalition Against Domestic Violence
P.O. Box 18749
Denver, CO 80218-0749
Toll-Free: (800) 799-7233
Phone: (303) 839-1852
Fax: (303) 831-9251
Website: http://www.ncadv.org
E-mail: sbaca@ncadv.org

National Council of Juvenile and Family Court Judges
P.O. Box 8970
Reno, NV 89507
Phone: (775) 784-6012
Fax: (775) 784-6628
Website: http://www.ncjfcj.org
E-mail: admin@ncjfcj.org

National Domestic Violence Hotline
Toll-Free: (800) 799-7233
TTY: (800) 787-3224
Website: http://www.ndvh.org

National Network to End Domestic Violence
660 Pennsylvania Avenue SE
Suite 303
Washington, DC 20003
Phone: (202) 543-5566
Fax: (202) 543-5626
Website: http://www.nnedv.org
E-mail: nnedv@nnedv.org

National Resource Center on Domestic Violence
383 Rhode Island Street
Suite 304
San Francisco, CA 94103-5133
Phone: (415) 252-8900
TTY: (800) 595-4889
Fax: (415) 252-8991
Website: http://endabuse.org
E-mail: info@endabuse.org

National Sexual Violence Resource Center
123 North Enola Drive
Enola, PA 17025
Toll-Free: (877) 739-3895
Phone: (717) 909-0710
TTY: (717) 909-0715
Fax: (717) 909-0714
Website: http://www.nsvrc.org
E-mail: resources@nsvrc.org

Native American Women's Health Education Resource Center
P.O. Box 572
Lake Andes, SD 57356-0572
Phone: (605) 487-7072
Fax: (605) 487-7964
Website: http://www.nativeshop
.org/nawherc.html
E-mail: nativewoman@igc .apc.org

NOW Legal Defense and Education Fund
395 Hudson Street
New York, NY 10014
Phone: (212) 925-6635
Fax: (212) 226-1066
Website: http://www.nowldef.org
E-mail: peo@nowldef.org

Office on Violence Against Women
810 7th Street, NW
Washington, DC 20531
Phone: (202) 307-6026
TTY: (202) 307-2277
Fax: (202) 307-3911
Website: http://
www.ojp.usdoj.gov/vawo

Partnerships Against Violence Network Online
Phone: (301) 504-5462
Website: http://www.pavnet.org
E-mail: pavnet@nal.usda.gov

Rape, Abuse, and Incest National Network
635-B Pennsylvania Avenue SE
Washington, DC 2003
Toll-Free: (800) 656-HOPE
Phone: (202) 544-1034
Fax: (202) 544-3556
Website: http://www.rainn.org
E-mail: info@rain.org

Survivors of Incest Anonymous
P.O. Box 190
Benson, MD 21018-9998
Phone: (410) 893-3322
Website: http://www.siawso.org
E-mail: info@siawso.org

Chapter 74

Directory of Organizations That Provide Public Health Assistance for Low-Income Women

American Civil Liberties Union
125 Broad Street
18th Floor
New York, NY 10004
Phone: (212) 549-2585
Website: http://www.aclu.org
E-mail: membership@aclu.org

American Public Human Services Association
810 First Street NE
Suite 500
Washington, DC 20002
Phone: (202) 682-0100
Fax: (202) 289-6555
Website: http://www.aphsa.org

Center for Health Care Strategies, Inc.
P.O. Box 3469
Princeton, NJ 08543-3469
Phone: (609) 895-8101
Fax: (609) 895-9648
Website: http://www.chcs.org
E-mail: mail@chcs.org

Centers for Medicare and Medicaid Services
7500 Security Boulevard
Baltimore, MD 21244-1850
Toll-Free: (877) 267-2323
TTY Toll-Free: (866) 226-1819
Phone: (410) 786-3000
TTY: (410) 786-0727
TTY: (866) 226-1819
Website: http://cms.hhs.gov

Resources in this chapter were compiled from many sources deemed accurate; all contact information was verified and updated in July 2003.

Commonwealth Fund
1 East 75th Street
New York, NY 10021
Phone: (212) 606-3800
Fax: (212) 606-3500
Website: http://www.cmwf.org
E-mail: cmwf@cmwf.org

Health Resources and Services Administration
5600 Fishers Lane
Rockville, MD 20857-0001
Toll-Free: (888) Ask HRSA (275-4772)
Phone: (301) 443-3376
Website: http://www.hrsa.gov
E-mail: ask@hrsa.gov

Institute for Health Policy Solutions
1444 I Street NW
Suite 900
Washington, DC 20005
Phone: (202) 789-1491
Fax: (202) 789-1879
Website: http://www.ihps.org

Institute for Reproductive Health Access
462 Broadway
Suite 540
New York, NY 10013
Phone: (212) 343-0114
Website: http://www.naralny.org/institute.htm
E-mail: irha@naralny.org

Lyon-Martin Women's Health Services
1748 Market Street, Suite 201
San Francisco, CA 94102
Phone: (415) 565-7667
Fax: (415) 252-7490
Website: http://www.sfccc.org/clinics/lmwhs.htm

National Academy for State Health Policy
50 Monument Square, Suite 502
Portland, ME 04101
Phone: (207) 874-6524
Fax: (207) 874-6527
Website: http://www.nashp.org
E-mail: info@nashp.org

National Alliance of Breast Cancer Organizations
9 East 37th Street, 10th Floor
New York, NY 10016
Toll-Free: (888) 806-2226
Phone: (212) 889-0606
Fax: (212) 689-1213
Website: http://www.nabco.org
E-mail: nabcoinfo@aol.com

National Association of Public Hospitals and Health Systems
1301 Pennsylvania Avenue NW
Washington, DC 20004
Phone: (202) 585-0100
Fax: (202) 585-0101
Website: http://www.naph.org
E-mail: naph@naph.org

National Coalition on Health Care
1200 G Street NW, Suite 750
Washington, DC 20005
Phone: (202) 638-7151
Website: http://www.nchc.org
E-mail: info@nchc.org

National Health Law Program
2639 South La Cienega Blvd.
Los Angeles, CA 90034-2675
Phone: (310) 204-6010
Fax: (310) 204-0891
Website: http://
www.healthlaw.org
E-mail: nhelp@healthlaw.org

National Health Policy Forum
2131 K Street NW, Suite 500
Washington DC 20037
Phone: (202) 872-1390
Fax: (202) 962-9837
Website: http://www.nhpf.org
E-mail: nhpf@gwu.edu

National Latina Institute for Reproductive Health
162 Montague Street, 3rd Floor
Brooklyn, NY 11201
Phone: (718) 260-8811
Fax: (718) 260-9941
Website: http://
www.latinainstitute.org
E-mail: nlirh@latinainstitute.org

National Rural Health Association
1 West Armour Boulevard
Suite 203
Kansas City, MO 64111-2087
Phone: (816) 756-3140
Website: http://
www.nrharural.org
E-mail: mail@nrharural.org

Office of Rural Health Policy
5600 Fishers Lane, 9A55
Rockville, MD 20857
Phone: (301) 443-0835
Fax: (301) 443-2803
Website: http://
www.ruralhealth.hrsa.gov

Planned Parenthood Federation of America
434 West 33rd Street
New York, NY 10001
Phone: (212) 541-7800
Fax: (212) 245-1845
Website: http://
www.plannedparenthood.org
E-mail:
communications@ppfa.org

Robert Wood Johnson Foundation
P.O. Box 2316
Princeton, NJ 08543
Phone: (888) 631-9989
Website: http://www.rwjf.org

Smiles for Success
645 North Michigan Avenue
#800
Chicago, IL 60611
Phone: (312) 280-9296
Fax: (312) 280-9893
Website: http://
www.smilesforsuccess.org
E-mail:
info@smilesforsuccess.org

State Coverage Initiatives
1801 K Street NW, #701-L
Washington, DC 20006
Phone: (202) 292-6700
Fax: (202) 292-6800
Website: http://
www.statecoverage.net
E-mail: sci@academyhealth.org

Stree Foundation
1804 Emarcadero Road, Suite 200
Palo Alto, CA 94303
Phone: (650) 849-9890
Fax: (650) 354-1603
Website: http://
www.streegiw.com
E-mail: info@streegiw.com

The Medicine Program
P.O. Box 515
Doniphan, MO 63935-0515
Phone: (573) 996-7300
Website: http://www.themedicine
program.com
E-mail: help@themedicine
program.com

Third Wave Foundation
511 West 25th Street
Suite 301
New York, NY 10001
Phone: (212) 255-6653
Fax: (212) 255-6653
Website: http://www.thirdwave
foundation.org
E-mail: info@thirdwave
foundation.org

Urban Institute
2100 M Street NW
Washington, DC 20037
Phone: (202) 833-7200
Website: http://www.urban.org
E-mail: paffairs@ui.urban.org

WISEWOMAN
4770 Buford Highway NE
MS/K-24
Atlanta, GA 30341-3717
Toll-Free: (888) 232-4674
Website: http://www.cdc.gov/
wisewoman
E-mail: ccdinfo@cdc.gov

Women, Infants, and Children
3101 Park Center Drive
Room 926
Alexandria, VA 22302
Phone: (703) 305-2746
Fax: (703) 305-2106
Website: http://
www.fns.usda.gov/wic
E-mail: wichq-web@fns.usda.gov

Chapter 75

Directory of Government Agencies and National Organizations Providing Help and Information to Women

Government Agencies

Agency for Healthcare Policy and Research
540 Gaither Road
Rockville, MD 20850
Phone: (301) 594-1364
Website: http://www.ahrq.gov
E-mail: info@ahrq.gov

Center for the Evaluation of Risks to Human Reproduction
NIEHS EC-32
P.O. Box 12233
Research Triangle Park
NC 27709
Phone: (919) 541-3455
Fax: (919) 316-4511
Website: http://cerhr.niehs.nih.gov

Centers for Disease Control and Prevention
1600 Clifton Road
Atlanta, GA 30333
Phone: (404) 639-3311
TTY: (404) 639-3312
Website: http://www.cdc.gov
E-mail: ccdinfo@cdc.gov

National Cancer Institute
6116 Executive Boulevard, MSC8322
Suite 3036A
Bethesda, MD 20892-8322
Toll-Free: (800) 422-6237
Toll-Free TTY: (800) 332-8615
Website: http://www.cancer.gov

Resources in this chapter were compiled from many sources deemed accurate; all contact information was verified and updated in July 2003.

National Center for Complementary and Alternative Medicine
P.O. Box 7923
Gaithersburg, MD 20898-7923
Toll-Free: (888) 644-6226
Phone: (301) 519-3153
TTY: (866) 464-3615
Fax: (866) 464-3616
Website: http://nccam.nih.gov
E-mail: info@nccam.nih.gov

National Center for Health Statistics
3311 Toledo Road
Metro IV Building
Hyattsville, MD 20782
Phone: (301) 458-4636
Website: http://www.cdc.gov/nchs
E-mail: nchsquery@cdc.gov

National Heart, Lung, and Blood Institute
P.O. Box 30105
Bethesda, MD 20824-0105
Phone: (301) 592 8573
TTY: (240) 629-3255
Fax: (301) 592-8563
Website: http://www.nhlbi.nih.gov
E-mail: nhlbiinfo@rover.nhlbi
.nih.gov

National Institute for Occupational Safety and Health
200 Independence Avenue SW
Hubert H. Humphrey Building,
Room 715H
Washington, DC 20201
Toll-Free: (800) 35-NIOSH (800-356-4674)
Phone: (513) 533-8328
Website: http://www.cdc.gov/niosh

National Institute of Allergy and Infectious Diseases
31 Center Drive, MSC 2520
Building 31, Room 7A50
Bethesda, MD 20892-2520
Phone: (301) 402-1663
Website: http://www.niaid.nih.gov

National Institute of Child Health and Human Development
P.O. Box 3006
Rockville, MD 20847
Toll-Free: (800) 370-2943
Phone: (301) 496-7101
Website: http://
www.nichd.nih.gov
E-mail: nichdinformation
resourcecenter@mail.nih.gov

National Institute of Diabetes and Digestive and Kidney Diseases
31 Center Drive, MSC 2560
Building 31, Room 9A04
Bethesda, MD 20892-2520
Phone: (301) 496-3583
Website: http://www.niddk.nih
.gov

National Institute of Environmental Health Sciences
P.O. Box 12233
Research Triangle Park, NC
27709
Phone: (919) 541-3345
TTY: (919) 541-0731
Website: http://www.niehs.nih.gov
E-mail: webcenter@niehs.nih.gov

National Institute of Mental Health
6001 Executive Boulevard
MSC 9663, Room 8184
Bethesda, MD 20892-9663
Toll Free: (866) 615-6464
Phone: (301) 443-4513
TTY: (301) 443-8431
Fax: (301) 433-4279
Website: http://www.nimh.nih.gov
E-mail: nimhinfo@nih.gov

National Institute on Aging
31 Center Drive, MSC 2292
Building 31, Room 5C27
Bethesda, MD 20892-2520
Toll-Free: (800) 222-2225
Toll Free TTY: (800) 222-4225
Phone: (301) 496-1752
Website: http://www.nia.nih.gov

National Institute on Drug Abuse
6001 Executive Boulevard
Room 5213
Bethesda, MD 20892-9561
Phone: (301) 443-1124
Website: http://www.nida.nih.gov
E-mail: information@lists.nida.nih.gov

National Institutes of Health
9000 Rockville Pike
Bethesda, MD 20892
Phone: (301) 496-4000
Website: http://www.nih.gov
E-mail: nihinfo@od.nih.gov

National Library of Medicine
8600 Rockville Pike
Bethesda, MD 20894
Toll-Free: (888) FIND-NLM
(888-346-3656)
Phone: (301) 594-5983
Fax: (301) 402-1384
Website: http://www.nlm.nih.gov
E-mail: custserv@nlm.nih.gov

National Women's Health Information Center
8550 Arlington Boulevard
Suite 300
Fairfax, VA 22031
Toll-Free: (800) 994-WOMAN
TTY: (888) 220-5446
Website: http://www.4woman.gov

Office of Disease Prevention and Health Promotion
200 Independence Avenue SW
Room 738G
Washington, DC 20201
Phone: (202) 205-8611
Fax: (202) 205-9478
Website: http://odphp.osophs.dhhs.gov

Office of Women's Health
5600 Fishers Lane
Rockville, MD 20857-0001
Phone: (301) 827-0350
Website: http://www.fda.gov/womens

U.S. Department of Health and Human Services

200 Independence Avenue SW
Washington, DC 20201
Toll-Free: (877) 696-6775
Phone: (877) 696-6775
Website: http://www.hhs.gov

U.S. Food and Drug Administration

5600 Fishers Lane
Rockville, MD 20857-0001
Toll-Free: (888) 463-6332
Website: http://www.fda.gov

Weight-Control Information Network

1 WIN Way
Bethesda, MD 20892-3665
Toll-Free: (877) 946-4627
Phone: (202) 828-1025
Fax: (202) 828-1028
Website: http://www.niddk.nih
.gov/health/nutrit/win.htm
E-mail: win@info.niddk.nih.gov

National Organizations

American Academy of Asthma, Allergy, and Immunology

611 East Wells Street
Milwaukee, WI 53202
Toll-Free: (800) 822-2762
Phone: (414) 272-6071
Website: http://www.aaaai.org
E-mail: info@aaaai.org

American Academy of Dermatology

930 East Woodfield Road
P.O. Box 4014
Schaumburg, IL 60168-4014
Toll Free: (888) 462-DERM
Phone: (847) 330-0230
Fax: (847) 330-0050
Website: http://www.aad.org

American Academy of Family Physicians

11400 Tomahawk Creek Parkway
Leawood, KS 66211-2672
Toll-Free: (800) 274-2237
Phone: (913) 906-6000
Website: http://www.aafp.org
E-mail: fp@aafp.org

American Academy of Orthopaedic Surgeons

6300 North River Road
Rosemont, IL 60018-4262
Toll-Free: (800) 346-AAOS
Phone: (847) 823-7186
Fax: (847) 823-8125
Fax-on-Demand: (800) 999-2939
Website: http://www.aaos.org
E-mail: pemr@aaos.org

American Association for Clinical Chemistry

2101 L Street NW, Suite 202
Washington, DC 20037-1558
Toll-Free: (800) 892-1400
Phone: (202) 857-0717
Fax: (202) 887-5083
Website: http://www.aacc.org
E-mail: info@aacc.org

American Association for Marriage and Family Therapy
112 South Alfred Street
Alexandria, VA 22314
Phone: (703) 838-9808
Fax: (703) 838-9805
Website: http://www.aamft.org

American Cancer Society
P.O. Box 102454
Atlanta, GA 30368-2454
Toll-Free: (800) ACS-2345
Website: http://www.cancer.org

American College of Obstetricians and Gynecologists (ACOG)
409 12th Street SW
P.O. Box 96920
Washington, DC 20090
Phone: (202) 863-2518
Fax: (202) 484-1595
Website: http://www.acog.org
E-mail: resources@acog.org

American College of Surgeons
633 North Saint Clair Street
Chicago, IL 60611-3211
Toll Free: (800) 621-4111
Phone: (312) 202-5000
Fax: (312) 202-5001
Website: http://www.facs.org
E-mail: postmaster@facs.org

American Council for Headache Education
19 Mantua Road
Mt. Royal, NJ 08061
Phone: (856) 423-0258
Fax: (856) 423-0082
Website: http://www.achenet.org
E-mail: achehq@talley.com

American Diabetes Association
1701 North Beauregard Street
Alexandria, VA 22311
Toll-Free: (800) DIABETES
Website: http://www.diabetes.org
E-mail: askada@diabetes.org

American Dietetic Association
120 South Riverside Plaza
Suite 2000
Chicago, IL 60606-6995
Toll-Free: (800) 877-1600
Website: http://www.eatright.org

American Heart Association
7272 Greenville Avenue
Dallas, TX 75231
Toll-Free: (800) AHA-USA1
(800-242-8721)
Website: http://www.americanheart.org

American Infertility Association
666 Fifth Avenue
Suite 278
New York, NY 10103
Toll-Free: (888) 917-3777
Phone: (718) 621-5083
Fax: (718) 601-7722
Website: http://www.americanin
fertility.org
E-mail: info@americaninfertility
.org

American Lung Association
61 Broadway, 6th Floor
New York, NY 10006
Toll Free: (800) 586-4872
Phone: (212) 315-8700
Website: http://www.lungusa.org

American Medical Association
515 North State Street
Chicago, IL 60610
Toll-Free: (800) AMA-3211
Phone: (312) 464-5000
Website: http://www.ama-assn.org

American Medical Women's Association
801 North Fairfax Street
Suite 400
Alexandria, VA 22314
Phone: (703) 838-0500
Fax: (703) 549-3864
Website: http://www.amwa-doc
.org
E-mail: info@amwa-doc.org

American Menopause Foundation
350 Fifth Avenue
Suite 2822
New York, NY 10118
Phone: (212) 714-2398
Fax: (212) 714-1252
Website: http://www.american
menopause.org
E-mail: menopause@american
menopause.org

American Obesity Association
1250 24th Street NW
Washington, DC 20037
Phone: (202) 776-7711
Fax: (202) 776-7712
Website: http://www.obesity.org
E-mail: pr@obesity.org

American Podiatric Medical Association
9312 Old Georgetown Road
Bethesda, MD 20814
Toll-Free: (800) ASK-APMA
Phone: (301) 571-9200
Fax: (301) 530-2752
Website: http://www.apma.org

American Psychiatric Association
1000 Wilson Boulevard
Suite 1825
Arlington, VA 22209-3901
Phone: (703) 907-7300
Website: http://www.psych.org
E-mail: apa@psych.org

American Society for Dermatologic Surgery
5550 Meadowbrook Drive
Suite 102
Rolling Meadows, IL 60008
Toll-Free: (800) 441-2737
Phone: (847) 956-0900
Website: http://www.asds-net.org
E-mail: info@aboutskinsurgery
.com

American Society for Reproductive Medicine
1209 Montgomery Highway
Birmingham, AL 35216-2809
Phone: (205) 978-5000
Fax: (205) 978-5005
Website: http://www.asrm.org
E-mail: asrm@asrm.org

American Society of Plastic Surgeons
444 East Algonquin Road
Arlington Heights, IL 60005
Toll-Free: (888) 475-2784
Phone: (847) 228-9900
Website: http://
www.plasticsurgery.org
E-mail: hr@plasticsurgery.org

American Stroke Association
7272 Greenville Avenue
Dallas, TX 75231
Toll-Free: (888) 4-STROKE (888-478-7653)
Website: http://www.stroke
association.org

Breastcancer.org
P.O. Box 222
Narberth, PA 19072-0222
Website: http://
www.breastcancer.org
E-mail: info@breastcancer.org

Brigham and Women's Hospital Center for Uterine Fibroids
Departments of Obstetrics /
Gynecology and Pathology
20 Shattuck Street
623 Thorn Building
Boston, MA 02115
Toll-Free: (800) 722-5520
Website: http://www.fibroids.net
E-mail: fibroids@rics.bwh
.harvard.edu

Cancer Research and Prevention Foundation
1600 Duke Street, Suite 110
Arlington, VA 22314
Toll-Free: (800) 227-2732
Phone: (703) 836-4412
Fax: (703) 836-4413
Website: http://www.prevent
cancer.org
E-mail: info@preventcancer.org

CancerSource
263 Summer Street
Boston, MA 02210-1506
Phone: (617) 399-4483
Website: http://
www.cancersource.com
E-mail: info@cancersource.com

Center for Research on Women with Disabilities
3440 Richmond Avenue
Suite B
Houston, TX 77046
Toll-Free: (800) 44-CROWD
Phone: (713) 960-0505
Fax: (713) 961-3555
Website: http://
www.bcm.tmc.edu/crowd
E-mail: crowd@bcm.tmc.edu

Childbirth Solutions, Inc.
P.O. Box 2220
Middleburg, VA 20118
Phone: (540) 364-9023
Fax: (540) 364-0481
Website: http://www.childbirth
solutions.com
E-mail: questions@childbirth
solutions.com

Cleveland Clinic Foundation
9500 Euclid Avenue
Cleveland, OH 44195
Toll-Free: (800) 223-2273
Website: http://www.cleveland
clinic.org

Community Breast Health Project
545 Bryant Street
Palo Alto, CA 94301
Phone: (650) 326-6686
Fax: (650) 326-6673
Website: http://www.cbhp.org
E-mail: info@cbhp.org

Endometriosis Association
8585 North 76th Place
Milwaukee, WI 53223
Phone: (414) 355-2200
Fax: (414) 355-6065
Website: http://www
.endometriosisassn .org
E-mail: endo@endometriosisassn
.org

Gay and Lesbian Medical Association
459 Fulton Street, Suite 107
San Francisco, CA 94102
Phone: (415) 255-4547
Fax: (415) 255-4784
Website: http://www.glma.org
E-mail: info@glma.org

HeartCenterOnline
1 South Ocean Boulevard
Suite 201
Boca Raton, FL 33432
Fax: (561) 620-9799
Website: http://
www.heartcenteronline.com

Henry J. Kaiser Family Foundation
2400 Sand Hill Road
Menlo Park, CA 94025
Phone: (650) 854-9400
Fax: (650) 854-4800
Website: http://www.kff.org

Hormone Foundation
8401 Connecticut Avenue
Suite 900
Chevy Chase, MD 20815-5817
Toll-Free: (800) HORMONE
Website: http://www.hormone.org

*International Council
on Infertility Information
Dissemination*
P.O. Box 6836
Arlington, VA 22206
Phone: (703) 379-9178
Fax: (703) 379-1593
Website: http://www.inciid.org
E-mail: inciidinfo@inciid.org

*Interstitial Cystitis
Association*
110 North Washington Street
Suite 340
Rockville, MD 20850
Toll-Free: (800) HELP-ICA
Phone: (301) 610-5300
Fax: (301) 610-5308
Website: http://www.ichelp.org
E-mail: icamail@ichelp.org

IVF.com
5445 Meridian Mark Drive
Suite 270
Atlanta, GA 30342
Phone: (404) 843-2229
Website: http://www.ivf.com
E-mail: info@ivf.com

Joslin Diabetes Center
1 Joslin Place
Boston, MA 02215
Phone: (617) 732-2415
Website: http://
www.joslin.harvard.edu

LungCancer.org
Toll-Free: (877) 646-LUNG (877-
646-5864)
Website: http://lungcancer.org

March of Dimes
1275 Mamaroneck Avenue
White Plains, NY 10605
Toll-Free: (800) 996-2724
Website: http://www.modimes
.org

*Mayo Foundation for
Medical Education and
Research*
200 First Street SW
Rochester, MN 55905
Phone: (507) 284-2511
TDD: (507) 284-9786
Fax: (507) 284-0161
Website: http://www.mayo.edu

*National Alliance of Breast
Cancer Organizations*
9 East 37th Street
10th Floor
New York, NY 10016
Toll-Free: (888) 806-2226
Phone: (212) 889-0606
Fax: (212) 689-1213
Website: http://www.nabco.org
E-mail: nabcoinfo@aol.com

*National Anemia Action
Council*
6300 Wilshire Boulevard
Suite 670
Los Angeles, CA 90048
Website: http://www.anemia.org

National Asian Women's Health Organization
250 Montgomery Street
Suite 900
San Francisco, CA 94104
Phone: (415) 989-9747
Fax: (415) 989-9758
Website: http://www.nawho.org
E-mail: nawho@nawho.org

National Breast Cancer Foundation
1 Hanover Park
16633 North Dallas Parkway
Suite 600
Addison, TX 75001
Website: http://
www.nationalbreastcancer.org
E-mail: info@nationalbreast
cancer.org

National Mental Health Association
2001 North Beauregard Street
12th Floor
Alexandria, VA 22311
Toll-Free: (800) 969-NMHA
Toll Free TTY: (800) 433-5959
Phone: (703) 684-7722
Fax: (703) 684-5968
Website: http://www.nmha.org

National Osteoporosis Foundation
1232 22nd Street NW
Washington, DC 20037-1292
Phone: (202) 223-2226
Website: http://www.nof.org
E-mail: webmaster@nof.org

National Sleep Foundation
1522 K Street NW
Suite 500
Washington, DC 20005
Phone: (202) 347-3471
Fax: (202) 347-3472
Website: http://
www.sleepfoundation.org
E-mail: nsf@sleepfoundation.org

National Uterine Fibroids Foundation
P.O. Box 9688
Colorado Springs, CO 80932-0688
Toll Free: (877) 553-6833
Phone: (719) 633-3454
Website: http://www.nuff.org
E-mail: info@nuff.org

National Women's Health Network
514 10th Street NW
Suite 400
Washington, DC 20004
Phone: (202) 347-1140
Fax: (202) 347-1168
Website: http://www.womens
healthnetwork.org

National Women's Health Resource Center
120 Albany Street
Suite 820
New Brunswick, NJ 08901
Toll-Free: (877) 986-9472
Website: http://
www.healthywomen.org
E-mail: info@healthywomen.org

*Nemours Foundation
Center for Children's
Health Media*
1600 Rockland Road
Wilmington, DE 19803
Phone: (302) 651-4046
Website: http://
www.kidshealth.org
E-mail: info@kidshealth.org

*North American Menopause
Society*
5900 Landerbrook Drive
Suite 195
Mayfield Heights, OH 44124
Toll-Free: (800) 774-5342
Phone: (440) 442-7550
Fax: (440) 442-2660
Website: http://www.menopause
.org
E-mail: info@menopause.org

*Oncolink: University of
Pennsylvania Cancer Center*
3400 Spruce Street
2 Donner
Philadelphia, PA 19104-4283
Fax: (215) 349-5445
Website: http://www.oncolink.com
E-mail: webmaster@oncollink
.com

*Planned Parenthood
Federation of America*
434 West 33rd Street
New York, NY 10001
Phone: (212) 541-7800
Fax: (212) 245-1845
Website: http://www.planned
parenthood.org
E-mail: communications@ppfa.org

*Resolve: The National
Infertility Association*
1310 Broadway
Somerville, MA 02144
Toll-Free: (888) 623-0744
Website: http://www.resolve.org
E-mail: info@resolve.org

*Society for Reproductive
Endocrinology and Fertility*
1209 Montgomery Highway
Birmingham, AL 35216-2809
Phone: (205) 978-5000, ext. 131
Fax: (205) 978-5005
Website: http://www.socrei.org

*Society for Women's Health
Research*
1828 L Street NW
Suite 625
Washington, DC 20036
Phone: (202) 223-8224
Fax: (202) 833-3472
Website: http://www.womens-
health.org
E-mail: info@womens-health.org

*Susan G. Komen Breast
Cancer Foundation*
5005 LBJ Freeway
Suite 250
Dallas, TX 75244
Toll Free: (800) 462-9273
Phone: (972) 855-1600
Fax: (972) 855-1605
Website: http://www.komen.org

SusanLoveMD.org
P.O. Box 846
Pacific Palisades, CA 90272
Phone: (310) 230-1712
Fax: (310) 230-1612
Website: http://www.susanlove
md.com

**WomenHeart: The National
Coalition for Women with
Heart Disease**
818 18th Street NW, Suite 7
Washington, DC 20006
Phone: (202) 728-7199
Fax: (202) 728-7238
Website: http://www
.womenheart.org
E-mail: mail@womenheart.org

Women's Heart Foundation
P.O. Box 7827
West Trenton, NJ 08628
Phone: (609) 771-9600
Fax: (609) 771-9427
Website: http://www.womens
heart foundation.org

**Women's Information
Network Against Breast
Cancer**
536 South Second Avenue
Suite K
Covina, CA 91723-3043
Toll-Free: (866) 2WIN-ABC
Phone: (626) 332-2255
Website: http://www.winabc.org
E-mail: mail@winabc.org

Index

Index

Page numbers followed by 'n' indicate a footnote. Page numbers in *italics* indicate a table or illustration.

A

ABCD rule, described 414
abdominal hysterectomy, described 226–27
abnormal uterine bleeding
  adenomyosis 183
  described 160–62
  dilation and curettage 220
  see also dysfunctional uterine bleeding
abortion, overview 312–20
"About D&C for Uterine Bleeding Problems" (American College of Surgeons) 219n
"About Hysterectomy" (American College of Surgeons) 223n
abstinence (sexual)
  contraception *309*
  described 35
acetaminophen 169, 313
Achilles tendinitis 590
ACLU *see* American Civil Liberties Union

ACOG *see* American College of Obstetricians and Gynecologists
acquired immune deficiency syndrome (AIDS)
  African Americans 127
  described *291*
  Hispanic Americans 133
  screening test frequency *54*
  statistics 475
  substance abuse 656
  women of color 126
Actiq (fentanyl citrate) 432
acupuncture, migraine headache 538–39
adenocarcinoma 402, *403*
adenomyosis
  chronic pain 172
  described 182–83
adhesions, laparoscopy 216
Adipex-P (phentermine) 92
adolescents
  depression 603
  diabetes mellitus 497
  puberty 32–36
  tobacco use 5, 508
Adriamycin (doxorubicin) 432
Adrucil (fouorouracil) 432
Advil 313
aerobic activity, described 87

Health Reference Series
COMPLETE CATALOG

Adolescent Health Sourcebook

Basic Consumer Health Information about Common Medical, Mental, and Emotional Concerns in Adolescents, Including Facts about Acne, Body Piercing, Mononucleosis, Nutrition, Eating Disorders, Stress, Depression, Behavior Problems, Peer Pressure, Violence, Gangs, Drug Use, Puberty, Sexuality, Pregnancy, Learning Disabilities, and More

Along with a Glossary of Terms and Other Resources for Further Help and Information

Edited by Chad T. Kimball. 658 pages. 2002. 0-7808-0248-9. $78.

"It is written in clear, nontechnical language aimed at general readers. . . . Recommended for public libraries, community colleges, and other agencies serving health care consumers."
— *American Reference Books Annual, 2003*

"Recommended for school and public libraries. Parents and professionals dealing with teens will appreciate the easy-to-follow format and the clearly written text. This could become a 'must have' for every high school teacher." — *E-Streams, Jan '03*

"A good starting point for information related to common medical, mental, and emotional concerns of adolescents." — *School Library Journal, Nov '02*

"This book provides accurate information in an easy to access format. It addresses topics that parents and caregivers might not be aware of and provides practical, useable information." — *Doody's Health Sciences Book Review Journal, Sep-Oct '02*

"Recommended reference source."
— *Booklist, American Library Association, Sep '02*

AIDS Sourcebook, 3rd Edition

Basic Consumer Health Information about Acquired Immune Deficiency Syndrome (AIDS) and Human Immunodeficiency Virus (HIV) Infection, Including Facts about Transmission, Prevention, Diagnosis, Treatment, Opportunistic Infections, and Other Complications, with a Section for Women and Children, Including Details about Associated Gynecological Concerns, Pregnancy, and Pediatric Care

Along with Updated Statistical Information, Reports on Current Research Initiatives, a Glossary, and Directories of Internet, Hotline, and Other Resources

Edited by Dawn D. Matthews. 664 pages. 2003. 0-7808-0631-X. $78.

ALSO AVAILABLE: AIDS Sourcebook, 1st Edition. Edited by Karen Bellenir and Peter D. Dresser. 831 pages. 1995. 0-7808-0031-1. $78.

AIDS Sourcebook, 2nd Edition. Edited by Karen Bellenir. 751 pages. 1999. 0-7808-0225-X. $78.

"Highly recommended."
— *American Reference Books Annual, 2000*

"Excellent sourcebook. This continues to be a highly recommended book. There is no other book that provides as much information as this book provides."
— *AIDS Book Review Journal, Dec-Jan 2000*

"Recommended reference source."
— *Booklist, American Library Association, Dec '99*

"A solid text for college-level health libraries."
— *The Bookwatch, Aug '99*

Cited in *Reference Sources for Small and Medium-Sized Libraries, American Library Association, 1999*

Alcoholism Sourcebook

Basic Consumer Health Information about the Physical and Mental Consequences of Alcohol Abuse, Including Liver Disease, Pancreatitis, Wernicke-Korsakoff Syndrome (Alcoholic Dementia), Fetal Alcohol Syndrome, Heart Disease, Kidney Disorders, Gastrointestinal Problems, and Immune System Compromise and Featuring Facts about Addiction, Detoxification, Alcohol Withdrawal, Recovery, and the Maintenance of Sobriety

Along with a Glossary and Directories of Resources for Further Help and Information

Edited by Karen Bellenir. 613 pages. 2000. 0-7808-0325-6. $78.

"This title is one of the few reference works on alcoholism for general readers. For some readers this will be a welcome complement to the many self-help books on the market. Recommended for collections serving general readers and consumer health collections."
— *E-Streams, Mar '01*

"This book is an excellent choice for public and academic libraries."
— *American Reference Books Annual, 2001*

"Recommended reference source."
— *Booklist, American Library Association, Dec '00*

"Presents a wealth of information on alcohol use and abuse and its effects on the body and mind, treatment, and prevention." — *SciTech Book News, Dec '00*

"Important new health guide which packs in the latest consumer information about the problems of alcoholism." — *Reviewer's Bookwatch, Nov '00*

SEE ALSO Drug Abuse Sourcebook, Substance Abuse Sourcebook

Allergies Sourcebook, 2nd Edition

Basic Consumer Health Information about Allergic Disorders, Triggers, Reactions, and Related Symptoms, Including Anaphylaxis, Rhinitis, Sinusitis, Asthma, Dermatitis, Conjunctivitis, and Multiple Chemical Sensitivity

Along with Tips on Diagnosis, Prevention, and Treatment, Statistical Data, a Glossary, and a Directory of Sources for Further Help and Information

Edited by Annemarie S. Muth. 598 pages. 2002. 0-7808-0376-0. $78.

ALSO AVAILABLE: *Allergies Sourcebook, 1st Edition.* Edited by Allan R. Cook. 611 pages. 1997. 0-7808-0036-2. $78.

"This book brings a great deal of useful material together. . . . This is an excellent addition to public and consumer health library collections."
— *American Reference Books Annual, 2003*

"This second edition would be useful to laypersons with little or advanced knowledge of the subject matter. This book would also serve as a resource for nursing and other health care professions students. It would be useful in public, academic, and hospital libraries with consumer health collections." — *E-Streams, Jul '02*

Alternative Medicine Sourcebook, 2nd Edition

Basic Consumer Health Information about Alternative and Complementary Medical Practices, Including Acupuncture, Chiropractic, Herbal Medicine, Homeopathy, Naturopathic Medicine, Mind-Body Interventions, Ayurveda, and Other Non-Western Medical Traditions

Along with Facts about such Specific Therapies as Massage Therapy, Aromatherapy, Qigong, Hypnosis, Prayer, Dance, and Art Therapies, a Glossary, and Resources for Further Information

Edited by Dawn D. Matthews. 618 pages. 2002. 0-7808-0605-0. $78.

ALSO AVAILABLE: *Alternative Medicine Sourcebook, 1st Edition.* Edited by Allan R. Cook. 737 pages. 1999. 0-7808-0200-4. $78.

"Recommended for public, high school, and academic libraries that have consumer health collections. Hospital libraries that also serve the public will find this to be a useful resource." — *E-Streams, Feb '03*

"Recommended reference source."
— *Booklist, American Library Association, Jan '03*

"An important alternate health reference."
— *MBR Bookwatch, Oct '02*

"A great addition to the reference collection of every type of library." — *American Reference Books Annual, 2000*

Alzheimer's Disease Sourcebook, 3rd Edition

Basic Consumer Health Information about Alzheimer's Disease, Other Dementias, and Related Disorders, Including Multi-Infarct Dementia, AIDS Dementia Complex, Dementia with Lewy Bodies, Huntington's Disease, Wernicke-Korsakoff Syndrome (Alcohol-Reated Dementia), Delirium, and Confusional States

Along with Information for People Newly Diagnosed with Alzheimer's Disease and Caregivers, Reports Detailing Current Research Efforts in Prevention, Diagnosis, and Treatment, Facts about Long-Term Care Issues, and Listings of Sources for Additional Information

Edited by Karen Bellenir. 645 pages. 2003. 0-7808-0666-2. $78.

ALSO AVAILABLE: *Alzheimer's, Stroke & 29 Other Neurological Disorders Sourcebook, 1st Edition.* Edited by Frank E. Bair. 579 pages. 1993. 1-55888-748-2. $78.

ALSO AVAILABLE: *Alzheimer's Disease Sourcebook, 2nd Edition.* Edited by Karen Bellenir. 524 pages. 1999. 0-7808-0223-3. $78.

"Provides a wealth of useful information not otherwise available in one place. This resource is recommended for all types of libraries."
— *American Reference Books Annual, 2000*

"Recommended reference source."
— *Booklist, American Library Association, Oct '99*

SEE ALSO *Brain Disorders Sourcebook*

Arthritis Sourcebook

Basic Consumer Health Information about Specific Forms of Arthritis and Related Disorders, Including Rheumatoid Arthritis, Osteoarthritis, Gout, Polymyalgia Rheumatica, Psoriatic Arthritis, Spondyloarthropathies, Juvenile Rheumatoid Arthritis, and Juvenile Ankylosing Spondylitis

Along with Information about Medical, Surgical, and Alternative Treatment Options, and Including Strategies for Coping with Pain, Fatigue, and Stress

Edited by Allan R. Cook. 550 pages. 1998. 0-7808-0201-2. $78.

". . . accessible to the layperson."
— *Reference and Research Book News, Feb '99*

Asthma Sourcebook

Basic Consumer Health Information about Asthma, Including Symptoms, Traditional and Nontraditional Remedies, Treatment Advances, Quality-of-Life Aids, Medical Research Updates, and the Role of Allergies, Exercise, Age, the Environment, and Genetics in the Development of Asthma

Along with Statistical Data, a Glossary, and Directories of Support Groups, and Other Resources for Further Information

Edited by Annemarie S. Muth. 628 pages. 2000. 0-7808-0381-7. $78.

"A worthwhile reference acquisition for public libraries and academic medical libraries whose readers desire a quick introduction to the wide range of asthma information." — *Choice, Association of College & Research Libraries, Jun '01*

"Recommended reference source."
— *Booklist, American Library Association, Feb '01*

"Highly recommended." — *The Bookwatch, Jan '01*

"There is much good information for patients and their families who deal with asthma daily."
— *American Medical Writers Association Journal, Winter '01*

"This informative text is recommended for consumer health collections in public, secondary school, and community college libraries and the libraries of universities with a large undergraduate population."
— *American Reference Books Annual, 2001*

Attention Deficit Disorder Sourcebook

Basic Consumer Health Information about Attention Deficit/Hyperactivity Disorder in Children and Adults, Including Facts about Causes, Symptoms, Diagnostic Criteria, and Treatment Options Such as Medications, Behavior Therapy, Coaching, and Homeopathy

Along with Reports on Current Research Initiatives, Legal Issues, and Government Regulations, and Featuring a Glossary of Related Terms, Internet Resources, and a List of Additional Reading Material

Edited by Dawn D. Matthews. 470 pages. 2002. 0-7808-0624-7. $78.

"Recommended reference source."
— *Booklist, American Library Association, Jan '03*

"This book is recommended for all school libraries and the reference or consumer health sections of public libraries." — *American Reference Books Annual, 2003*

Back & Neck Disorders Sourcebook

Basic Information about Disorders and Injuries of the Spinal Cord and Vertebrae, Including Facts on Chiropractic Treatment, Surgical Interventions, Paralysis, and Rehabilitation

Along with Advice for Preventing Back Trouble

Edited by Karen Bellenir. 548 pages. 1997. 0-7808-0202-0. $78.

"The strength of this work is its basic, easy-to-read format. Recommended."
— *Reference and User Services Quarterly, American Library Association, Winter '97*

Blood & Circulatory Disorders Sourcebook

Basic Information about Blood and Its Components, Anemias, Leukemias, Bleeding Disorders, and Circulatory Disorders, Including Aplastic Anemia, Thalassemia, Sickle-Cell Disease, Hemochromatosis, Hemophilia, Von Willebrand Disease, and Vascular Diseases

Along with a Special Section on Blood Transfusions and Blood Supply Safety, a Glossary, and Source Listings for Further Help and Information

Edited by Karen Bellenir and Linda M. Shin. 554 pages. 1998. 0-7808-0203-9. $78.

"Recommended reference source."
— *Booklist, American Library Association, Feb '99*

"An important reference sourcebook written in simple language for everyday, non-technical users. "
— *Reviewer's Bookwatch, Jan '99*

Brain Disorders Sourcebook

Basic Consumer Health Information about Strokes, Epilepsy, Amyotrophic Lateral Sclerosis (ALS/Lou Gehrig's Disease), Parkinson's Disease, Brain Tumors, Cerebral Palsy, Headache, Tourette Syndrome, and More

Along with Statistical Data, Treatment and Rehabilitation Options, Coping Strategies, Reports on Current Research Initiatives, a Glossary, and Resource Listings for Additional Help and Information

Edited by Karen Bellenir. 481 pages. 1999. 0-7808-0229-2. $78.

"Belongs on the shelves of any library with a consumer health collection." — *E-Streams, Mar '00*

"Recommended reference source."
— *Booklist, American Library Association, Oct '99*

SEE ALSO Alzheimer's Disease Sourcebook

Breast Cancer Sourcebook

Basic Consumer Health Information about Breast Cancer, Including Diagnostic Methods, Treatment Options, Alternative Therapies, Self-Help Information, Related Health Concerns, Statistical and Demographic Data, and Facts for Men with Breast Cancer

Along with Reports on Current Research Initiatives, a Glossary of Related Medical Terms, and a Directory of Sources for Further Help and Information

Edited by Edward J. Prucha and Karen Bellenir. 580 pages. 2001. 0-7808-0244-6. $78.

"It would be a useful reference book in a library or on loan to women in a support group."
— *Cancer Forum, Mar '03*

"Recommended reference source."
— *Booklist, American Library Association, Jan '02*

"This reference source is highly recommended. It is quite informative, comprehensive and detailed in nature, and yet it offers practical advice in easy-to-read language. It could be thought of as the 'bible' of breast cancer for the consumer."
— *E-Streams, Jan '02*

"The broad range of topics covered in lay language make the *Breast Cancer Sourcebook* an excellent addition to public and consumer health library collections."
— *American Reference Books Annual 2002*

"From the pros and cons of different screening methods and results to treatment options, *Breast Cancer Sourcebook* provides the latest information on the subject."
— *Library Bookwatch, Dec '01*

"This thoroughgoing, very readable reference covers all aspects of breast health and cancer. . . . Readers will find much to consider here. Recommended for all public and patient health collections."
— *Library Journal, Sep '01*

SEE ALSO Cancer Sourcebook for Women, Women's Health Concerns Sourcebook

■

Breastfeeding Sourcebook

Basic Consumer Health Information about the Benefits of Breastmilk, Preparing to Breastfeed, Breastfeeding as a Baby Grows, Nutrition, and More, Including Information on Special Situations and Concerns Such as Mastitis, Illness, Medications, Allergies, Multiple Births, Prematurity, Special Needs, and Adoption

Along with a Glossary and Resources for Additional Help and Information

Edited by Jenni Lynn Colson. 388 pages. 2002. 0-7808-0332-9. $78.

SEE ALSO Pregnancy & Birth Sourcebook

"Particularly useful is the information about professional lactation services and chapters on breastfeeding when returning to work. . . . *Breastfeeding Sourcebook* will be useful for public libraries, consumer health libraries, and technical schools offering nurse assistant training, especially in areas where Internet access is problematic."
— *American Reference Books Annual, 2003*

■

Burns Sourcebook

Basic Consumer Health Information about Various Types of Burns and Scalds, Including Flame, Heat, Cold, Electrical, Chemical, and Sun Burns

Along with Information on Short-Term and Long-Term Treatments, Tissue Reconstruction, Plastic Surgery, Prevention Suggestions, and First Aid

Edited by Allan R. Cook. 604 pages. 1999. 0-7808-0204-7. $78.

"This is an exceptional addition to the series and is highly recommended for all consumer health collections, hospital libraries, and academic medical centers."
— *E-Streams, Mar '00*

"This key reference guide is an invaluable addition to all health care and public libraries in confronting this ongoing health issue."
— *American Reference Books Annual, 2000*

"Recommended reference source."
— *Booklist, American Library Association, Dec '99*

SEE ALSO Skin Disorders Sourcebook

■

Cancer Sourcebook, 4th Edition

Basic Consumer Health Information about Major Forms and Stages of Cancer, Featuring Facts about Head and Neck Cancers, Lung Cancers, Gastrointestinal Cancers, Genitourinary Cancers, Lymphomas, Blood Cell Cancers, Endocrine Cancers, Skin Cancers, Bone Cancers, Sarcomas, and Others, and Including Information about Cancer Treatments and Therapies, Identifying and Reducing Cancer Risks, and Strategies for Coping with Cancer and the Side Effects of Treatment

Along with a Cancer Glossary, Statistical and Demographic Data, and a Directory of Sources for Additional Help and Information

Edited by Karen Bellenir. 1,119 pages. 2003. 0-7808-0633-6. $78.

ALSO AVAILABLE: Cancer Sourcebook, 1st Edition. Edited by Frank E. Bair. 932 pages. 1990. 1-55888-888-8. $78.

New Cancer Sourcebook, 2nd Edition. Edited by Allan R. Cook. 1,313 pages. 1996. 0-7808-0041-9. $78.

Cancer Sourcebook, 3rd Edition. Edited by Edward J. Prucha. 1,069 pages. 2000. 0-7808-0227-6. $78.

"This title is recommended for health sciences and public libraries with consumer health collections."
— *E-Streams, Feb '01*

". . . can be effectively used by cancer patients and their families who are looking for answers in a language they can understand. Public and hospital libraries should have it on their shelves."
— *American Reference Books Annual, 2001*

"Recommended reference source."
— *Booklist, American Library Association, Dec '00*

Cited in *Reference Sources for Small and Medium-Sized Libraries, American Library Association, 1999*

"The amount of factual and useful information is extensive. The writing is very clear, geared to general readers. Recommended for all levels." — *Choice, Association of College & Research Libraries, Jan '97*

SEE ALSO Breast Cancer Sourcebook, Cancer Sourcebook for Women, Pediatric Cancer Sourcebook, Prostate Cancer Sourcebook

Cancer Sourcebook for Women, 2nd Edition

Basic Consumer Health Information about Gynecologic Cancers and Related Concerns, Including Cervical Cancer, Endometrial Cancer, Gestational Trophoblastic Tumor, Ovarian Cancer, Uterine Cancer, Vaginal Cancer, Vulvar Cancer, Breast Cancer, and Common Non-Cancerous Uterine Conditions, with Facts about Cancer Risk Factors, Screening and Prevention, Treatment Options, and Reports on Current Research Initiatives

Along with a Glossary of Cancer Terms and a Directory of Resources for Additional Help and Information

Edited by Karen Bellenir. 604 pages. 2002. 0-7808-0226-8. $78.

ALSO AVAILABLE: *Cancer Sourcebook for Women, 1st Edition.* Edited by Allan R. Cook and Peter D. Dresser. 524 pages. 1996. 0-7808-0076-1. $78.

"An excellent addition to collections in public, consumer health, and women's health libraries."
— *American Reference Books Annual, 2003*

"Overall, the information is excellent, and complex topics are clearly explained. As a reference book for the consumer it is a valuable resource to assist them to make informed decisions about cancer and its treatments." — *Cancer Forum, Nov '02*

"Highly recommended for academic and medical reference collections." — *Library Bookwatch, Sep '02*

"This is a highly recommended book for any public or consumer library, being reader friendly and containing accurate and helpful information."
— *E-Streams, Aug '02*

"Recommended reference source."
— *Booklist, American Library Association, Jul '02*

SEE ALSO *Breast Cancer Sourcebook, Women's Health Concerns Sourcebook*

Cardiovascular Diseases & Disorders Sourcebook, 1st Edition

SEE *Heart Diseases & Disorders Sourcebook, 2nd Edition*

Caregiving Sourcebook

Basic Consumer Health Information for Caregivers, Including a Profile of Caregivers, Caregiving Responsibilities and Concerns, Tips for Specific Conditions, Care Environments, and the Effects of Caregiving

Along with Facts about Legal Issues, Financial Information, and Future Planning, a Glossary, and a Listing of Additional Resources

Edited by Joyce Brennfleck Shannon. 600 pages. 2001. 0-7808-0331-0. $78.

"Essential for most collections."
— *Library Journal, Apr 1, 2002*

"An ideal addition to the reference collection of any public library. Health sciences information professionals may also want to acquire the *Caregiving Sourcebook* for their hospital or academic library for use as a ready reference tool by health care workers interested in aging and caregiving." — *E-Streams, Jan '02*

"Recommended reference source."
— *Booklist, American Library Association, Oct '01*

Childhood Diseases & Disorders Sourcebook

Basic Consumer Health Information about Medical Problems Often Encountered in Pre-Adolescent Children, Including Respiratory Tract Ailments, Ear Infections, Sore Throats, Disorders of the Skin and Scalp, Digestive and Genitourinary Diseases, Infectious Diseases, Inflammatory Disorders, Chronic Physical and Developmental Disorders, Allergies, and More

Along with Information about Diagnostic Tests, Common Childhood Surgeries, and Frequently Used Medications, with a Glossary of Important Terms and Resource Directory

Edited by Chad T. Kimball. 662 pages. 2003. 0-7808-0458-9. $78.

Colds, Flu & Other Common Ailments Sourcebook

Basic Consumer Health Information about Common Ailments and Injuries, Including Colds, Coughs, the Flu, Sinus Problems, Headaches, Fever, Nausea and Vomiting, Menstrual Cramps, Diarrhea, Constipation, Hemorrhoids, Back Pain, Dandruff, Dry and Itchy Skin, Cuts, Scrapes, Sprains, Bruises, and More

Along with Information about Prevention, Self-Care, Choosing a Doctor, Over-the-Counter Medications, Folk Remedies, and Alternative Therapies, and Including a Glossary of Important Terms and a Directory of Resources for Further Help and Information

Edited by Chad T. Kimball. 638 pages. 2001. 0-7808-0435-X. $78.

"A good starting point for research on common illnesses. It will be a useful addition to public and consumer health library collections."
— *American Reference Books Annual 2002*

"Will prove valuable to any library seeking to maintain a current, comprehensive reference collection of health resources. . . . Excellent reference."
— *The Bookwatch, Aug '01*

"Recommended reference source."
— *Booklist, American Library Association, July '01*

Communication Disorders Sourcebook

Basic Information about Deafness and Hearing Loss, Speech and Language Disorders, Voice Disorders, Balance and Vestibular Disorders, and Disorders of Smell, Taste, and Touch

Edited by Linda M. Ross. 533 pages. 1996. 0-7808-0077-X. $78.

"This is skillfully edited and is a welcome resource for the layperson. It should be found in every public and medical library." — *Booklist Health Sciences Supplement, American Library Association, Oct '97*

Congenital Disorders Sourcebook

Basic Information about Disorders Acquired during Gestation, Including Spina Bifida, Hydrocephalus, Cerebral Palsy, Heart Defects, Craniofacial Abnormalities, Fetal Alcohol Syndrome, and More

Along with Current Treatment Options and Statistical Data

Edited by Karen Bellenir. 607 pages. 1997. 0-7808-0205-5. $78.

"Recommended reference source."
— *Booklist, American Library Association, Oct '97*

SEE ALSO Pregnancy & Birth Sourcebook

Consumer Issues in Health Care Sourcebook

Basic Information about Health Care Fundamentals and Related Consumer Issues, Including Exams and Screening Tests, Physician Specialties, Choosing a Doctor, Using Prescription and Over-the-Counter Medications Safely, Avoiding Health Scams, Managing Common Health Risks in the Home, Care Options for Chronically or Terminally Ill Patients, and a List of Resources for Obtaining Help and Further Information

Edited by Karen Bellenir. 618 pages. 1998. 0-7808-0221-7. $78.

"Both public and academic libraries will want to have a copy in their collection for readers who are interested in self-education on health issues."
— *American Reference Books Annual, 2000*

"The editor has researched the literature from government agencies and others, saving readers the time and effort of having to do the research themselves. Recommended for public libraries."
— *Reference and User Services Quarterly, American Library Association, Spring '99*

"Recommended reference source."
— *Booklist, American Library Association, Dec '98*

Contagious & Non-Contagious Infectious Diseases Sourcebook

Basic Information about Contagious Diseases like Measles, Polio, Hepatitis B, and Infectious Mononucleosis, and Non-Contagious Infectious Diseases like Tetanus and Toxic Shock Syndrome, and Diseases Occurring as Secondary Infections Such as Shingles and Reye Syndrome

Along with Vaccination, Prevention, and Treatment Information, and a Section Describing Emerging Infectious Disease Threats

Edited by Karen Bellenir and Peter D. Dresser. 566 pages. 1996. 0-7808-0075-3. $78.

Death & Dying Sourcebook

Basic Consumer Health Information for the Layperson about End-of-Life Care and Related Ethical and Legal Issues, Including Chief Causes of Death, Autopsies, Pain Management for the Terminally Ill, Life Support Systems, Insurance, Euthanasia, Assisted Suicide, Hospice Programs, Living Wills, Funeral Planning, Counseling, Mourning, Organ Donation, and Physician Training

Along with Statistical Data, a Glossary, and Listings of Sources for Further Help and Information

Edited by Annemarie S. Muth. 641 pages. 1999. 0-7808-0230-6. $78.

"Public libraries, medical libraries, and academic libraries will all find this sourcebook a useful addition to their collections."
— *American Reference Books Annual, 2001*

"An extremely useful resource for those concerned with death and dying in the United States."
— *Respiratory Care, Nov '00*

"Recommended reference source."
— *Booklist, American Library Association, Aug '00*

"This book is a definite must for all those involved in end-of-life care." — *Doody's Review Service, 2000*

Dental Care & Oral Health Sourcebook, 2nd Edition

Basic Consumer Health Information about Dental Care, Including Oral Hygiene, Dental Visits, Pain Management, Cavities, Crowns, Bridges, Dental Implants, and Fillings, and Other Oral Health Concerns, Such as Gum Disease, Bad Breath, Dry Mouth, Genetic and Developmental Abnormalities, Oral Cancers, Orthodontics, and Temporomandibular Disorders

Along with Updates on Current Research in Oral Health, a Glossary, a Directory of Dental and Oral Health Organizations, and Resources for People with Dental and Oral Health Disorders

Edited by Amy L. Sutton. 609 pages. 2003. 0-7808-0634-4. $78.

Depression Sourcebook

Basic Consumer Health Information about Unipolar Depression, Bipolar Disorder, Postpartum Depression, Seasonal Affective Disorder, and Other Types of Depression in Children, Adolescents, Women, Men, the Elderly, and Other Selected Populations

Along with Facts about Causes, Risk Factors, Diagnostic Criteria, Treatment Options, Coping Strategies, Suicide Prevention, a Glossary, and a Directory of Sources for Additional Help and Information

Edited by Karen Belleni. 602 pages. 2002. 0-7808-0611-5. $78.

Diabetes Sourcebook, 3rd Edition

Basic Consumer Health Information about Type 1 Diabetes (Insulin-Dependent or Juvenile-Onset Diabetes), Type 2 Diabetes (Noninsulin-Dependent or Adult-Onset Diabetes), Gestational Diabetes, Impaired Glucose Tolerance (IGT), and Related Complications, Such as Amputation, Eye Disease, Gum Disease, Nerve Damage, and End-Stage Renal Disease, Including Facts about Insulin, Oral Diabetes Medications, Blood Sugar Testing, and the Role of Exercise and Nutrition in the Control of Diabetes

Along with a Glossary and Resources for Further Help and Information

Edited by Dawn D. Matthews. 622 pages. 2003. 0-7808-0629-8. $78.

ALSO AVAILABLE: *Diabetes Sourcebook, 1st Edition.* Edited by Karen Bellenir and Peter D. Dresser. 827 pages. 1994. 1-55888-751-2. $78.

Diabetes Sourcebook, 2nd Edition. Edited by Karen Bellenir. 688 pages. 1998. 0-7808-0224-1. $78.

Diet & Nutrition Sourcebook, 2nd Edition

Basic Consumer Health Information about Dietary Guidelines, Recommended Daily Intake Values, Vitamins, Minerals, Fiber, Fat, Weight Control, Dietary Supplements, and Food Additives

Along with Special Sections on Nutrition Needs throughout Life and Nutrition for People with Such Specific Medical Concerns as Allergies, High Blood Cholesterol, Hypertension, Diabetes, Celiac Disease, Seizure Disorders, Phenylketonuria (PKU), Cancer, and Eating Disorders, and Including Reports on Current Nutrition Research and Source Listings for Additional Help and Information

Edited by Karen Bellenir. 650 pages. 1999. 0-7808-0228-4. $78.

ALSO AVAILABLE: *Diet & Nutrition Sourcebook, 1st Edition.* Edited by Dan R. Harris. 662 pages. 1996. 0-7808-0084-2. $78.

SEE ALSO *Digestive Diseases & Disorders Sourcebook, Eating Disorders Sourcebook, Gastrointestinal Diseases & Disorders Sourcebook, Vegetarian Sourcebook*

Digestive Diseases & Disorders Sourcebook

Basic Consumer Health Information about Diseases and Disorders that Impact the Upper and Lower Digestive System, Including Celiac Disease, Constipation,

Crohn's Disease, Cyclic Vomiting Syndrome, Diarrhea, Diverticulosis and Diverticulitis, Gallstones, Heartburn, Hemorrhoids, Hernias, Indigestion (Dyspepsia), Irritable Bowel Syndrome, Lactose Intolerance, Ulcers, and More

Along with Information about Medications and Other Treatments, Tips for Maintaining a Healthy Digestive Tract, a Glossary, and Directory of Digestive Diseases Organizations

Edited by Karen Bellenir. 335 pages. 2000. 0-7808-0327-2. $78.

"This title would be an excellent addition to all public or patient-research libraries."
—American Reference Books Annual, 2001

"This title is recommended for public, hospital, and health sciences libraries with consumer health collections."
—E-Streams, Jul-Aug '00

"Recommended reference source."
—Booklist, American Library Association, May '00

SEE ALSO Diet & Nutrition Sourcebook, Eating Disorders Sourcebook, Gastrointestinal Diseases & Disorders Sourcebook

■

Disabilities Sourcebook

Basic Consumer Health Information about Physical and Psychiatric Disabilities, Including Descriptions of Major Causes of Disability, Assistive and Adaptive Aids, Workplace Issues, and Accessibility Concerns

Along with Information about the Americans with Disabilities Act, a Glossary, and Resources for Additional Help and Information

Edited by Dawn D. Matthews. 616 pages. 2000. 0-7808-0389-2. $78.

"It is a must for libraries with a consumer health section."
—American Reference Books Annual 2002

"A much needed addition to the Omnigraphics Health Reference Series. A current reference work to provide people with disabilities, their families, caregivers or those who work with them, a broad range of information in one volume, has not been available until now. . . . It is recommended for all public and academic library reference collections."
—E-Streams, May '01

"An excellent source book in easy-to-read format covering many current topics; highly recommended for all libraries."
—Choice, Association of College and Research Libraries, Jan '01

"Recommended reference source."
—Booklist, American Library Association, Jul '00

■

Domestic Violence & Child Abuse Sourcebook

Basic Consumer Health Information about Spousal/Partner, Child, Sibling, Parent, and Elder Abuse, Covering Physical, Emotional, and Sexual Abuse, Teen Dating Violence, and Stalking; Includes Information

about Hotlines, Safe Houses, Safety Plans, and Other Resources for Support and Assistance, Community Initiatives, and Reports on Current Directions in Research and Treatment

Along with a Glossary, Sources for Further Reading, and Governmental and Non-Governmental Organizations Contact Information

Edited by Helene Henderson. 1,064 pages. 2001. 0-7808-0235-7. $78.

"Interested lay persons should find the book extremely beneficial. . . . A copy of Domestic Violence and Child Abuse Sourcebook should be in every public library in the United States."
—Social Science & Medicine, No. 56, 2003

"This is important information. The Web has many resources but this sourcebook fills an important societal need. I am not aware of any other resources of this type."
—Doody's Review Service, Sep '01

"Recommended for all libraries, scholars, and practitioners."
—Choice, Association of College & Research Libraries, Jul '01

"Recommended reference source."
—Booklist, American Library Association, Apr '01

"Important pick for college-level health reference libraries."
—The Bookwatch, Mar '01

"Because this problem is so widespread and because this book includes a lot of issues within one volume, this work is recommended for all public libraries."
—American Reference Books Annual, 2001

■

Drug Abuse Sourcebook

Basic Consumer Health Information about Illicit Substances of Abuse and the Diversion of Prescription Medications, Including Depressants, Hallucinogens, Inhalants, Marijuana, Narcotics, Stimulants, and Anabolic Steroids

Along with Facts about Related Health Risks, Treatment Issues, and Substance Abuse Prevention Programs, a Glossary of Terms, Statistical Data, and Directories of Hotline Services, Self-Help Groups, and Organizations Able to Provide Further Information

Edited by Karen Bellenir. 629 pages. 2000. 0-7808-0242-X. $78.

"Containing a wealth of information . . . . This resource belongs in libraries that serve a lower-division undergraduate or community college clientele as well as the general public."
—Choice, Association of College and Research Libraries, Jun '01

"Recommended reference source."
—Booklist, American Library Association, Feb '01

"Highly recommended."
—The Bookwatch, Jan '01

"Even though there is a plethora of books on drug abuse, this volume is recommended for school, public, and college libraries."
—American Reference Books Annual, 2001

SEE ALSO Alcoholism Sourcebook, Substance Abuse Sourcebook

Ear, Nose & Throat Disorders Sourcebook

Basic Information about Disorders of the Ears, Nose, Sinus Cavities, Pharynx, and Larynx, Including Ear Infections, Tinnitus, Vestibular Disorders, Allergic and Non-Allergic Rhinitis, Sore Throats, Tonsillitis, and Cancers That Affect the Ears, Nose, Sinuses, and Throat

Along with Reports on Current Research Initiatives, a Glossary of Related Medical Terms, and a Directory of Sources for Further Help and Information

Edited by Karen Bellenir and Linda M. Shin. 576 pages. 1998. 0-7808-0206-3. $78.

"Overall, this sourcebook is helpful for the consumer seeking information on ENT issues. It is recommended for public libraries."
— *American Reference Books Annual, 1999*

"Recommended reference source."
— *Booklist, American Library Association, Dec '98*

■

Eating Disorders Sourcebook

Basic Consumer Health Information about Eating Disorders, Including Information about Anorexia Nervosa, Bulimia Nervosa, Binge Eating, Body Dysmorphic Disorder, Pica, Laxative Abuse, and Night Eating Syndrome

Along with Information about Causes, Adverse Effects, and Treatment and Prevention Issues, and Featuring a Section on Concerns Specific to Children and Adolescents, a Glossary, and Resources for Further Help and Information

Edited by Dawn D. Matthews. 322 pages. 2001. 0-7808-0335-3. $78.

"Recommended for health science libraries that are open to the public, as well as hospital libraries. This book is a good resource for the consumer who is concerned about eating disorders." — *E-Streams, Mar '02*

"This volume is another convenient collection of excerpted articles. Recommended for school and public library patrons; lower-division undergraduates; and two-year technical program students." — *Choice, Association of College & Research Libraries, Jan '02*

"Recommended reference source." — *Booklist, American Library Association, Oct '01*

SEE ALSO *Diet & Nutrition Sourcebook, Digestive Diseases & Disorders Sourcebook, Gastrointestinal Diseases & Disorders Sourcebook*

■

Emergency Medical Services Sourcebook

Basic Consumer Health Information about Preventing, Preparing for, and Managing Emergency Situations, When and Who to Call for Help, What to Expect in the Emergency Room, the Emergency Medical Team, Patient Issues, and Current Topics in Emergency Medicine

Along with Statistical Data, a Glossary, and Sources of Additional Help and Information

Edited by Jenni Lynn Colson. 494 pages. 2002. 0-7808-0420-1. $78.

"Handy and convenient for home, public, school, and college libraries. Recommended."
— *Choice, Association of College and Research Libraries, Apr '03*

"This reference can provide the consumer with answers to most questions about emergency care in the United States, or it will direct them to a resource where the answer can be found."
— *American Reference Books Annual, 2003*

"Recommended reference source."
— *Booklist, American Library Association, Feb '03*

■

Endocrine & Metabolic Disorders Sourcebook

Basic Information for the Layperson about Pancreatic and Insulin-Related Disorders Such as Pancreatitis, Diabetes, and Hypoglycemia; Adrenal Gland Disorders Such as Cushing's Syndrome, Addison's Disease, and Congenital Adrenal Hyperplasia; Pituitary Gland Disorders Such as Growth Hormone Deficiency, Acromegaly, and Pituitary Tumors; Thyroid Disorders Such as Hypothyroidism, Graves' Disease, Hashimoto's Disease, and Goiter; Hyperparathyroidism; and Other Diseases and Syndromes of Hormone Imbalance or Metabolic Dysfunction

Along with Reports on Current Research Initiatives

Edited by Linda M. Shin. 574 pages. 1998. 0-7808-0207-1. $78.

"Omnigraphics has produced another needed resource for health information consumers."
— *American Reference Books Annual, 2000*

"Recommended reference source."
— *Booklist, American Library Association, Dec '98*

■

Environmental Health Sourcebook, 2nd Edition

Basic Consumer Health Information about the Environment and Its Effect on Human Health, Including the Effects of Air Pollution, Water Pollution, Hazardous Chemicals, Food Hazards, Radiation Hazards, Biological Agents, Household Hazards, Such as Radon, Asbestos, Carbon Monoxide, and Mold, and Information about Associated Diseases and Disorders, Including Cancer, Allergies, Respiratory Problems, and Skin Disorders

Along with Information about Environmental Concerns for Specific Populations, a Glossary of Related Terms, and Resources for Further Help and Information

Edited by Dawn D. Matthews. 673 pages. 2003. 0-7808-0632-8. $78.

ALSO AVAILABLE: *Environmentally Induced Disorders Sourcebook, 1st Edition.* Edited by Allan R. Cook. 620 pages. 1997. 0-7808-0083-4. $78.

■

Environmentally Induced Disorders Sourcebook, 1st Edition

SEE *Environmental Health Sourcebook, 2nd Edition*

■

Ethnic Diseases Sourcebook

Basic Consumer Health Information for Ethnic and Racial Minority Groups in the United States, Including General Health Indicators and Behaviors, Ethnic Diseases, Genetic Testing, the Impact of Chronic Diseases, Women's Health, Mental Health Issues, and Preventive Health Care Services

Along with a Glossary and a Listing of Additional Resources

Edited by Joyce Brennfleck Shannon. 664 pages. 2001. 0-7808-0336-1. $78.

■

Eye Care Sourcebook, 2nd Edition

Basic Consumer Health Information about Eye Care and Eye Disorders, Including Facts about the Diag-

nosis, Prevention, and Treatment of Common Refractive Problems Such as Myopia, Hyperopia, Astigmatism, and Presbyopia, and Eye Diseases, Including Glaucoma, Cataract, Age-Related Macular Degeneration, and Diabetic Retinopathy

Along with a Section on Vision Correction and Refractive Surgeries, Including LASIK and LASEK, a Glossary, and Directories of Resources for Additional Help and Information

Edited by Amy L. Sutton. 543 pages. 2003. 0-7808-0635-2. $78.

ALSO AVAILABLE: *Ophthalmic Disorders Sourcebook, 1st Edition.* Edited by Linda M. Ross. 631 pages. 1996. 0-7808-0081-8. $78.

■

Family Planning Sourcebook

Basic Consumer Health Information about Planning for Pregnancy and Contraception, Including Traditional Methods, Barrier Methods, Hormonal Methods, Permanent Methods, Future Methods, Emergency Contraception, and Birth Control Choices for Women at Each Stage of Life

Along with Statistics, a Glossary, and Sources of Additional Information

Edited by Amy Marcaccio Keyzer. 520 pages. 2001. 0-7808-0379-5. $78.

SEE ALSO *Pregnancy & Birth Sourcebook*

■

Fitness & Exercise Sourcebook, 2nd Edition

Basic Consumer Health Information about the Fundamentals of Fitness and Exercise, Including How to Begin and Maintain a Fitness Program, Fitness as a Lifestyle, the Link between Fitness and Diet, Advice for Specific Groups of People, Exercise as It Relates to Specific Medical Conditions, and Recent Research in Fitness and Exercise

Along with a Glossary of Important Terms and Resources for Additional Help and Information

Edited by Kristen M. Gledhill. 646 pages. 2001. 0-7808-0334-5. $78.

■

Food & Animal Borne Diseases Sourcebook

Basic Information about Diseases That Can Be Spread to Humans through the Ingestion of Contaminated Food or Water or by Contact with Infected Animals and Insects, Such as Botulism, E. Coli, Hepatitis A, Trichinosis, Lyme Disease, and Rabies

Along with Information Regarding Prevention and Treatment Methods, and Including a Special Section for International Travelers Describing Diseases Such as Cholera, Malaria, Travelers' Diarrhea, and Yellow Fever, and Offering Recommendations for Avoiding Illness

Edited by Karen Bellenir and Peter D. Dresser. 535 pages. 1995. 0-7808-0033-8. $78.

■

Food Safety Sourcebook

Basic Consumer Health Information about the Safe Handling of Meat, Poultry, Seafood, Eggs, Fruit Juices, and Other Food Items, and Facts about Pesticides, Drinking Water, Food Safety Overseas, and the Onset, Duration, and Symptoms of Foodborne Illnesses,

Including Types of Pathogenic Bacteria, Parasitic Protozoa, Worms, Viruses, and Natural Toxins

Along with the Role of the Consumer, the Food Handler, and the Government in Food Safety; a Glossary, and Resources for Additional Help and Information

Edited by Dawn D. Matthews. 339 pages. 1999. 0-7808-0326-4. $78.

■

Forensic Medicine Sourcebook

Basic Consumer Information for the Layperson about Forensic Medicine, Including Crime Scene Investigation, Evidence Collection and Analysis, Expert Testimony, Computer-Aided Criminal Identification, Digital Imaging in the Courtroom, DNA Profiling, Accident Reconstruction, Autopsies, Ballistics, Drugs and Explosives Detection, Latent Fingerprints, Product Tampering, and Questioned Document Examination

Along with Statistical Data, a Glossary of Forensics Terminology, and Listings of Sources for Further Help and Information

Edited by Annemarie S. Muth. 574 pages. 1999. 0-7808-0232-2. $78.

Gastrointestinal Diseases & Disorders Sourcebook

Basic Information about Gastroesophageal Reflux Disease (Heartburn), Ulcers, Diverticulosis, Irritable Bowel Syndrome, Crohn's Disease, Ulcerative Colitis, Diarrhea, Constipation, Lactose Intolerance, Hemorrhoids, Hepatitis, Cirrhosis, and Other Digestive Problems, Featuring Statistics, Descriptions of Symptoms, and Current Treatment Methods of Interest for Persons Living with Upper and Lower Gastrointestinal Maladies

Edited by Linda M. Ross. 413 pages. 1996. 0-7808-0078-8. $78.

". . . very readable form. The successful editorial work that brought this material together into a useful and understandable reference makes accessible to all readers information that can help them more effectively understand and obtain help for digestive tract problems."
— *Choice, Association of College & Research Libraries, Feb '97*

SEE ALSO *Diet & Nutrition Sourcebook, Digestive Diseases & Disorders, Eating Disorders Sourcebook*

◾

Genetic Disorders Sourcebook, 2nd Edition

Basic Consumer Health Information about Hereditary Diseases and Disorders, Including Cystic Fibrosis, Down Syndrome, Hemophilia, Huntington's Disease, Sickle Cell Anemia, and More; Facts about Genes, Gene Research and Therapy, Genetic Screening, Ethics of Gene Testing, Genetic Counseling, and Advice on Coping and Caring

Along with a Glossary of Genetic Terminology and a Resource List for Help, Support, and Further Information

Edited by Kathy Massimini. 768 pages. 2001. 0-7808-0241-1. $78.

ALSO AVAILABLE: *Genetic Disorders Sourcebook, 1st Edition.* Edited by Karen Bellenir. 642 pages. 1996. 0-7808-0034-6. $78.

"Recommended for public libraries and medical and hospital libraries with consumer health collections."
— *E-Streams, May '01*

"Recommended reference source."
— *Booklist, American Library Association, Apr '01*

"Important pick for college-level health reference libraries." — *The Bookwatch, Mar '01*

"Provides essential medical information to both the general public and those diagnosed with a serious or fatal genetic disease or disorder." —*Choice, Association of College and Research Libraries, Jan '97*

Head Trauma Sourcebook

Basic Information for the Layperson about Open-Head and Closed-Head Injuries, Treatment Advances, Recovery, and Rehabilitation

Along with Reports on Current Research Initiatives

Edited by Karen Bellenir. 414 pages. 1997. 0-7808-0208-X. $78.

◾

Headache Sourcebook

Basic Consumer Health Information about Migraine, Tension, Cluster, Rebound and Other Types of Headaches, with Facts about the Cause and Prevention of Headaches, the Effects of Stress and the Environment, Headaches during Pregnancy and Menopause, and Childhood Headaches

Along with a Glossary and Other Resources for Additional Help and Information

Edited by Dawn D. Matthews. 362 pages. 2002. 0-7808-0337-X. $78.

"Highly recommended for academic and medical reference collections." — *Library Bookwatch, Sep '02*

◾

Health Insurance Sourcebook

Basic Information about Managed Care Organizations, Traditional Fee-for-Service Insurance, Insurance Portability and Pre-Existing Conditions Clauses, Medicare, Medicaid, Social Security, and Military Health Care

Along with Information about Insurance Fraud

Edited by Wendy Wilcox. 530 pages. 1997. 0-7808-0222-5. $78.

"Particularly useful because it brings much of this information together in one volume. This book will be a handy reference source in the health sciences library, hospital library, college and university library, and medium to large public library."
— *Medical Reference Services Quarterly, Fall '98*

Awarded "Books of the Year Award"
— *American Journal of Nursing, 1997*

"The layout of the book is particularly helpful as it provides easy access to reference material. A most useful addition to the vast amount of information about health insurance. The use of data from U.S. government agencies is most commendable. Useful in a library or learning center for healthcare professional students."
— *Doody's Health Sciences Book Reviews, Nov '97*

◾

Health Reference Series Cumulative Index 1999

A Comprehensive Index to the Individual Volumes of the Health Reference Series, Including a Subject Index, Name Index, Organization Index, and Publication Index

Along with a Master List of Acronyms and Abbreviations

Edited by Edward J. Prucha, Anne Holmes, and Robert Rudnick. 990 pages. 2000. 0-7808-0382-5. $78.

"This volume will be most helpful in libraries that have a relatively complete collection of the Health Reference Series." —*American Reference Books Annual, 2001*

"Essential for collections that hold any of the numerous *Health Reference Series* titles." — *Choice, Association of College and Research Libraries, Nov '00*

Healthy Aging Sourcebook

Basic Consumer Health Information about Maintaining Health through the Aging Process, Including Advice on Nutrition, Exercise, and Sleep, Help in Making Decisions about Midlife Issues and Retirement, and Guidance Concerning Practical and Informed Choices in Health Consumerism

Along with Data Concerning the Theories of Aging, Different Experiences in Aging by Minority Groups, and Facts about Aging Now and Aging in the Future; and Featuring a Glossary, a Guide to Consumer Help, Additional Suggested Reading, and Practical Resource Directory

Edited by Jenifer Swanson. 536 pages. 1999. 0-7808-0390-6. $78.

"Recommended reference source." —*Booklist, American Library Association, Feb '00*

SEE ALSO *Physical & Mental Issues in Aging Sourcebook*

Healthy Children Sourcebook

Basic Consumer Health Information about the Physical and Mental Development of Children between the Ages of 3 and 12, Including Routine Health Care, Preventative Health Services, Safety and First Aid, Healthy Sleep, Dental Care, Nutrition, and Fitness, and Featuring Parenting Tips on Such Topics as Bedwetting, Choosing Day Care, Monitoring TV and Other Media, and Establishing a Foundation for Substance Abuse Prevention

Along with a Glossary of Commonly Used Pediatric Terms and Resources for Additional Help and Information.

Edited by Chad T. Kimball. 647 pages. 2003. 0-7808-0247-0. $78.

Healthy Heart Sourcebook for Women

Basic Consumer Health Information about Cardiac Issues Specific to Women, Including Facts about Major Risk Factors and Prevention, Treatment and Control Strategies, and Important Dietary Issues

Along with a Special Section Regarding the Pros and Cons of Hormone Replacement Therapy and Its Impact on Heart Health, and Additional Help, Including Recipes, a Glossary, and a Directory of Resources

Edited by Dawn D. Matthews. 336 pages. 2000. 0-7808-0329-9. $78.

"A good reference source and recommended for all public, academic, medical, and hospital libraries." — *Medical Reference Services Quarterly, Summer '01*

"Because of the lack of information specific to women on this topic, this book is recommended for public libraries and consumer libraries." —*American Reference Books Annual, 2001*

"Contains very important information about coronary artery disease that all women should know. The information is current and presented in an easy-to-read format. The book will make a good addition to any library." — *American Medical Writers Association Journal, Summer '00*

"Important, basic reference." — *Reviewer's Bookwatch, Jul '00*

SEE ALSO *Heart Diseases & Disorders Sourcebook, Women's Health Concerns Sourcebook*

Heart Diseases & Disorders Sourcebook, 2nd Edition

Basic Consumer Health Information about Heart Attacks, Angina, Rhythm Disorders, Heart Failure, Valve Disease, Congenital Heart Disorders, and More, Including Descriptions of Surgical Procedures and Other Interventions, Medications, Cardiac Rehabilitation, Risk Identification, and Prevention Tips

Along with Statistical Data, Reports on Current Research Initiatives, a Glossary of Cardiovascular Terms, and Resource Directory

Edited by Karen Bellenir. 612 pages. 2000. 0-7808-0238-1. $78.

ALSO AVAILABLE: *Cardiovascular Diseases & Disorders Sourcebook, 1st Edition.* Edited by Karen Bellenir and Peter D. Dresser. 683 pages. 1995. 0-7808-0032-X. $78.

"This work stands out as an imminently accessible resource for the general public. It is recommended for the reference and circulating shelves of school, public, and academic libraries." —*American Reference Books Annual, 2001*

"Recommended reference source." —*Booklist, American Library Association, Dec '00*

"Provides comprehensive coverage of matters related to the heart. This title is recommended for health sciences and public libraries with consumer health collections." —*E-Streams, Oct '00*

SEE ALSO *Healthy Heart Sourcebook for Women*

Household Safety Sourcebook

Basic Consumer Health Information about Household Safety, Including Information about Poisons, Chemicals, Fire, and Water Hazards in the Home

Along with Advice about the Safe Use of Home Maintenance Equipment, Choosing Toys and Nursery Furni-

ture, Holiday and Recreation Safety, a Glossary, and Resources for Further Help and Information

Edited by Dawn D. Matthews. 606 pages. 2002. 0-7808-0338-8. $78.

"This work will be useful in public libraries with large consumer health and wellness departments."
— *American Reference Books Annual, 2003*

"As a sourcebook on household safety this book meets its mark. It is encyclopedic in scope and covers a wide range of safety issues that are commonly seen in the home." — *E-Streams, Jul '02*

■

Immune System Disorders Sourcebook

Basic Information about Lupus, Multiple Sclerosis, Guillain-Barré Syndrome, Chronic Granulomatous Disease, and More

Along with Statistical and Demographic Data and Reports on Current Research Initiatives

Edited by Allan R. Cook. 608 pages. 1997. 0-7808-0209-8. $78.

■

Infant & Toddler Health Sourcebook

Basic Consumer Health Information about the Physical and Mental Development of Newborns, Infants, and Toddlers, Including Neonatal Concerns, Nutrition Recommendations, Immunization Schedules, Common Pediatric Disorders, Assessments and Milestones, Safety Tips, and Advice for Parents and Other Caregivers

Along with a Glossary of Terms and Resource Listings for Additional Help

Edited by Jenifer Swanson. 585 pages. 2000. 0-7808-0246-2. $78.

"As a reference for the general public, this would be useful in any library." — *E-Streams, May '01*

"Recommended reference source."
— *Booklist, American Library Association, Feb '01*

"This is a good source for general use."
— *American Reference Books Annual, 2001*

■

Injury & Trauma Sourcebook

Basic Consumer Health Information about the Impact of Injury, the Diagnosis and Treatment of Common and Traumatic Injuries, Emergency Care, and Specific Injuries Related to Home, Community, Workplace, Transportation, and Recreation

Along with Guidelines for Injury Prevention, a Glossary, and a Directory of Additional Resources

Edited by Joyce Brennfleck Shannon. 696 pages. 2002. 0-7808-0421-X. $78.

"This publication is the most comprehensive work of its kind about injury and trauma."
— *American Reference Books Annual, 2003*

"This sourcebook provides concise, easily readable, basic health information about injuries. . . . This book is well organized and an easy to use reference resource suitable for hospital, health sciences and public libraries with consumer health collections."
— *E-Streams, Nov '02*

"Practitioners should be aware of guides such as this in order to facilitate their use by patients and their families." — *Doody's Health Sciences Book Review Journal, Sep-Oct '02*

"Recommended reference source."
— *Booklist, American Library Association, Sep '02*

"Highly recommended for academic and medical reference collections." — *Library Bookwatch, Sep '02*

■

Kidney & Urinary Tract Diseases & Disorders Sourcebook

Basic Information about Kidney Stones, Urinary Incontinence, Bladder Disease, End Stage Renal Disease, Dialysis, and More

Along with Statistical and Demographic Data and Reports on Current Research Initiatives

Edited by Linda M. Ross. 602 pages. 1997. 0-7808-0079-6. $78.

■

Learning Disabilities Sourcebook, 2nd Edition

Basic Consumer Health Information about Learning Disabilities, Including Dyslexia, Developmental Speech and Language Disabilities, Non-Verbal Learning Disorders, Developmental Arithmetic Disorder, Developmental Writing Disorder, and Other Conditions That Impede Learning Such as Attention Deficit/ Hyperactivity Disorder, Brain Injury, Hearing Impairment, Klinefelter Syndrome, Dyspraxia, and Tourette Syndrome

Along with Facts about Educational Issues and Assistive Technology, Coping Strategies, a Glossary of Related Terms, and Resources for Further Help and Information

Edited by Dawn D. Matthews. 621 pages. 2003. 0-7808-0626-3. $78.

ALSO AVAILABLE: *Learning Disabilities Sourcebook, 1st Edition. Edited by Linda M. Shin. 579 pages. 1998. 0-7808-0210-1. $78.*

"Teachers as well as consumers will find this an essential guide to understanding various syndromes and their latest treatments. [An] invaluable reference for public and school library collections alike."
— *Library Bookwatch, Apr '03*

Named "Outstanding Reference Book of 1999."
— *New York Public Library, Feb 2000*

"An excellent candidate for inclusion in a public library reference section. It's a great source of information. Teachers will also find the book useful. Definitely worth reading."
— *Journal of Adolescent & Adult Literacy, Feb 2000*

"Readable . . . provides a solid base of information regarding successful techniques used with individuals who have learning disabilities, as well as practical suggestions for educators and family members. Clear language, concise descriptions, and pertinent information for contacting multiple resources add to the strength of this book as a useful tool." — *Choice, Association of College and Research Libraries, Feb '99*

"Recommended reference source."
— *Booklist, American Library Association, Sep '98*

"A useful resource for libraries and for those who don't have the time to identify and locate the individual publications." — *Disability Resources Monthly, Sep '98*

Leukemia Sourcebook

Basic Consumer Health Information about Adult and Childhood Leukemias, Including Acute Lymphocytic Leukemia (ALL), Chronic Lymphocytic Leukemia (CLL), Acute Myelogenous Leukemia (AML), Chronic Myelogenous Leukemia (CML), and Hairy Cell Leukemia, and Treatments Such as Chemotherapy, Radiation Therapy, Peripheral Blood Stem Cell and Marrow Transplantation, and Immunotherapy

Along with Tips for Life During and After Treatment, a Glossary, and Directories of Additional Resources

Edited by Joyce Brennfleck Shannon. 587 pages. 2003. 0-7808-0627-1. $78.

Liver Disorders Sourcebook

Basic Consumer Health Information about the Liver and How It Works; Liver Diseases, Including Cancer, Cirrhosis, Hepatitis, and Toxic and Drug Related Diseases; Tips for Maintaining a Healthy Liver; Laboratory Tests, Radiology Tests, and Facts about Liver Transplantation

Along with a Section on Support Groups, a Glossary, and Resource Listings

Edited by Joyce Brennfleck Shannon. 591 pages. 2000. 0-7808-0383-3. $78.

"A valuable resource."
— *American Reference Books Annual, 2001*

"This title is recommended for health sciences and public libraries with consumer health collections." — *E-Streams, Oct '00*

"Recommended reference source."
— *Booklist, American Library Association, Jun '00*

Lung Disorders Sourcebook

Basic Consumer Health Information about Emphysema, Pneumonia, Tuberculosis, Asthma, Cystic Fibrosis, and Other Lung Disorders, Including Facts about Diagnostic Procedures, Treatment Strategies, Disease Prevention Efforts, and Such Risk Factors as Smoking, Air Pollution, and Exposure to Asbestos, Radon, and Other Agents

Along with a Glossary and Resources for Additional Help and Information

Edited by Dawn D. Matthews. 678 pages. 2002. 0-7808-0339-6. $78.

"This title is a great addition for public and school libraries because it provides concise health information on the lungs."
— *American Reference Books Annual, 2003*

"Highly recommended for academic and medical reference collections." — *Library Bookwatch, Sep '02*

Medical Tests Sourcebook

Basic Consumer Health Information about Medical Tests, Including Periodic Health Exams, General Screening Tests, Tests You Can Do at Home, Findings of the U.S. Preventive Services Task Force, X-ray and Radiology Tests, Electrical Tests, Tests of Blood and Other Body Fluids and Tissues, Scope Tests, Lung Tests, Genetic Tests, Pregnancy Tests, Newborn Screening Tests, Sexually Transmitted Disease Tests, and Computer Aided Diagnoses

Along with a Section on Paying for Medical Tests, a Glossary, and Resource Listings

Edited by Joyce Brennfleck Shannon. 691 pages. 1999. 0-7808-0243-8. $78.

"Recommended for hospital and health sciences libraries with consumer health collections."
— *E-Streams, Mar '00*

"This is an overall excellent reference with a wealth of general knowledge that may aid those who are reluctant to get vital tests performed."
— *Today's Librarian, Jan 2000*

"A valuable reference guide."
— *American Reference Books Annual, 2000*

Men's Health Concerns Sourcebook, 2nd Edition

Basic Consumer Health Information about the Medical and Mental Concerns of Men, Including Theories about the Shorter Male Lifespan, the Leading Causes of Death and Disability, Physical Concerns of Special Significance to Men, Reproductive and Sexual Concerns, Sexually Transmitted Diseases, Men's Mental and Emotional Health, and Lifestyle Choices That Affect Wellness, Such as Nutrition, Fitness, and Substance Use

Along with a Glossary of Related Terms and a Directory of Organizational Resources in Men's Health

Edited by Robert Aquinas McNally. 644 pages. 2004. 0-7808-0671-9. $78.

ALSO AVAILABLE: *Men's Health Concerns Sourcebook, 1st Edition.* Edited by Allan R. Cook. 738 pages. 1998. 0-7808-0212-8. $78.

"This comprehensive resource and the series are highly recommended."
— *American Reference Books Annual, 2000*

■

Mental Health Disorders Sourcebook, 2nd Edition

Basic Consumer Health Information about Anxiety Disorders, Depression and Other Mood Disorders, Eating Disorders, Personality Disorders, Schizophrenia, and More, Including Disease Descriptions, Treatment Options, and Reports on Current Research Initiatives

Along with Statistical Data, Tips for Maintaining Mental Health, a Glossary, and Directory of Sources for Additional Help and Information

Edited by Karen Bellenir. 605 pages. 2000. 0-7808-0240-3. $78.

ALSO AVAILABLE: *Mental Health Disorders Sourcebook, 1st Edition.* Edited by Karen Bellenir. 548 pages. 1995. 0-7808-0040-0. $78.

■

Mental Retardation Sourcebook

Basic Consumer Health Information about Mental Retardation and Its Causes, Including Down Syndrome, Fetal Alcohol Syndrome, Fragile X Syndrome, Genetic Conditions, Injury, and Environmental Sources

Along with Preventive Strategies, Parenting Issues, Educational Implications, Health Care Needs, Employment and Economic Matters, Legal Issues, a Glossary, and a Resource Listing for Additional Help and Information

Edited by Joyce Brennfleck Shannon. 642 pages. 2000. 0-7808-0377-9. $78.

■

Movement Disorders Sourcebook

Basic Consumer Health Information about Neurological Movement Disorders, Including Essential Tremor,

Parkinson's Disease, Dystonia, Cerebral Palsy, Huntington's Disease, Myasthenia Gravis, Multiple Sclerosis, and Other Early-Onset and Adult-Onset Movement Disorders, Their Symptoms and Causes, Diagnostic Tests, and Treatments

Along with Mobility and Assistive Technology Information, a Glossary, and a Directory of Additional Resources

Edited by Joyce Brennfleck Shannon. 655 pages. 2003. 0-7808-0628-X. $78.

■

Obesity Sourcebook

Basic Consumer Health Information about Diseases and Other Problems Associated with Obesity, and Including Facts about Risk Factors, Prevention Issues, and Management Approaches

Along with Statistical and Demographic Data, Information about Special Populations, Research Updates, a Glossary, and Source Listings for Further Help and Information

Edited by Wilma Caldwell and Chad T. Kimball. 376 pages. 2001. 0-7808-0333-7. $78.

■

Ophthalmic Disorders Sourcebook, 1st Edition

SEE *Eye Care Sourcebook, 2nd Edition*

■

Oral Health Sourcebook

SEE *Dental Care & Oral Health Sourcebook, 2nd Edition*

■

Osteoporosis Sourcebook

Basic Consumer Health Information about Primary and Secondary Osteoporosis and Juvenile Osteoporosis and Related Conditions, Including Fibrous Dysplasia, Gaucher Disease, Hyperthyroidism, Hypophosphatasia, Myeloma, Osteopetrosis, Osteogenesis Imperfecta, and Paget's Disease

Along with Information about Risk Factors, Treatments, Traditional and Non-Traditional Pain Management, a Glossary of Related Terms, and a Directory of Resources

Edited by Allan R. Cook. 584 pages. 2001. 0-7808-0239-X. $78.

"This would be a book to be kept in a staff or patient library. The targeted audience is the layperson, but the therapist who needs a quick bit of information on a particular topic will also find the book useful."
— *Physical Therapy, Jan '02*

"This resource is recommended as a great reference source for public, health, and academic libraries, and is another triumph for the editors of Omnigraphics."
— *American Reference Books Annual 2002*

"Recommended for all public libraries and general health collections, especially those supporting patient education or consumer health programs."
— *E-Streams, Nov '01*

"Will prove valuable to any library seeking to maintain a current, comprehensive reference collection of health resources. . . . From prevention to treatment and associated conditions, this provides an excellent survey."
— *The Bookwatch, Aug '01*

"Recommended reference source."
— *Booklist, American Library Association, July '01*

SEE ALSO *Women's Health Concerns Sourcebook*

Pain Sourcebook, 2nd Edition

Basic Consumer Health Information about Specific Forms of Acute and Chronic Pain, Including Muscle and Skeletal Pain, Nerve Pain, Cancer Pain, and Disorders Characterized by Pain, Such as Fibromyalgia, Shingles, Angina, Arthritis, and Headaches

Along with Information about Pain Medications and Management Techniques, Complementary and Alternative Pain Relief Options, Tips for People Living with Chronic Pain, a Glossary, and a Directory of Sources for Further Information

Edited by Karen Bellenir. 670 pages. 2002. 0-7808-0612-3. $78.

ALSO AVAILABLE: *Pain Sourcebook, 1st Edition.* Edited by Allan R. Cook. 667 pages. 1997. 0-7808-0213-6. $78.

"A source of valuable information. . . . This book offers help to nonmedical people who need information about pain and pain management. It is also an excellent reference for those who participate in patient education."
— *Doody's Review Service, Sep '02*

"The text is readable, easily understood, and well indexed. This excellent volume belongs in all patient education libraries, consumer health sections of public libraries, and many personal collections."
— *American Reference Books Annual, 1999*

"A beneficial reference." — *Booklist Health Sciences Supplement, American Library Association, Oct '98*

"The information is basic in terms of scholarship and is appropriate for general readers. Written in journalistic style . . . intended for non-professionals. Quite thorough in its coverage of different pain conditions and summarizes the latest clinical information regarding pain treatment." — *Choice, Association of College and Research Libraries, Jun '98*

"Recommended reference source."
— *Booklist, American Library Association, Mar '98*

Pediatric Cancer Sourcebook

Basic Consumer Health Information about Leukemias, Brain Tumors, Sarcomas, Lymphomas, and Other Cancers in Infants, Children, and Adolescents, Including Descriptions of Cancers, Treatments, and Coping Strategies

Along with Suggestions for Parents, Caregivers, and Concerned Relatives, a Glossary of Cancer Terms, and Resource Listings

Edited by Edward J. Prucha. 587 pages. 1999. 0-7808-0245-4. $78.

"An excellent source of information. Recommended for public, hospital, and health science libraries with consumer health collections." — *E-Streams, Jun '00*

"Recommended reference source."
— *Booklist, American Library Association, Feb '00*

"A valuable addition to all libraries specializing in health services and many public libraries."
— *American Reference Books Annual, 2000*

Physical & Mental Issues in Aging Sourcebook

Basic Consumer Health Information on Physical and Mental Disorders Associated with the Aging Process, Including Concerns about Cardiovascular Disease, Pulmonary Disease, Oral Health, Digestive Disorders, Musculoskeletal and Skin Disorders, Metabolic Changes, Sexual and Reproductive Issues, and Changes in Vision, Hearing, and Other Senses

Along with Data about Longevity and Causes of Death, Information on Acute and Chronic Pain, Descriptions of Mental Concerns, a Glossary of Terms, and Resource Listings for Additional Help

Edited by Jenifer Swanson. 660 pages. 1999. 0-7808-0233-0. $78.

"This is a treasure of health information for the layperson." — *Choice Health Sciences Supplement, Association of College & Research Libraries, May 2000*

"Recommended for public libraries."
— *American Reference Books Annual, 2000*

"Recommended reference source."
— *Booklist, American Library Association, Oct '99*

SEE ALSO *Healthy Aging Sourcebook*

Podiatry Sourcebook

Basic Consumer Health Information about Foot Conditions, Diseases, and Injuries, Including Bunions, Corns, Calluses, Athlete's Foot, Plantar Warts, Hammertoes and Clawtoes, Clubfoot, Heel Pain, Gout, and More

Along with Facts about Foot Care, Disease Prevention, Foot Safety, Choosing a Foot Care Specialist, a Glossary of Terms, and Resource Listings for Additional Information

Edited by M. Lisa Weatherford. 380 pages. 2001. 0-7808-0215-2. $78.

"Recommended reference source."
— *Booklist, American Library Association, Feb '02*

"There is a lot of information presented here on a topic that is usually only covered sparingly in most larger comprehensive medical encyclopedias."
— *American Reference Books Annual 2002*

■

Pregnancy & Birth Sourcebook, 2nd Edition

Basic Consumer Health Information about Conception and Pregnancy, Including Facts about Fertility, Infertility, Pregnancy Symptoms and Complications, Fetal Growth and Development, Labor, Delivery, and the Postpartum Period, as Well as Information about Maintaining Health and Wellness during Pregnancy and Caring for a Newborn

Along with Information about Public Health Assistance for Low-Income Pregnant Women, a Glossary, and Directories of Agencies and Organizations Providing Help and Support

Edited by Amy L. Sutton. 600 pages. 2004. 0-7808-0672-7. $78.

ALSO AVAILABLE: *Pregnancy & Birth Sourcebook, 1st Edition.* Edited by Heather E. Aldred. 737 pages. 1997. 0-7808-0216-0. $78.

"A well-organized handbook. Recommended."
— *Choice, Association of College and Research Libraries, Apr '98*

"Recommended reference source."
— *Booklist, American Library Association, Mar '98*

"Recommended for public libraries."
— *American Reference Books Annual, 1998*

SEE ALSO *Congenital Disorders Sourcebook, Family Planning Sourcebook*

■

Prostate Cancer Sourcebook

Basic Consumer Health Information about Prostate Cancer, Including Information about the Associated Risk Factors, Detection, Diagnosis, and Treatment of Prostate Cancer

Along with Information on Non-Malignant Prostate Conditions, and Featuring a Section Listing Support and Treatment Centers and a Glossary of Related Terms

Edited by Dawn D. Matthews. 358 pages. 2001. 0-7808-0324-8. $78.

"Recommended reference source."
— *Booklist, American Library Association, Jan '02*

"A valuable resource for health care consumers seeking information on the subject. . . .All text is written in a clear, easy-to-understand language that avoids technical jargon. Any library that collects consumer health resources would strengthen their collection with the addition of the *Prostate Cancer Sourcebook*."
— *American Reference Books Annual 2002*

■

Public Health Sourcebook

Basic Information about Government Health Agencies, Including National Health Statistics and Trends, Healthy People 2000 Program Goals and Objectives, the Centers for Disease Control and Prevention, the Food and Drug Administration, and the National Institutes of Health

Along with Full Contact Information for Each Agency

Edited by Wendy Wilcox. 698 pages. 1998. 0-7808-0220-9. $78.

"Recommended reference source."
— *Booklist, American Library Association, Sep '98*

"This consumer guide provides welcome assistance in navigating the maze of federal health agencies and their data on public health concerns."
— *SciTech Book News, Sep '98*

■

Reconstructive & Cosmetic Surgery Sourcebook

Basic Consumer Health Information on Cosmetic and Reconstructive Plastic Surgery, Including Statistical Information about Different Surgical Procedures, Things to Consider Prior to Surgery, Plastic Surgery Techniques and Tools, Emotional and Psychological Considerations, and Procedure-Specific Information

Along with a Glossary of Terms and a Listing of Resources for Additional Help and Information

Edited by M. Lisa Weatherford. 374 pages. 2001. 0-7808-0214-4. $78.

"An excellent reference that addresses cosmetic and medically necessary reconstructive surgeries. . . . The style of the prose is calm and reassuring, discussing the many positive outcomes now available due to advances in surgical techniques."
— *American Reference Books Annual 2002*

"Recommended for health science libraries that are open to the public, as well as hospital libraries that are open to the patients. This book is a good resource for the consumer interested in plastic surgery."
— *E-Streams, Dec '01*

"Recommended reference source."
— *Booklist, American Library Association, July '01*

Rehabilitation Sourcebook

Basic Consumer Health Information about Rehabilitation for People Recovering from Heart Surgery, Spinal Cord Injury, Stroke, Orthopedic Impairments, Amputation, Pulmonary Impairments, Traumatic Injury, and More, Including Physical Therapy, Occupational Therapy, Speech/ Language Therapy, Massage Therapy, Dance Therapy, Art Therapy, and Recreational Therapy

Along with Information on Assistive and Adaptive Devices, a Glossary, and Resources for Additional Help and Information

Edited by Dawn D. Matthews. 531 pages. 1999. 0-7808-0236-5. $78.

"This is an excellent resource for public library reference and health collections."
— *American Reference Books Annual, 2001*

"Recommended reference source."
— *Booklist, American Library Association, May '00*

Respiratory Diseases & Disorders Sourcebook

Basic Information about Respiratory Diseases and Disorders, Including Asthma, Cystic Fibrosis, Pneumonia, the Common Cold, Influenza, and Others, Featuring Facts about the Respiratory System, Statistical and Demographic Data, Treatments, Self-Help Management Suggestions, and Current Research Initiatives

Edited by Allan R. Cook and Peter D. Dresser. 771 pages. 1995. 0-7808-0037-0. $78.

"Designed for the layperson and for patients and their families coping with respiratory illness. . . . an extensive array of information on diagnosis, treatment, management, and prevention of respiratory illnesses for the general reader." — *Choice, Association of College and Research Libraries, Jun '96*

"A highly recommended text for all collections. It is a comforting reminder of the power of knowledge that good books carry between their covers."
— *Academic Library Book Review, Spring '96*

"A comprehensive collection of authoritative information presented in a nontechnical, humanitarian style for patients, families, and caregivers."
— *Association of Operating Room Nurses, Sep/Oct '95*

SEE ALSO *Lung Disorders Sourcebook*

Sexually Transmitted Diseases Sourcebook, 2nd Edition

Basic Consumer Health Information about Sexually Transmitted Diseases, Including Information on the Diagnosis and Treatment of Chlamydia, Gonorrhea, Hepatitis, Herpes, HIV, Mononucleosis, Syphilis, and Others

Along with Information on Prevention, Such as Condom Use, Vaccines, and STD Education; And Featuring a Section on Issues Related to Youth and Adolescents, a Glossary, and Resources for Additional Help and Information

Edited by Dawn D. Matthews. 538 pages. 2001. 0-7808-0249-7. $78.

ALSO AVAILABLE: *Sexually Transmitted Diseases Sourcebook, 1st Edition.* Edited by Linda M. Ross. 550 pages. 1997. 0-7808-0217-9. $78.

"Recommended for consumer health collections in public libraries, and secondary school and community college libraries."
— *American Reference Books Annual 2002*

"Every school and public library should have a copy of this comprehensive and user-friendly reference book."
— *Choice, Association of College & Research Libraries, Sep '01*

"This is a highly recommended book. This is an especially important book for all school and public libraries." — *AIDS Book Review Journal, Jul-Aug '01*

"Recommended reference source."
— *Booklist, American Library Association, Apr '01*

"Recommended pick both for specialty health library collections and any general consumer health reference collection." — *The Bookwatch, Apr '01*

Skin Disorders Sourcebook

Basic Information about Common Skin and Scalp Conditions Caused by Aging, Allergies, Immune Reactions, Sun Exposure, Infectious Organisms, Parasites, Cosmetics, and Skin Traumas, Including Abrasions, Cuts, and Pressure Sores

Along with Information on Prevention and Treatment

Edited by Allan R. Cook. 647 pages. 1997. 0-7808-0080-X. $78.

". . . comprehensive, easily read reference book."
— *Doody's Health Sciences Book Reviews, Oct '97*

SEE ALSO *Burns Sourcebook*

Sleep Disorders Sourcebook

Basic Consumer Health Information about Sleep and Its Disorders, Including Insomnia, Sleepwalking, Sleep Apnea, Restless Leg Syndrome, and Narcolepsy

Along with Data about Shiftwork and Its Effects, Information on the Societal Costs of Sleep Deprivation, Descriptions of Treatment Options, a Glossary of Terms, and Resource Listings for Additional Help

Edited by Jenifer Swanson. 439 pages. 1998. 0-7808-0234-9. $78.

"This text will complement any home or medical library. It is user-friendly and ideal for the adult reader."
— *American Reference Books Annual, 2000*

"A useful resource that provides accurate, relevant, and accessible information on sleep to the general public. Health care providers who deal with sleep disorders patients may also find it helpful in being prepared to answer some of the questions patients ask."
— *Respiratory Care, Jul '99*

"Recommended reference source."
— *Booklist, American Library Association, Feb '99*

Sports Injuries Sourcebook, 2nd Edition

Basic Consumer Health Information about the Diagnosis, Treatment, and Rehabilitation of Common Sports-Related Injuries in Children and Adults

Along with Suggestions for Conditioning and Training, Information and Prevention Tips for Injuries Frequently Associated with Specific Sports and Special Populations, a Glossary, and a Directory of Additional Resources

Edited by Joyce Brennfleck Shannon. 614 pages. 2002. 0-7808-0604-2. $78.

ALSO AVAILABLE: Sports Injuries Sourcebook, 1st Edition. Edited by Heather E. Aldred. 624 pages. 1999. 0-7808-0218-7. $78.

"This is an excellent reference for consumers and it is recommended for public, community college, and undergraduate libraries."
— *American Reference Books Annual, 2003*

"Recommended reference source."
— *Booklist, American Library Association, Feb '03*

Stress-Related Disorders Sourcebook

Basic Consumer Health Information about Stress and Stress-Related Disorders, Including Stress Origins and Signals, Environmental Stress at Work and Home, Mental and Emotional Stress Associated with Depression, Post-Traumatic Stress Disorder, Panic Disorder, Suicide, and the Physical Effects of Stress on the Cardiovascular, Immune, and Nervous Systems

Along with Stress Management Techniques, a Glossary, and a Listing of Additional Resources

Edited by Joyce Brennfleck Shannon. 610 pages. 2002. 0-7808-0560-7. $78.

"Well written for a general readership, the *Stress-Related Disorders Sourcebook* is a useful addition to the health reference literature."
— *American Reference Books Annual, 2003*

"I am impressed by the amount of information. It offers a thorough overview of the causes and consequences of stress for the layperson. . . . A well-done and thorough reference guide for professionals and nonprofessionals alike."
— *Doody's Review Service, Dec '02*

Stroke Sourcebook

Basic Consumer Health Information about Stroke, Including Ischemic, Hemorrhagic, Transient Ischemic Attack (TIA), and Pediatric Stroke, Stroke Triggers and Risks, Diagnostic Tests, Treatments, and Rehabilitation Information

Along with Stroke Prevention Guidelines, Legal and Financial Information, a Glossary, and a Directory of Additional Resources

Edited by Joyce Brennfleck Shannon. 606 pages. 2003. 0-7808-0630-1. $78.

Substance Abuse Sourcebook

Basic Health-Related Information about the Abuse of Legal and Illegal Substances Such as Alcohol, Tobacco, Prescription Drugs, Marijuana, Cocaine, and Heroin; and Including Facts about Substance Abuse Prevention Strategies, Intervention Methods, Treatment and Recovery Programs, and a Section Addressing the Special Problems Related to Substance Abuse during Pregnancy

Edited by Karen Bellenir. 573 pages. 1996. 0-7808-0038-9. $78.

"A valuable addition to any health reference section. Highly recommended."
— *The Book Report, Mar/Apr '97*

". . . a comprehensive collection of substance abuse information that's both highly readable and compact. Families and caregivers of substance abusers will find the information enlightening and helpful, while teachers, social workers and journalists should benefit from the concise format. Recommended."
— *Drug Abuse Update, Winter '96/'97*

SEE ALSO Alcoholism Sourcebook, Drug Abuse Sourcebook

Surgery Sourcebook

Basic Consumer Health Information about Inpatient and Outpatient Surgeries, Including Cardiac, Vascular, Orthopedic, Ocular, Reconstructive, Cosmetic, Gynecologic, and Ear, Nose, and Throat Procedures and More

Along with Information about Operating Room Policies and Instruments, Laser Surgery Techniques, Hospital Errors, Statistical Data, a Glossary, and Listings of Sources for Further Help and Information

Edited by Annemarie S. Muth and Karen Bellenir. 596 pages. 2002. 0-7808-0380-9. $78.

"Invaluable reference for public and school library collections alike."
— *Library Bookwatch, Apr '03*

Transplantation Sourcebook

Basic Consumer Health Information about Organ and Tissue Transplantation, Including Physical and Financial Preparations, Procedures and Issues Relating to Specific Solid Organ and Tissue Transplants, Rehabilitation, Pediatric Transplant Information, the Future

744

of Transplantation, and Organ and Tissue Donation

Along with a Glossary and Listings of Additional Resources

Edited by Joyce Brennfleck Shannon. 628 pages. 2002. 0-7808-0322-1. $78.

"Along with these advances [in transplantation technology] have come a number of daunting questions for potential transplant patients, their families, and their health care providers. This reference text is the best single tool to address many of these questions. . . . It will be a much-needed addition to the reference collections in health care, academic, and large public libraries."
—American Reference Books Annual, 2003

"Recommended for libraries with an interest in offering consumer health information." —E-Streams, Jul '02

"This is a unique and valuable resource for patients facing transplantation and their families."
—Doody's Review Service, Jun '02

Traveler's Health Sourcebook

Basic Consumer Health Information for Travelers, Including Physical and Medical Preparations, Transportation Health and Safety, Essential Information about Food and Water, Sun Exposure, Insect and Snake Bites, Camping and Wilderness Medicine, and Travel with Physical or Medical Disabilities

Along with International Travel Tips, Vaccination Recommendations, Geographical Health Issues, Disease Risks, a Glossary, and a Listing of Additional Resources

Edited by Joyce Brennfleck Shannon. 613 pages. 2000. 0-7808-0384-1. $78.

"Recommended reference source."
—Booklist, American Library Association, Feb '01

"This book is recommended for any public library, any travel collection, and especially any collection for the physically disabled."
—American Reference Books Annual, 2001

Vegetarian Sourcebook

Basic Consumer Health Information about Vegetarian Diets, Lifestyle, and Philosophy, Including Definitions of Vegetarianism and Veganism, Tips about Adopting Vegetarianism, Creating a Vegetarian Pantry, and Meeting Nutritional Needs of Vegetarians, with Facts Regarding Vegetarianism's Effect on Pregnant and Lactating Women, Children, Athletes, and Senior Citizens

Along with a Glossary of Commonly Used Vegetarian Terms and Resources for Additional Help and Information

Edited by Chad T. Kimball. 360 pages. 2002. 0-7808-0439-2. $78.

"Organizes into one concise volume the answers to the most common questions concerning vegetarian diets and lifestyles. This title is recommended for public and secondary school libraries." —E-Streams, Apr '03

"Invaluable reference for public and school library collections alike." — Library Bookwatch, Apr '03

"The articles in this volume are easy to read and come from authoritative sources. The book does not necessarily support the vegetarian diet but instead provides the pros and cons of this important decision. The *Vegetarian Sourcebook* is recommended for public libraries and consumer health libraries."
—American Reference Books Annual, 2003

Women's Health Concerns Sourcebook, 2nd Edition

Basic Consumer Health Information about the Medical and Mental Concerns of Women, Including Maintaining Health and Wellness, Gynecological Concerns, Breast Health, Sexuality and Reproductive Issues, Menopause, Cancer in Women, the Leading Causes of Death and Disability among Women, Physical Concerns of Special Significance to Women, and Women's Mental and Emotional Health

Along with a Glossary of Related Terms and Directories of Resources for Additional Help and Information

Edited by Amy L. Sutton. 748 pages. 2004. 0-7808-0673-5. $78.

ALSO AVAILABLE: Women's Health Concerns Sourcebook, 1st Edition. Edited by Heather E. Aldred. 567 pages. 1997. 0-7808-0219-5. $78.

"Handy compilation. There is an impressive range of diseases, devices, disorders, procedures, and other physical and emotional issues covered . . . well organized, illustrated, and indexed." —Choice, Association of College and Research Libraries, Jan '98

SEE ALSO Breast Cancer Sourcebook, Cancer Sourcebook for Women, Healthy Heart Sourcebook for Women, Osteoporosis Sourcebook

Workplace Health & Safety Sourcebook

Basic Consumer Health Information about Workplace Health and Safety, Including the Effect of Workplace Hazards on the Lungs, Skin, Heart, Ears, Eyes, Brain, Reproductive Organs, Musculoskeletal System, and Other Organs and Body Parts

Along with Information about Occupational Cancer, Personal Protective Equipment, Toxic and Hazardous Chemicals, Child Labor, Stress, and Workplace Violence

Edited by Chad T. Kimball. 626 pages. 2000. 0-7808-0231-4. $78.

"As a reference for the general public, this would be useful in any library." —E-Streams, Jun '01

"Provides helpful information for primary care physicians and other caregivers interested in occupational medicine. . . . General readers; professionals."
— Choice, Association of College & Research Libraries, May '01

"Recommended reference source."
—Booklist, American Library Association, Feb '01

"Highly recommended." —The Bookwatch, Jan '01

Worldwide Health Sourcebook

Basic Information about Global Health Issues, Including Malnutrition, Reproductive Health, Disease Dispersion and Prevention, Emerging Diseases, Risky Health Behaviors, and the Leading Causes of Death

Along with Global Health Concerns for Children, Women, and the Elderly, Mental Health Issues, Research and Technology Advancements, and Economic, Environmental, and Political Health Implications, a Glossary, and a Resource Listing for Additional Help and Information

Edited by Joyce Brennfleck Shannon. 614 pages. 2001. 0-7808-0330-2. $78.

"Named an Outstanding Academic Title."
—Choice, Association of College & Research Libraries, Jan '02

"Yet another handy but also unique compilation in the extensive Health Reference Series, this is a useful work because many of the international publications reprinted or excerpted are not readily available. Highly recommended." *—Choice, Association of College & Research Libraries, Nov '01*

"Recommended reference source."
—Booklist, American Library Association, Oct '01

Teen Health Series

Helping Young Adults Understand, Manage, and Avoid Serious Illness

Diet Information for Teens

Health Tips about Diet and Nutrition

Including Facts about Nutrients, Dietary Guidelines, Breakfasts, School Lunches, Snacks, Party Food, Weight Control, Eating Disorders, and More

Edited by Karen Bellenir. 399 pages. 2001. 0-7808-0441-4. $58.

"Full of helpful insights and facts throughout the book. . . . An excellent resource to be placed in public libraries or even in personal collections."
—*American Reference Books Annual 2002*

"Recommended for middle and high school libraries and media centers as well as academic libraries that educate future teachers of teenagers. It is also a suitable addition to health science libraries that serve patrons who are interested in teen health promotion and education." —*E-Streams, Oct '01*

"This comprehensive book would be beneficial to collections that need information about nutrition, dietary guidelines, meal planning, and weight control. . . . This reference is so easy to use that its purchase is recommended." —*The Book Report, Sep-Oct '01*

"This book is written in an easy to understand format describing issues that many teens face every day, and then provides thoughtful explanations so that teens can make informed decisions. This is an interesting book that provides important facts and information for today's teens." —*Doody's Health Sciences Book Review Journal, Jul-Aug '01*

"A comprehensive compendium of diet and nutrition. The information is presented in a straightforward, plain-spoken manner. This title will be useful to those working on reports on a variety of topics, as well as to general readers concerned about their dietary health."
—*School Library Journal, Jun '01*

Drug Information for Teens

Health Tips about the Physical and Mental Effects of Substance Abuse

Including Facts about Alcohol, Anabolic Steroids, Club Drugs, Cocaine, Depressants, Hallucinogens, Herbal Products, Inhalants, Marijuana, Narcotics, Stimulants, Tobacco, and More

Edited by Karen Bellenir. 452 pages. 2002. 0-7808-0444-9. $58.

"The chapters are quick to make a connection to their teenage reading audience. The prose is straightforward and the book lends itself to spot reading. It should be useful both for practical information and for research, and it is suitable for public and school libraries."
—*American Reference Books Annual, 2003*

"Recommended reference source."
—*Booklist, American Library Association, Feb '03*

"This is an excellent resource for teens and their parents. Education about drugs and substances is key to discouraging teen drug abuse and this book provides this much needed information in a way that is interesting and factual." —*Doody's Review Service, Dec '02*

Mental Health Information for Teens

Health Tips about Mental Health and Mental Illness

Including Facts about Anxiety, Depression, Suicide, Eating Disorders, Obsessive-Compulsive Disorders, Panic Attacks, Phobias, Schizophrenia, and More

Edited by Karen Bellenir. 406 pages. 2001. 0-7808-0442-2. $58.

"In both language and approach, this user-friendly entry in the *Teen Health Series* is on target for teens needing information on mental health concerns." —*Booklist, American Library Association, Jan '02*

"Readers will find the material accessible and informative, with the shaded notes, facts, and embedded glossary insets adding appropriately to the already interesting and succinct presentation."
—*School Library Journal, Jan '02*

"This title is highly recommended for any library that serves adolescents and parents/caregivers of adolescents." —*E-Streams, Jan '02*

"Recommended for high school libraries and young adult collections in public libraries. Both health professionals and teenagers will find this book useful."
—*American Reference Books Annual 2002*

"This is a nice book written to enlighten the society, primarily teenagers, about common teen mental health issues. It is highly recommended to teachers and parents as well as adolescents."
—*Doody's Review Service, Dec '01*

Sexual Health Information for Teens

Health Tips about Sexual Development, Human Reproduction, and Sexually Transmitted Diseases

Including Facts about Puberty, Reproductive Health, Chlamydia, Human Papillomavirus, Pelvic Inflam-

matory Disease, Herpes, AIDS, Contraception, Pregnancy, and More

Edited by Deborah A. Stanley. 391 pages. 2003. 0-7808-0445-7. $58.

Skin Health Information
For Teens
Health Tips about Dermatological Concerns and Skin Cancer Risks

Including Facts about Acne, Warts, Hives, and Other Conditions and Lifestyle Choices, Such as Tanning, Tattooing, and Piercing, That Affect the Skin, Nails, Scalp, and Hair

Edited by Robert Aquinas McNally. 430 pages. 2003. 0-7808-0446-5. $58.

Sports Injuries Information
For Teens
Health Tips about Sports Injuries and Injury Protection

Including Facts about Specific Injuries, Emergency Treatment, Rehabilitation, Sports Safety, Competition Stress, Fitness, Sports Nutrition, Steroid Risks, and More

Edited by Joyce Brennfleck Shannon. 425 pages. 2003. 0-7808-0447-3. $58.

748

Health Reference Series